Fundamentals of Anaesthesia and Acute Medicine

Clinical Cardiovascular Medicine in Anaesthesia

Edited by
Pierre Coriat
Professor and Head of Department, Department of Anaesthesia and Intensive Care, Hôpital Pitié-Salpêtrière, Paris, France

Series editors
Ronald M Jones
Professor of Anaesthetics, St Mary's Hospital Medical School, London

Alan R Aitkenhead
Professor of Anaesthesia, University of Nottingham

and

Pierre Foëx
Nuffield Professor of Anaesthetics, University of Oxford

BMJ
Publishing
Group

First published in 1997
by the BMJ Publishing Group, BMA House, Tavistock Square,
London WC1H 9JR

British Library Cataloguing in Publication Data

A catalogue record for this book is available
from the British Library

ISBN 0-7279-1127-9

Typeset by Apek Typesetters Ltd, Nailsea, Bristol
Printed and bound in Great Britain by Latimer Trend Ltd, Plymouth

Clinical Cardiovascular Medicine in Anaesthesia

Contents

Contributors   vii

Preface   ix

Part One   Interaction of cardiovascular drugs and anaesthesia

1   Beta-adrenoceptor antagonists   3
SIMON HOWELL, PIERRE FOËX
2   Calcium-channel blockers   29
JEAN-JAQUES LEHOT, PIERRE-GEORGES DURAND, VINCENT PIRIOU
3   Angiotensin-converting enzyme inhibitors   52
PASCAL COLSON
4   Antiarrhythmic agents   74
JEAN EMMANUEL DE LA COUSSAYE, JEAN-JACQUES ELEDJAM
5   Alpha$_2$-adrenoceptor agonists   108
PIERRE-LOUIS DARMON, FRANCIS BONNET

Part Two   Use of cardiovascular agents in anaesthesia and intensive care

6   Treatment of intraoperative hypotension   123
AXEL W. GOERTZ
7   Treatment of acute postoperative hypertension   137
CHRIS DECLERCK, PIERRE CORIAT
8   Perioperative management of myocardial ischaemia and coronary artery bypass graft spasm   159
PHILIPPE OLIVIER, NICOLA D'ATTELLIS, JEAN-FRANÇOIS BARON
9   Treatment of perioperative left ventricular dysfunction   177
JOACHIM BOLDT
10   Treatment of perioperative arrhythmias   201
HELFRIED METZLER
11   Treatment of pulmonary hypertension   213
JOSE OTAVIO AULER JR, PEDRO POSO RUIZ-NETO

12 Pharmacological treatment of hypoxaemia in patients with
   acute respiratory distress syndrome   241
   LOUIS PUYBASSET, JEAN-JACQUES ROUBY
13 Cardioactive drugs: future directions   284
   PHILLIPE LECHAT
   Index   291

Contributors

Nicola D'Attellis, MD
Staff Anaethesiologist, Department of Anaesthesia and Intensive Care, Hôpital Broussais, Paris, France

Jose Otavio Auler Jr, MD, PhD
Full Professor, Director of Anaesthesia and Intensive Care Unit, Instituto do Coração do Hospital das Clínicas da FMUSP, Saõ Paulo, Brazil

Jean-François Baron, MD, PhD
Professor and Head of Department, Department of Anaesthesia and Intensive Care, Hôpital Broussais, Paris, France

Joachim Boldt, MD, PhD
Professor and Head of Department, Department of Anaesthesiology and Intensive Care Medicine, Klinikum der Stadt Ludwigshafen, Germany

Francis Bonnet, MD
Professor and Head of Department, Surgical Intensive Care and Traumatology Unit, Department of Anaesthesia and Intensive Care, Hôpital Henri Mondor, Creteil, France

Pascal Colson, MD, PhD
Professor and Head of Department, Department of Anaesthesiology and Intensive Care, Centre Hospitalo-Universitaire, Montpellier, France

Pierre Coriat, MD
Professor and Head of Department, Department of Anaesthesia and Intensive Care, Hôpital Pitié-Salpétrière, Paris, France

Jean Emmanuel de la Coussaye, MD, PhD
Professor of Anaesthesia, Departments of Anaesthesiology, Intensive Care, and Emergency Medicine, Hôpital Universitaire de Nîmes, Nîmes, France

Pierre-Louis Darmon, MD
Staff Anaesthesiologist, Department of Anaesthesia and Intensive Care, Hôpital Pitié-Salpétrière, Paris, France

Chris Declerck, MD
Research Fellow, Department of Anaesthesia and Intensive Care, Hôpital Pitié-Salpétrière, Paris, France

Pierre-Georges Durand, MD
Consultant Anaesthetist, Department of Anaesthesia and Intensive Care, Hôpital Cardio-vasculaire et Pneumologique Louis Pradel, Lyons, France

Jean-Jacques Eledjam, MD
Professor and Head of Department, Departments of Anaesthesiology, Intensive Care, and Emergency Medicine, Hôpital Universitaire de Nîmes, Nîmes, France

Pierre Foëx, DM, DPhil, FRCA, FANZCA
Professor of Anaesthetics, Nuffield Department of Anaesthetics, Radcliffe Infirmary, Oxford, UK

Axel W. Goertz, MD
Professor, Department of Anaesthesiology, Klinikum der Universität Ulm, Ulm, Germany

Simon Howell, BA, MB, BS, MSc, FRCA
Clinical Lecturer, Nuffield Department of Anaesthetics, Radcliffe Infirmary, Oxford, UK

Philippe Lechat, MD, PhD
Professor of Pharmacology, Pharmacology Department, Hôpital Pitié-Salpétrière, Paris, France

Jean-Jacques Lehot, MD, PhD
Professor and Head of Department, Department of Anaesthesia and Intensive Care, Hôpital Cardiovasculaire et Pneumologique Louis Pradel, Lyons, France

Helfried Metzler, MD
Professor and Head of Department, Department of Anaesthesiology and Intensive Care Medicine, University of Graz, Graz, Austria

Philippe Olivier, MD
Assistant Professor, Department of Anaesthesia and Intensive Care, Hôpital Broussais, Paris, France

Vincent Piriou, MD
Assistant Professor, Department of Anaesthesia and Intensive Care, Hôpital Cardio-vasculaire et Pneumologique Louis Pradel, Lyons, France

Louis Puybasset, MD, PhD
Assistant Professor of Anaesthesia, Surgical Intensive Care Unit, Department of Anaesthesiology, Hôpital Pitié-Salpétrière, Paris, France

Pedro Poso Ruiz-Neto, MD, PhD
Assistant Professor, Department of Anaesthesia, Instituto Central do Hospital das Clínicas da FMUSP, São Paulo, Brazil

Jean-Jacques Rouby, MD, PhD
Professor of Anaesthesia, Surgical Intensive Care Unit, Department of Anaesthesiology, Hôpital Pitié-Salpétrière, Paris, France

Preface

This book came into being because we perceived a definite need for a text dedicated to the interactions between cardiovascular medicine and anaesthesia. This is a subject which makes one look at cardiovascular physiology and pharmacology in a new light and allows a better understanding of the compensatory mechanisms activated to limit the circulatory stress of the perioperative period.

The book is divided into two parts. The first (Chapters 1 to 5) describes the effects of cardiovascular drugs on patients undergoing operations, and explains how these treatments, can, when used in conjunction with anaesthetic agents, put the circulatory balance in jeopardy. The second (Chapters 6 to 13) discusses the use of cardiovascular drugs to treat intra and postoperative circulatory and cardiac disorders.

It is imperative that circulatory stability is maintained in patients at cardiovascular risk, most of whom benefit from cardiac treatment designed to improve both their symptoms and life expectancy. Such cardiovascular agents either interfere with regulatory mechanisms of blood pressure and regional circulations, or they affect the cardiac electrophysiology or contractility. The direct effects of the anaesthetic agents on the loading conditions of the heart and on contractility are moderate. This explains why most perioperative circulatory anomalies are not due to the effect of anaesthetic agents on the circulation, but to the interactions between cardiovascular and anaesthetic agents, both of which alter the functioning of several physiological systems (renin-angiotensin, sympathetic) and limit the body's compensatory mechanisms that come into force to maintain circulatory balance when the loading conditions of the heart deteriorate. On the other hand, surgical stimulation and postoperative stress often cause violent increases in heart rate and systemic vascular resistance, both of which can be effectively overcome by the use of intravenously administered cardiovascular drugs.

Finally, on a more personal note, I would like to express what a pleasure and privilege it has been to coordinate the work of colleagues from several European countries. I hope that this book will be an excellent reflection of the quality of European medical thought in the field of anaesthesia and intensive care.

PIERRE CORIAT

ix

Part One

Interaction of cardiovascular drugs and anaesthesia

1: Beta-adrenoceptor antagonists

SIMON HOWELL AND PIERRE FOËX

Beta-blockers (β-blockers) are used mainly in the management of coronary heart disease, hypertensive heart disease, obstructive cardiomyopathies and, recently, have been introduced in the management of cardiac failure, a condition that was hitherto regarded as a contraindication to these drugs.

Beta-blockers act as antagonists or partial agonists at the β-adrenoceptors. Membrane β-receptors are stimulated by catecholamines released by postganglionic sympathetic neurones or the adrenal glands. Beta-adrenoceptors are membrane receptors with seven membrane spanning domains linked to guanine nucleotide binding regulatory (G) proteins.[1] The G proteins are involved in the activation of one or more second messenger-effector systems such as adenylate cyclase, phospholipases, potassium and calcium ion channels, and the sodium/proton (Na^+/H^+) antiport.

Beta-receptors have two main characteristics: (a) affinity for a specific molecule (the transmitter) and (b) the triggering of a chain of reactions leading to a physiological response. Chemicals other than the natural transmitters may bind to the receptor and cause either activation (agonists) or inactivation (antagonists). Receptors may be located on the cell membrane, in the cytoplasm or at the surface of intracellular organelles. The wide variety of locations of β-adrenoceptors (Table 1.1) explains the

Table 1.1 Location of β-adrenoceptors

Location	Subtype of receptor
Heart	β_1, β_2
Blood vessels	β_1, β_2
Lungs (bronchi)	β_2
Gut	β_1
Uterus	β_2
Eye	β_2
Kidney	β_1
Pancreas	β_2
Adipose tissue	β_1

multiplicity of the effects of adrenergic stimulation or blockade.

Beta-adrenoceptors are subject to regulation and desensitisation. Desensitisation causes a reduction of the efficacy of an agonist for the receptor. It may occur because of uncoupling of the receptor G-protein, sequestration of the receptors into intracellular vesicles, or destruction of the receptors. Prolonged sympathetic overactivity and even short periods of exposure to pharmacological doses of β-adrenoceptor agonists may lead to β_1-receptor down-regulation and, therefore, to a reduction in the efficacy of β-agonists. This is well demonstrated in patients with terminal cardiac failure because of the long-standing sympathetic overactivity observed in this condition. Similarly, in patients with phaeochromocytoma, exposure to high catecholamine concentrations decreases the number of receptors. Beta-adrenoceptor up-regulation is observed in hyperthyroidism. It is also a feature of the prolonged administration of β-adrenoceptor blockers. This increase in receptor density explains the adverse effects of the abrupt withdrawal of β-blockers. As the β-receptor density is increased, even a modest degree of sympathetic overactivity is capable of causing large β-receptor-mediated effects. This may explain the rebound angina that has been well documented after withdrawal of β-blocker therapy, as well as other complications such as unstable angina, myocardial infarction, sudden death, and rebound hypertension.

Post-synaptic β_1-receptors are sensitive to noradrenaline and behave as transmitter receptors, while β_2-receptors behave mostly as hormonal receptors responding to circulating catecholamines.

The cardiovascular effects of β-adrenoceptor stimulation include β_1 effects such as tachycardia, increased contractility and cardiac output, improved conduction, and enhanced excitability, that is to say, positive chronotropy, inotropy, dromotropy, and bathmotropy. The latter may facilitate the development of dysrhythmias. Stimulation of the β_2-receptors results in vasodilatation and contributes to the positive chronotropy and inotropy of non-selective β-adrenergic agonists as β_2-receptors represent approximately 25% of the heart's β-receptors. Beta$_2$-adrenoceptor stimulation is responsible for many metabolic effects of adrenergic stimulation, and for bronchodilatation.

Three types of drugs interact with the receptors: the agonists, partial agonists and antagonists. Most of the interactions are competitive. In the presence of an antagonist, the dose–response curve to the agonist is displaced to the right (Figure 1.1). Partial agonists exert a stimulating effect on the receptors and prevent the association of agonist with the receptors.

Characteristics of the β-adrenoceptor antagonists

As a group, β-adrenoceptor antagonists exhibit the five main characteristics:

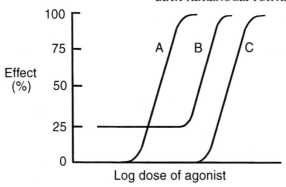

Fig 1.1   Diagrammatic representation of the interaction between an agonist and a partial agonist (agonist–antagonist), or a pure antagonist. **A** denotes the dose-response curve to the agonist in the absence of antagonist; **B** denotes the dose–response in the presence of an agonist–antagonist; **C** denotes the dose-response in the presence of a pure antagonist. Note that in this example the agonist–antagonist exerts 25% of the maximal effect of a pure agonist

1 they are competitive antagonists at the β-receptors;
2 they may exhibit receptor subtype selectivity;
3 they may exhibit partial agonist activity;
4 they possess, at very high doses, 'quinidine-like activity';
5 they may cause an increase in the number of β-receptors, when administered over a prolonged period of time.

Competitive antagonism   Beta-blockers displace the dose–response curve to isoprenaline or dobutamine to the right. Because they are competitive, their effects can be reversed by the administration of large doses of β-adrenoceptor agonists

Receptor subtype selectivity   The structure of the β-adrenoceptor antago-nists is relatively similar to that of the sympathomimetic amines. Some β-adrenoceptor antagonists have greater affinity for the cardiac (β_1) than for the peripheral (β_2) adrenoceptors. Propranolol is considered non-selective, since it is almost equally as effective in blocking β_1- and β_2-adrenoceptors. Similarly, nadolol, oxprenolol, pindolol, and timolol are non-selective β-adrenoceptor antagonists. Cardioselective antagonists (ace-butolol, atenolol, metoprolol) act predominantly on the β_1-adrenoceptors, reducing the positive inotropic and chronotropic responses to isoprenaline without inhibiting peripheral vasodilatation and bronchodilatation. Never-theless, when large doses of β_1-adrenoceptor blockers are administered, they eventually block both β_1- and β_2-receptors.

Partial agonist activity   Partial agonists stimulate β_1- or β_1- and β_2-adrenoceptors, an effect previously called intrinsic sympathomimetic

5

activity (ISA). However, their presence at receptor sites prevents the effect of other agonists.[2] Partial agonists increase heart rate and contractility. Typical examples include acebutolol, oxprenolol, pindolol, and xamoterol. They cause less resting bradycardia and, in the case of borderline heart failure, may be better tolerated than pure antagonists.

Membrane stabilisation   Membrane stabilisation is caused by inhibition of sodium transport. With the exception of atenolol and nadolol, the β-adrenoceptor antagonists cause some membrane stabilisation in the heart and, therefore, resemble quinidine but only at concentrations that are considerably greater than those required to obtain adequate clinical β-adrenoceptor blockade.

Up-regulation of β-adrenoceptors   Prolonged administration of β-adrenoceptor blockers causes an increase in the number of β-adrenoceptors. This up-regulation may be partly responsible for the adverse effects of the abrupt withdrawal of β-adrenoceptor blockers.

Antiarrhythmic action

The major antiarrhythmic effect of β-adrenoceptor blockade is the prevention of the arrhythmogenic effect of the endogenous and exogenous catecholamines. Membrane stabilisation is probably of little importance. However, increased duration of the action potential contributes to the antidysrhythmic efficacy of solatol.[3] As β-adrenoceptor blockers decrease heart rate and contractility, thereby reducing myocardial oxygen consumption, they are also effective in the treatment of ischaemia-related dysrhythmias.

Complex β-blockers

Some β-blockers, in addition to their effects on β-adrenoceptors exert antagonistic effects on α-adrenoceptors, or possess vasodilating and/or diuretic properties. These additional properties may widen their indications, particularly in the management of arterial hypertension and cardiac failure.

Classification of β-blockers

By combining the properties of receptor selectivity and partial agonist characteristics, it is possible to classify β-blockers in subgroups with similar characteristics and, therefore, similar pharmacodynamic properties (Table 1.2).

Absorption and elimination

Lipophilic β-blockers (metoprolol, pindolol, propranolol, timolol) are almost completely absorbed from the gastrointestinal tract. The more hydrophilic β-blockers (atenolol, nadolol) are absorbed to a much lesser

Table 1.2   Classification of β-blockers

Type	Cardioselective (β_1)	Non-selective (β_1 and β_2)	Non-selective (α, β_1 and β_2)
Pure agonists	Atenolol Metroprolol Esmolol	Propranolol Nadolol Sotalol Timolol	Labetalol Carvedilol
Partial agonists	Acebutolol Xamoterol	Oxprenolol Pindolol	
Partial agonist at β_2-receptors	Dilevalol		

extent (25–50%). Because of degradation in gut wall and liver (first-pass effect), bioavailability may be as low as 25% (nadolol) or between 50 and 100% (pindolol). The most lipophilic drugs have the highest bio-availability.[4, 5] Though data on bioavailability are very important when oral administration is to be replaced by intravenous administration, it is necessary to titrate the intravenous administration to obtain the desired effect (Table 1.3).

Effects of β-adrenoceptor blockers

Haemodynamic effects of β-adrenoceptor blockade

All β-adrenoceptor blockers reduce heart rate and cardiac output because they reduce the effect of β_1-receptor stimulation on the heart. Their effects are more pronounced when sympathetic activity is exaggerated and less pronounced when it is depressed. In addition, non-selective blockers cause an increase in peripheral vascular resistance because they abolish the β_2 vasodilator effect of sympathetic activation, leaving α-mediated vasoconstriction unopposed. Changes in heart rate and cardiac output are of

Table 1.3   Absorption and bioavailability of β-blockers after oral administration

	Absorption (% of dose)	Bioavailability (% of dose)
Acebutolol	≈70	≈40
Atenolol	≈50	≈40
Celiprolol	≈30	≈30
Dilevalol	>90	≈30
Labetalol	>90	≈33
Metoprolol	>90	≈50
Nadolol	≈30	≈30
Oxprenolol	≈90	≈40
Pindolol	>90	≈90
Propranolol	>90	≈30
Sotalol	≈70	≈60
Timolol	>90	≈75
Xamoterol	≈10	≈5

smaller magnitude with partial agonists. During exercise, the heart rate response is minimised and cardiac output increases less than in the absence of β-blockade. It is often thought that β_1-blockade depresses myocardial contractility. This is true in as much as removal of β_1-adrenergic support brings contractility back to a basal level. However, depression of contractility by the drugs themselves, over and above the removal of β_1 support, only occurs with doses considerably in excess of the therapeutic range.

Because of the reduction of heart rate and the return of contractility to a more basal level, β-blockers decrease myocardial oxygen consumption. At the same time they increase the duration of diastole; this may enhance coronary perfusion.

Cardiac protection by β-adrenoceptor blockers

Beta-receptor blockers improve the stability of the cardiovascular system and protect the myocardium in patients with coronary heart disease, hypertensive heart disease, dysrhythmias, or obstructive cardiomyopathies.

Blockade of β_2-receptors decreases the release of renin. This may contribute to the efficacy of β-blockade in the management of arterial hypertension as plasma levels of angiotensin II and aldosterone decrease.[6]

Effect on respiratory function

Beta–adrenoceptor blockade may worsen airway obstruction, especially when non-selective antagonists are used. In addition, they may decrease the ventilatory response to CO_2.

Reversal of β-adrenoceptor blockade

Reversing the effect of β-adrenoceptor blockade is seldom warranted. However, bradycardia may cause concern and this may be treated with atropine. If it becomes necessary to increase the inotropic state of the myocardium, β-adrenoceptor agonists are effective, but the doses required may be 5–20 times the usual doses. When non-selective β-adrenoceptor antagonists have been administered, large doses of the non-selective agonist isoprenaline are effective. When cardioselective β_1-adrenoceptor antagonists have been administered, a β_1-agonist, such as dobutamine, should be administered.

Withdrawal syndrome

Sudden withdrawal of adrenergic blockade may be dangerous.[7] The syndrome of withdrawal comprises development of ventricular dysrhythmias, worsening of angina, myocardial infarction and even sudden death. This may reflect β-adrenoceptor up-regulation. Another risk is rebound hypertension.

Medical indication of β-blockers

Beta-blockers continue to be used extensively in the management of coronary artery disease and hypertensive heart disease. Their benefits have been clearly demonstrated in the early and long-term management of acute myocardial infarction where they reduce the early mortality and decrease the infarct size. In the longer term they are effective in the secondary prevention of reinfarction. Their efficacy in the control of angina stems mainly from the control of heart rate.

In the management of arterial hypertension β-blockers remain one of the first-line drugs and their long-term administration has been shown to decrease morbidity. Over the recent past they have been used less extensively because of the perceived better drug compliance to calcium channel blockers, notably nifedipine. However, recent evidence suggests that calcium channel blockers, whilst clinically very effective in the management of hypertension and angina, may increase the risk of sudden death. It is, therefore, likely that β-blockers and ACE inhibitors, together with diuretics, will become the most important drugs in the management of arterial hypertension.

Other indications for β-blockade include obstructive cardiomyopathies (the major effect is to control the inotropic state and prevent increases in contractility in response to sympathetic stimulation), thyroid crisis (control of the metabolic and cardiac effects, partly mediated by sympathetic overactivity), and phaeochromocytoma (after α-adrenoceptor blockade has been established, β-blockade increases the haemodynamic stability of these patients). Acute β-adrenoceptor blockade is also effective in controlling the cardiovascular effects of sympathetic overactivity observed in tetanus patients.

Beta-blockade in myocardial infarction

Agents which reduce myocardial oxygen demand can potentially reduce the extent of myocardial necrosis and thus preserve segmental and global cardiac function. Beta-blockers decrease heart rate, blood pressure, wall stress, and myocardial oxygen consumption. In addition, they minimise the effect of catecholamines of myocardial metabolism so that increases in free fatty acids (FFA) are prevented. They may also produce a redistribution of coronary blood flow to the subendocardium. Early treatment with β-blockers, experimentally and in clinical practice, has been shown to decrease infarct size. In the ISIS-1 (First International Study of Infarct Survival), mortality was reduced by about 15% during the seven days of trteatment (3·9% vs. 4·6%), without evidence of excess delayed mortality.[8] Other studies have confirmed the reduction in mortality in the first seven days. The risk of reinfarction is also reduced by about 15%. The reduction in mortality is due mainly to a reduction in the number of cardiac ruptures.

Long-term, β-blockers reduce mortality of acute myocardial infarction by about 22% (from 9·4% to 7·6%), the main benefit being a reduction in the number of sudden deaths. Mortality reduction appears to be greater (26%) with non-ISA than with ISA drugs (15%).[9] The benefits of early β-blockade are significantly greater in high-risk than in low-risk patients.[10]

Beta-blockade and regional ischaemic dysfunction

Beta-adrenoceptor blockade may improve regional function of ischaemic myocardial segments. Usually benefits are attributed to improved oxygen balance, increased diastolic filling time, and increased collateral flow. In experimental animals with fully developed collaterals, brief episodes of coronary occlusion cause less ischaemic dysfunction and less haemodynamic impairment in the presence than in the absence of β-blockade. In contrast, β-blockade was of no benefit in the absence of collaterals.[11] These results are in keeping with other studies reporting beneficial effects of β-blockade in the presence of coronary stenosis rather than occlusion, when there was some coronary blood flow to the compromised area.[12, 13] As improvement of function in the ischaemic, collateralised segment was more prominent with relatively fast cardiac pacing than at slower rates, prolonged diastolic time cannot be the major mechanism of protection by β-blockade. A shift of coronary blood flow towards the ischaemic segment is a more plausible explanation. Other factors, such as protection of mitochondrial function,[14] and depression of contractility, if they were of major importance in protecting against acute total occlusion, should have had the same effect before and after collateral flow development.

Beta-blockade in syndrome X

Many patients may experience angina in the absence of demonstrable coronary atherosclerosis or vasospam (syndrome X). Such patients may suffer from an inadequate capacity of the coronary microcirculation to dilate in response to increased myocardial oxygen demand.[15] As β-blockade minimises the extent of increases in myocardial oxygen consumption, it may be expected to reduce the number of episodes of angina. Indeed, Bugiardini and colleagues[16] have shown propranolol to be effective in this syndrome.

Beta-receptors in congestive heart failure

Abnormalities of the β-receptor system have been described in patients with congestive heart failure. They include a decrease in β-adrenoceptor density in human heart muscle associated with reduced responsiveness to β-agonists,[17, 18] associated with a reduction of β-receptor density in peripheral lymphocytes.[19] A correlation between β-receptor density and functional impairment has been postulated. Mancini and colleagues[20] found that the average lymphocytic β-receptor density was reduced at rest in patients with congestive heart failure. This was associated with a reduced adenylate cyclase activity and a reduced response of adenylcyclase to isoprenaline. During exercise, these patients exhibited an increase in β-receptor density that was only 58% of that of normal subjects, and no increase in isoprenaline-stimulated adenylate cyclase activity. This attenuated adenylcyclase activity may limit the capacity of drugs such as β-agonists and phosphodiesterase inhibitors to increase cyclic AMP.

Beta-blockade may be associated with a reduction of cardiac contractility and a consequent decline in ventricular performance. This may be a major risk in patients with congestive heart failure. However, β-blockers with ISA (partial agonists) such as pindolol, may be safer in such patients. Indeed, Binkley and colleagues,[21] have shown, in patients with a mean ejection fraction of $23 \pm 5\%$, that pindolol (five consecutive doses of 10 mg) caused small increases in cardiac contractility assessed in terms of end-systolic pressure-dimension relationships and velocity of fibre shortening.

Beta-blockers as antiarrhythmics

Beta-adrenoceptor blockers are effective in the treatment of dysrhythmias caused by increased sympathetic activity. They are also effective in the management of dysrhythmias associated with myocardial infarction. These dysrhythmias are due to a number of factors, including increases in plasma catecholamines, leakage of potassium due to hypoxia, rise in free fatty acids, and alterations in action potential duration (shortened by hypoxia; lengthened by acidosis), all of which enhance the heterogeneity of repolarisation.

Beta-blockers cause significant reductions in sinus rate and decrease the number of both supraventricular and ventricular dysrhythmias.[22] This is associated with a reduction in the incidence of ventricular fibrillation, and a reduction in mortality.[23]

Solatol, a non-selective β-blocker, exhibits both Class 2 and Class 3 antiarrhythmic properties and effectively controls life-threatening dysrhythmias, especially ventricular premature complexes, ventricular tachycardia, and ventricular fibrillation. Solatol reduces cardiac mortality in patients with life-threating ventricular dysrhythmias. It is also effective in supraventricular dysrhythmias. Solatol rarely causes worsening of congestive heart failure. Its administration may cause life-threatening dysrhythmias, including torsades de pointes.[24]

Contraindications for β-blockade

Beta-blockers are contraindicated in patients with overt cardiac failure or hypovolaemia. They are also contraindicated in major conduction disorders, unless patients have the benefits of cardiac pacing. Asthma, arteriopathies, including Raynaud's syndrome, and severe depression are also contraindications to β-blockade. Though β-blockers may be well tolerated by patients with chronic obstructive airways disease, no functional test allows tolerance to be predicted. Insulin-dependent diabetes is also a relative contraindication because of the possible masking of hypoglycaemic symptoms by β-blockers.

Beta-blockers and anaesthetic practice

Until the early 1970s it was widely accepted that β-adrenoceptor blockers should be stopped prior to elective surgery. The reason given for this approach was that blockade of the β-adrenoceptor could result in cardiac failure during anaesthesia and surgery, as both inotropic and chronotropic support to the heart would be removed at a time anaesthetic agents caused myocardial depression. There was anecdotal evidence of cardiovascular collapse in patients receiving β-blockers.

The first detailed haemodynamic studies of the interactions between β-adrenoceptor blockade and anaesthesia were published in 1973.[25] These studies showed that the administration of an intravenous dose of a β-blocker (practolol 0·4 mg/kg) after atropine (0·01 mg/kg) did not significantly alter the systemic haemodynamics during halothane anaesthesia. Similarly, preoperative oral treatment with practolol for three days prior to surgery did not significantly alter the response to anaesthesia except that heart rate was slower in β-blocked patients. In addition, these studies showed that intravenous or oral β-blockade minimised the increases in systolic pressure and heart rate that are usually observed in hypertensive patients in response to laryngoscopy and intubation. They also prevented ventricular dysrhthmias and ST segment depression. These observations, based on small numbers of patients, were enough to cause a complete change of policy. Since the mid-1970s it has become customary to maintain patients on their β-blocker therapy until the morning of surgery and throughout the perioperative period.

Further studies have confirmed the safety of anaesthesia in the face of high-grade β-blockade.[26] In addition, a number of experimental studies have explored the possibility of adverse interactions between β-blockade and anaesthesia by mimicking incidents such as haemorrhage, haemodilution, hypoxia, and hypo- or hypercarbia. The haemodynamic responses to such incidents were modified by β-blockade but not in a manner likely to cause significant haemodynamic impairment.[27-29]

A potential hazard of β-adrenoceptor blockade, however, is that the tachycardic response to hypovolaemia is blunted. Unless all those concerned with the care of the patient are aware of this effect of β-blockade, the absence of tachycardia may cause volume loss to be underestimated and, therefore, may delay volume replacement.

Noradrenergic pathways within the CNS are involved in producing anaesthesia. Catecholamine depletors such as α-methyldopa and reserpine are known to reduce anaesthetic requirements. Similarly, the α_2-adreno-ceptor agonists clonidine and dexmetedomidine reduce MAC for inhalational anaesthetics and potentiate the analgesic effects of opioids. Modulation of CNS noradrenergic pathways can also be achieved by blockade of the β-adrenoceptors. It has been long recognised that β-blockers are effective in the management of anxiety states, tremor and stage fright. While there is evidence of sedation by propranolol, there was no evidence that propranolol reduces MAC for halothane until a recent study showed that both esmolol and propranolol reduce MAC for halothane in a rat model.[30] However, most of the time, the addition of a β-blocker to any anaesthetic regime is made in order to reduce the incidence of tachycardia and hypertension in response to rapid changes in anaesthetic (laryngoscopy and intubation, extubation) or surgical stimulation, rather than to alter the anaesthetic requirements *per se*.

Another important consideration is the risk of withdrawal of β-blockade after surgery when patients are unable to take oral drugs. It is known that prolonged β-blockade causes an increase in the number of β-adrenocep-tors, termed up-regulation. This means that on the abrupt withdrawal of β-blockade exaggerated sympathetic response may be observed associated with rebound hypertension and myocardial ischaemia, myocardial infarc-tion or even cardiac deaths. The solution is to replace the oral drug by intravenous β-blockade up until the patient can absorb oral drugs again. In practice, however, β-blockade is often simply omitted. The most noticeable effect is tachycardia. Indeed, in the postoperative period, heart rate is usually faster than preoperatively. This trend is accentuated when β-blockers are omitted and this may cause myocardial ischaemia.

Indication for β-blockers in anaesthesia

Beta-blockers are effective in controlling some of the effects of the sympathetic overactivity caused by laryngoscopy, endotracheal intubation, and extubation. While tachycardia is either controlled or prevented, the increase in blood pressure is likely to be blunted rather than suppressed because it is due to α-adrenoceptor-mediated vasoconstriction. As tachy-cardia is the major risk factor for myocardial ischaemia, β-blockers are effective in decreasing the incidence of myocardial ischaemia at these particular phases of the perioperative period. Beta-blockers are equally effective in controlling the effects of the sympathetic overactivity observed during neurosurgical procedures, dental surgery, intrathoracic surgery, visceral manipulation, and urological surgery. Their efficacy against tachycardia is greater than against hypertension as α-adrenoceptor-mediated effects persist. When deliberately induced hypotension is required, the tachycardia that attends the administration of potent vasodilators is prevented by β-blockers and control of the level of hypotension is made easier.

Though very effective, β-blockers should not be used to treat the effects of sympathetic overactivity when the cause of the latter can be identified and treated. This would be the case of sympathetic overactivity caused by hypercapnia, hypoxia or severe haemodilution anaemia. In these instances, β-blockade could unmask circulatory depression and cause acute circulatory failure: correction of the primary disorder is essential.

Beta-blockers and preoperative anxiety

The primary aim of premedication is to relieve anxiety and produce sedation. Anxiety is associated with considerable increases in sympathetic tone, the effects of which may be minimised by β-adrenoceptor blockers. While benzodiazepines are sedative and anxiolytic, a comparison between diazepam–placebo and diazepam–metoprolol (15 mg and 100 mg respectively), showed better anxiolysis when the premedication included the β-blocker.[31] This was associated with some reduction in plasma catecholamines in both groups. However, poor correlation between catecholamines and anxiety scores indicates that catecholamines are only one of the factors of anxiety.

Beta-blockers in silent ischaemia

Most episodes of transient myocardial ischaemia are not accompanied by angina. Dynamic coronary artery narrowing or an increase in oxygen demand may contribute to episodes of silent ischaemia. As most episodes occur while patients are physically inactive but mentally active,[32] and as catecholamines play an important role in alertness, β-adrenergic mechanisms may be involved. A number of studies have shown the efficacy of non-ISA β-blockers in reducing the number of episodes of silent ischaemia in patients with effort angina.[33] In patients with rest angina, the benefits of β-blockers are less clear-cut.[34] Total silent ischaemic time and the frequency of episodes are reduced by metoprolol, as are average daily heart rate at onset of ischaemia.[35] Control of heart rate appears to be a major factor in the protection against silent ischaemia.[36]

A very important role for β-adrenoceptor blockers is the prevention of perioperative silent myocardial ischaemia. Silent ischaemia is known to be associated with adverse outcome and there is a strong association between preoperative silent ischaemia and postoperative complications such as myocardial infarction, unstable angina, life-threatening dysrhythmias and acute left ventricular failure. The association between postoperative silent ischaemia and adverse outcome is even stronger. Indeed, the presence of postoperative silent ischaemia is associated with a substantial reduction of survival at two to three years. This suggests that control of silent ischaemia could improve outcome in the short and possibly in the long term. Many studies have shown that acute β-blockade decreases the incidence of perioperative ischaemia. A single dose of β-blocker given with the premedication almost totally prevents silent ischaemia during the immediate perioperative period.[37] Moreover, this effect is still observed for the next 12 hours.[38] If β-blockade is continued, significant protection against silent myocardial ischaemia is observed for the next few days.[39] Though prevention of silent ischaemia is expected to be beneficial, there is little data, as yet, to demonstrate that prevention of perioperative ischaemia or early treatment of ischaemia improves outcome. Most of the studies, so far, have observed an excess morbidity in patients with silent ischaemia but have not addressed the crucial issue of the efficacy of β-blockade as a prophylatic or therapeutic intervention. In this respect it is worth noting that silent ischaemia is very common in poorly controlled or untreated hypertensive patients. It may be that this group of patients would benefit from perioperative β-blockade.

Beta-blockade and haemodilution

Isovolumic haemodilution is associated with a hyperdynamic response of the circulation due to sympathetic stimulation. Blockade of the β-adrenoceptors prevents increases in contractility but does not suppress the haemodynamic response completely because vascular resistance and blood viscosity are reduced, so that the left ventricle may empty more easily against a reduced aortic input impedance.[40-42] Regional blood flow responses are heterogenous and are altered by β-adrenoceptor blockade. Experimentally, haemodilution itself does modify blood flow to the renal cortex, liver and spleen, and increases flow to the pancreas, duodenum, brain and myocardium. Beta-blockade does not substantially alter the haemodilution-induced alterations in blood flow.[43] With or without β-blockade, it is essentially in brain and myocardium that increases in flow maintain adequate oxyen delivery. While the effect of haemodilution on regional function of myocardium supplied by a critically constricted coronary artery has been studied, and the increase in flow through the fixed stenosis shown to be unable to maintain adequate oxygen supply and normal function,[44] the interaction between β-adrenoceptor blockade, haemodilution, and critical coronary stenosis has not been studied. Whether β-blockade, by blunting the response of the circulation, and by improving oxygen usage, may protect the compromised myocardium remains to be elucidated.

Beta-blockers of special relevance to perioperative management

Esmolol

For many years, intravenous β-blockers have been used in the management of cardiovascular disorders, such as myocardial ischaemia, hypertension, tachycardia, and dysrhythmias, that develop in surgical patients. Conventional β-adrenoceptor blockers are relatively long-acting. This may be an advantage, as control of the disorder is established for many hours. Their intravenous administration must start with low doses, and it is impossible to titrate the degree of blockade to changing autonomic activity. In some patients adverse effects, such as exaggerated hypotension and reduced cardiac output, may develop and compromise outcome. If conventional blockers cause circulatory failure, recovery is slow and inotropic drugs may have to be given. Should this be necessary, the doses of adrenergic agonists may have to be much larger than usual and their side-effects may be enhanced, complicating treatment.

The concept of ultra-short-acting β-blockers stems from the need, in the intensive care situation, to titrate the level of blockade quickly and reversibly, and has been achieved by incorporation of enzymatic lability into the molecule.[45] Esmolol, a cardioselective β_1-adrenergic blocker, devoid of intrinsic sympathomimetic activity and of membrane stabilising activity, has an α-distribution half-life of 2 minutes, and a β-elimination half-life of 9 minutes. The reason for short duration of action is an ester group in the para-position which is rapidly hydrolysed by red blood cells.[46, 47] Esmolol is metabolised into two metabolites, methanol and ASL-8123. The latter is a very weak β-blocker. Protein binding is about 55%, and total body clearance is approximately 20 1/h. Esmolol is 50-fold less potent than propranolol and six-fold less potent than metoprolol.[45, 48]

Studies in humans have shown that over the range of 25–300 µg/kg/min, esmolol causes dose-dependent haemodynamic effects. On discontinuation of the infusion, significant recovery occurs in 10–20 minutes.[49] Depression of contractility is dose-dependent, and is associated with decreases in sinoatrial node activity, atrioventricular conduction and atrioventricular node refractoriness.

Hypotension may occur in patients and volunteers receiving esmolol infusions. The risk of developing systolic hypotension may be greater than the expected therapeutic benefits with infusion rates of greater than 100 µg/kg/min,[50] though infusion rates up to 750 µg/kg/min have been used.[51] If hypotension is due essentially to β-blockade, there should be essentially parallel reductions in stroke volume and heart rate. If hypotension occurs also without reduction in heart rate, a direct negative inotropic action of esmolol must be postulated. A detailed haemodynamic investigation of the effects of stepped infusion rates of esmolol has shown that esmolol causes a dose-related reduction in left ventricular performance (assessed by the relationship between stroke work and end-diastolic diameter) independent of a decline in heart rate.[52] This dissociation of inotropic and chronotropic effects may suggest that esmolol exerts, in clinically relevant dosages, some quinidine-like effect.

1 Tachycardia and hypertension

Esmolol is effective in preventing both the tachycardia and hypertension which occur in high-risk patients in response to laryngoscopy and intubation. Cucchiara and colleagues[53] have demonstrated that increases in heart rate are significantly reduced by esmolol infusion (9 beats/min as opposed to 24 beats/min in placebo controls) and that hypertensive responses are essentially suppressed (increases in systolic pressure: 2 mmHg as opposed to 45 mmHg in placebo controls), in patients presenting for carotid endarterectomy.

In studies of patients undergoing myocardial revascularisation, the blood pressure responses were better blunted than the rate responses. Moreover, ST segment changes were found to be less frequent in esmolol - than placebo-treated patients.[54] Esmolol is as effective in treating cardiovascular abnormalities as it is in preventing their development. This is particularly true of tachycardia, as reported by Gold et al.[55] and by Newsome et al.[56]

Postoperatively, esmolol is also effective in the management of hypertension. In a cross-over comparison with nitroprusside, comparable reductions in systolic pressure were obtained. However, nitroprusside decreased diastolic arterial pressure (-31%) more than esmolol (-8%); esmolol caused a reduction in heart rate, while nitroprusside caused tachycardia.[57] Similarly, esmolol is effective in the control of supraventricular dysrhythmias. As such dysrhythmias may be harmful in patients with coronary heart disease, control by a short-acting β-blocker offers the advantage of immediate action, without the drawback of prolonged effects.

In most studies, infusion rates up to 300 μg/kg/min have been used with return of haemodynamic parameters to base line within 30 minutes of discontinuation of the infusion. This makes esmolol very safe in the perioperative period.[58] However, the risk of hypotension must be borne in mind.[59]

2 Atrial fibrillation

Esmolol is effective in the treatment of a variety of supraventricular tachydysrhythmias,[60] and could be used instead of verapamil. In the management of atrial fibrillation and atrial flutter, esmolol is as effective as verapamil in reducing heart rate and produces a higher proportion (50% vs 12%) of conversion to sinus rhythm. The incidence of hypotension is similar with both drugs. After successful administration of esmolol, treatment may be continued with oral β-blockers or digoxin.[61]

3 Myocardial revascularisation

Patients undergoing coronary artery bypass grafting (CABG) are at risk for myocardial ischaemia, particularly if tachycardia is allowed to develop.[62, 63] Beta-blockers are effective to prevent or treat tachycardia. However, the long-lasting effects of most β-blockers may be a drawback in the acute perioperative management of tachycardia because of the potential for cardiac depression. Under high dose fentanyl anaesthesia, administration of esmolol does not cause exaggerated reductions in heart rate and mean arterial pressure in unstimulated patients, though cardiac index may be reduced by approximately 10%. During surgical stimulation, esmolol is effective in preventing the increase in heart rate due to intubation, but did not prevent the increase in blood pressure,[64] as the latter is caused predominantly by an increase in peripheral vascular resistance.[65]

Whether a prophylactic infusion of esmolol is necessarily justified has been questioned, as a bolus dose of approximately 1 mg/kg, followed by an infusion of 12 mg/min is effective in the treatment of increases in systolic pressure and heart rate observed during CABG in enflurane-anaesthetised patients.[66]

In neurosurgical patients, hypertension during emergence can be controlled by a loading dose (40 mg/min for 4 minutes) followed by an infusion (24 mg/min) continued until extubation. Only a small proportion of the esmolol-treated patients (1/20) as opposed to a large proportion (14/19) of the placebo-treated patients needed additional antihypertensive medication. In two patients esmolol had to be discontinued because of hypotension.[67]

4 Deliberate hypotension

Long-acting β-blockers are known to reduce the dose of nitroprusside required to produce deliberate hypotension. Similarly, esmolol increases the hypotensive effects of nitroprusside when given as a loading dose (500 μg/kg) followed by an infusion (300 μg/kg/min) in enflurane-anaesthetised dogs.[68]

5 Tetralogy of Fallot

Patients with tetralogy of Fallot are prone to severe hypoxic episodes ("hypercyanotic episodes"), often brought on by stress, anxiety, and exercise. Increased obstruction of the pulmonary outflow tract may be responsible for such episodes. Standard medical management includes the correction of acidosis (if present), morphine to alleviate stress and decrease catecholamine discharge, phenylephrine to increase systemic vascular resistance, thus enhancing flow through the pulmonary circulation, and β-blockers to reduce contractility,[69] thus minimising outflow tract obstruction. Particularly in the paediatric age group, β-blockade may cause bradycardia. This has led many clinicians to use only small doses of β-

blockers, or to avoid them altogether. With esmolol, a titrated response can be obtained, and all the advantages of β-blockade are available without the risks associated with prolonged adverse effects.[70]

6 Phaeochromocytoma

Preoperative α-blockade is a major factor in the reduction of perioperative morbidity of patients with phaeochromocytoma. Usually, β-blockade is associated with α-blockade to control tachycardia and dysrhythmias. Nevertheless, haemodynamic instability is common during handling of the tumour and further interventions are often necessary. Control of hypertension with sodium nitroprusside may cause tachycardia. The latter is well controlled by an infusion of esmolol, so that the combination of both, in titratable doses, appears particularly indicated in the management of these patients.[71]

7 Thyrotoxicosis

Optimal perioperative management of patients with thyrotoxicosis should render them euthyroid before surgery. However, this is not always possible. Beta-blockers have become standard therapy in such circumstances,[72, 73] yet some patients may appear to be refractory to conventional oral β-blockers. In such patients intravenous esmolol may be used intraoperatively as well as postoperatively to control both tachycardia and hypertension. The rapid titrability of esmolol is advantageous and relatively high infusion rates may be required.[74]

Labetalol

Labetalol is a competitive antagonist at β_1- and β_2-adrenoceptors and has some intrinsic activity at the β_2-adrenoceptors. In addition, labetalol is a competitive antagonist at postsynaptic α-adrenoceptors. It is four to eight times more potent at β- than α-receptors.

1 Perioperative hypertension

Labetalol can be used prophylactically to prevent hypertensive episodes; it is usually effective and well tolerated. Doses of labetalol between 0·25 and 0·75 mg/kg given prior to induction of anaesthesia do not cause significant haemodynamic changes in ASA Class I–III patients. However, they exert a dose-dependent blocking effect on the pressure and rate response to laryngoscopy and intubation. There is a risk of hypotension with doses in excess of 0·75 mg/kg.[75] More detailed haemodynamic studies have shown this blunting to be due to attenuation of cardiac function. Indeed, the reduction in stroke volume that attends laryngoscopy and intubation is accentuated by labetolol.[76] When smaller doses are used (less than 0·4 mg/kg), the rate but not the pressor response was minimised.[77, 78]

Labetalol is also often used when hypertension has developed. Given as repeated small boluses (5 mg), labetolol is effective in reducing blood pressure, while causing only moderate reductions in heart rate.[79] This suggests that labetalol causes more vasodilatation than β-blockade. When larger doses are given (0·75 mg/kg), however, the decrease in blood pressure reflects negative inotropy, as attested by studies showing an increase in end-diastolic area measured by transoesophageal echocardiography.[80] The management of perioperative hypertension is discussed in Chapter 7.

2   Deliberate hypotension

Deliberate hypotension reduces bleeding and provides a clear operative field; this is particularly valuable in microsurgery such as middle-ear surgery. Many drugs can be used for this purpose (sodium nitroprusside, trimetaphan, calcium antagonists), associated with inhalational anaesthetics. Often several drugs are used, for example sodium nitroprusside and β-blockers, the latter being used to minimise the infusion rate of sodium nitroprusside and to suppress the tachycardia. Labetalol in association with inhalational anaesthetics provides stable hypotension with tachycardia (or excessive bradycardia) and without rebound hypertension. The doses of labetalol necessary to achieve a mean arterial pressure of 50 mmHg, in the presence of 1 MAC halothane, enflurane or isoflurane, are approximately 0·55 mg/kg (initial dose) with extra doses of the order of 0·3 mg/kg/h.[81]

Newer β-adrenergic agonist–antagonists

Xamoterol

Xamoterol is a partial agonist at the β_1-adrenoceptors with little effect on vascular resistance. Its partial agonist activity amounts to 45% of the maximum activity of the full agonist isoprenaline.[82] Xamoterol has positive inotropic and chronotropic properties and attenuates the chronotropic response to exercise, thus demonstrating that it is an agonist–antagonist.[83] Xamoterol alters the relationship between sympathetic stimulation and the response of the heart so that at low level of sympathetic activity it behaves as an agonist, and at high levels, as an antagonist. The inotropic support associated with blunting of exercise-induced heart rate increases may benefit patients with left ventricular dysfunction, without necessarily increasing the risk of myocardial ischaemia.

With exercise, plasma noradrenaline levels increase and there is a linear relationship between heart rate and plasma noradrenaline. The slope of this relationship is depressed by xamoterol in patients with mild to moderate left ventricular dysfunction.[84] Similarly, the slope of the relationship between cardiac output and plasma noradrenaline is depressed by xamoterol. For both relationships, however, the cross-over point of the lines with and without xamoterol occurs at plasma noradrenaline concentrations which correspond to a low level of exercise (400–500 pg/ml noradrenaline). This indicates that xamoterol acts as an agonist at rest and mild exercise, and as an antagonist at higher sympathetic drive. Unexpectedly, PCWP decreases with xamoterol. As arteriolar dilatation has not been observed in response to xamoterol, improved diastolic function is more likely to explain this beneficial effect at rest and during exercise. This profile makes xamoterol particularly attractive in the treatment of effort angina associated with left ventricular dysfunction.[85]

In support of the hypothesis that xamoterol may improve the diastolic properties of the left ventricle, Pouleur and colleagues,[86] have shown an improvement of the diastolic pressure–volume relationship, and a reduction of myocardial stiffness in patients with documented anterior myocardial infarction given xamoterol. This suggests that impaired diastolic function after myocardial infarction is not entirely caused by scar tissue, but also by some functional, possibly drug-reversible alterations in the myocardium. While scar tissue is unlikely to be influenced by moderate β-adrenergic simulation, chronically ischaemic border zones may be responsive to drugs. The prolonged administration of xamoterol, by protecting against the adverse effects of exaggerated sympathetic stimulation, may prevent repeated ischaemic stunning of underperfused areas.[87] This in turn may improve diastolic function.

In patients with poor left ventricular function xamoterol causes significant increases in cardiac index, reduces the pulmonary wedge pressure, improves exercise tolerance and attenuates the exercise-induced increase in heart rate.[88] In chronic heart failure, xamoterol significantly increases exercise duration (bicycle ergometer) and improves both breathlessness and tiredness.[89] Recent studies of the use of β-blockers in heart failure after myocardial infarction suggest that xamoterol may have minor advantages over metoprolol in terms of functional improvements.[89] Combined with digoxin, xamoterol improves the control of atrial fibrillation and enhances exercise tolerance.[90]

In patients with exertional dyspnoea and low ejection fractions (28%) caused by myocardial infarction, xamoterol can improve resting haemodynamics and exercise tolerance. At rest, xamoterol increases stroke volume, stroke work index, and heart rate, and reduces the pulmonary capillary wedge pressure. Exercise tolerance is enhanced, and the increase in heart rate is less with xamoterol- than in placebo-treated patients.[91]

One of the final tests of drug therapy in heart failure is its efficacy in a prospective double-blind placebo-controlled trial. In a comparison of digoxin, xamoterol and placebo, xamoterol has been shown to increase exercise duration, and to reduce breathlessnes and tiredness during daily life in a study involving over 400 patients. As there is still controversy as to the efficacy of digoxin, it must be noted that digoxin's modest effect was not statistically different from placebo.[90]

Celiprolol

One of the problems of non-selective β-adrenoceptor blockers is their adverse effect on both peripheral vasculature and bronchial smooth muscle. These problems are only partly overcome with the selective β_1-blockers, as adverse effects may occur, particularly when high doses are administered. Recently, new drugs have been developed which combine β_1-blockade and stimulation of β_2-receptors.

Celiprolol is a β_1-selective adrenoceptor antagonist which acts as a weak agonist at the β_2-adrenoceptors, and is excreted unchanged.[92] Celiprolol has a bronchosparing effect in patients with reversible airways disease. The drug demonstrates vasodilator properties and has been shown to be effective in the management of arterial hypertension and in the treatment of stable effort angina.[93] The advantage of celiprolol over other β-blockers is the reduction of peripheral vascular resistance and the maintenance of resting heart rate.[94] Vasodilatation may be an advantage in the management of patients with heart failure. In hypertensive patients celiprolol is as effective as atenolol in terms of blood pressure reduction but has the advantage of not reducing cardiac output.[95]

Dilevalol

Dilevalol, a stereoisomer of labetalol, is an antagonist at the β_1-receptors and an agonist–antagonist at the β_2-receptors.[96] It has a high first-pass metabolism so that its bioavailability is only 12%. Its mean elimination half-life is 8–12 hours.[97] The β_2-agonist activity of dilevalol on peripheral vascular resistance is approximately 50% of that of isoprenaline. Blockade of β_1-receptors is as effective as that of propranolol. At variance with its isomer labetalol, dilevalol possesses little if any α-blocking activity. Dilevalol exerts potent antihypertensive activity in a variety of animal models. As this activity is blocked by propranolol (a pure β_1- and β_2-antagonist), the major antihypertensive action must reside in the agonist effect on β_2-adrenoceptor, causing peripheral vasodilatation. As could be expected from its pharmacological profile, dilevalol decreases myocardial contractility and increases cardiac output owing to peripheral vasodilatation. The latter effect is more apparent at rest than during exercise.[98]

Carvedilol

Carvedilol is a non-selective β-adrenoceptor blocking drug which exhibits α_1-blocking and anti-oxidant properties. Because of the vasodilatation that attends α-1 blockade, carvedilol has been shown to improve

22

cardiac function in patients with mild to moderate heart failure;[99] worsening of heart failure, life-threatening ventricular dysrhythmias, as well as risk of death are minimised by carvedilol. The improvement in resting cardiac function is associated with improvement of symptoms of failure.[100] In the management of hypertension, an advantage of carvedilol is that the reduction in peripheral vascular resistance does not cause reflexly induced tachycardia because of the blockade of the cardiac β-receptors.[101] An interesting observation is that carvedilol appears to protect vascular function by scavenging free radicals.[102]

Summary and conclusions

The distinction between α- and β-adrenergic receptors was made by Ahlquist in 1948.[103] Propranolol became available in the early 1960s. The subsequent years have witnessed a growing appreciation of the complexity of the autonomic nervous system, and of the role of β-adrenoceptors within this system. A range of drugs acting at adrenergic receptors have been developed and have found wide application.

Anaesthetists encounter large numbers of patients taking β-blockers for hypertension or angina, and the control of heart rate, blood pressure, and myocardial oxygen consumption is at the core of the use of these drugs. The importance of maintaining beta-blockade in these patients during the perioperative period is now well established. Beta-blockers may also be used in the treatment of ventricular and supraventricular dysrhythmias and to control the ventricular rate in intractable atrial fibrillation. A more recent development is the use of β-blockers with intrinsic sympathomimetic activity in the treatment of cardiac failure. Other cardiac applications of β-blockers include their use in hypertrophic cardiomyopathy and in the tetralogy of Fallot. They may also be used to control generalised sympathetic overactivity caused by anxiety or by hyperthyroidism.

Specific indications for β-blockers in anaesthesia include premedication, the blunting of the sympathomimetic response to laryngoscopy or vigorous surgical stimulation, the control of tachycardia and tachydysrhythmias, and as a component of hypotensive anaesthesia. Labetalol and esmolol have particular applications in anaesthesia. Both are administered parenterally. The combined α- and β-adrenergic blockade produced by labetalol allows blood pressure to be lowered without the production of a reflex tachycardia. The rapid onset and short duration of action of esmolol allow rapid control of heart rate and blood pressure with an agent which can be titrated to effect and discontinued rapidly when no longer required.

It seems certain that β-blockers will remain part of our practice for the foreseeable future. It also seems likely that the full potential of these drugs has not yet been fully realised and that the β-blockers available will become increasingly sophisticated in their design and diverse in their applications.

1 Schwinn DA. Adrenoceptors as models for G protein-coupled receptors: structure, function and regulation. *Br J Anaesth* 1993;**71**:77–85.
2 Ablad B, Brogard M, Ek L. Pharmacologic properties of H56/28 a beta-adrenergic receptor antagonist. *Acta Pharmacol Toxicol (Kopenhaven)* 1967;**25**,Suppl.2:9–40.
3 Bennett DH. Acute prolongation of myocardial refractoriness by sotalol. *Br Heart J* 1982;**47**:521–6.
4 Regardh C-G. Pharmacokinetics of β-adrenoceptor antagonists. In: Poppers PJ, van Dijk B, van Elzakker AHM, eds. *β-blockade and anaesthesia*. Rijswijk, The Netherlands: Astra Pharmaceutica, 1982:29–45.
5 Feely J, de Vane PJ, Maclean D. Beta-blockers and sympathomimetics. *Br Med J* 1983;**286**:1043–7.
6 Cruickshank JM. The clinical importance of cardioselectivity and liposolubility in beta-blockers. *Am Heart J* 1980;**100**:160–78.
7 Ponten J, Biber B, Bjuro T, Henriksson BA, Hjalmarson A, Lundberg D. β-receptor blockade and spinal anaesthesia. Withdrawal versus continuation of long-term therapy. *Acta Anaesthesiol Scand* 1982;**76**(Suppl):62–9.
8 ISIS-1 Collaborative Group. Randomised trial of intravenous atenolol among 16,027 cases of suspected acute myocardial infarction: ISIS-1. *Lancet* 1986;**1**:57–66.
9 Yusuf S. The use of beta-adrenergic blocking agents, iv nitrates and calcium channel blocking agents following acute myocardial infarction. *Chest* 1988; **93**: 25S–28S.
10 Hjalmarson A. International beta-blocker review in acute and postmyocardial infarction. *Am J Cardiol* 1988;**61**:26B–29B.
11 Morhi M, Tomoike H, Inoue T, Nakamura M. Amelioration by beta-adrenergic blockade of regional myocardial dysfunction induced by coronary occlusion after, but not before collateral development in conscious dogs. *Am Heart J* 1989;**117**:45–52.
12 Tomoike H, Ross J jr, Franklin D, Crozatier B, McKeown D, Kemper WS. Improvement by propranolol of regional myocardial dysfunction and abnormal coronary flow pattern in conscious dogs with coronary narrowing. *Am J Cardiol* 1978;**41**:689–96.
13 Matsuzaki M, Partitti J, Tajimi T, Miller M, Kemper WS, Ross J jr. Effects of beta blockade on regional myocardial flow and function during exercise. *Am J Physiol* 1984;**247**:H52–H60.
14 Kloner RA, Fishbein MC, Braunwald E, Maroko PR. Effect of propranolol on mitochondrial morphology during acute myocardial ischemia. *Am J Cardiol* 1978;**41**:880–6.
15 Cannon RO, Leon MB, Watson RM, Rosing DR, Epstein SE. Chest pain in patients with 'normal' coronary arteries. The role of small coronary arteries. *Am J Cardiol* 1985;**55**:50B–60B.
16 Bugiardini R, Borghi A, Biagetti L, Puddu P. Comparison of verapamil versus propranolol therapy in syndrome X. *Am J Cardiol* 1989;**63**:286–90.
17 Bristow M, Ginsburg R, Minobe W *et al.* Decreased catecholamine sensitivity and beta-adrenergic receptor density in failing human hearts. *N Engl J Med* 1982;**307**:205–11.
18 Fowler M, Laser J, Hopkins G, Minobe W, Bristow M. Assessment of beta-adrenergic receptor pathways in the intact failing human heart: progressive receptor down-regulation and subsensitivity to agonist response. *Circulation* 1986;**74**:1290–302.
19 Colucci W, Alexander RW, Williams G *et al.* Decreased lymphocyte beta-adrenergic density in patients with heart failure and tolerance to the beta agonist pirbuterol. *N Engl J Med* 1981;**305**:185–90.
20 Mancini DM, Frey MJ, Fishberg D, Molinoff PB, Wilson JR. Characterization of lymphocyte beta-adrenergic receptors at rest and during exercise in ambulatory patients with chronic congestive heart failure. *Am J Cardiol* 1989;**63**:307–12.
21 Binkley PF, Lewe RF, Unverferth DV, Leier CV. Preservation of the end-systolic pressure/end-systolic dimension relation following pindolol in congestive heart failure. *Am Heart J* 1988;**115**:1245–50.
22 Rossi PRF, Yusuf S, Ramsdale D, Furze L, Sleight P. Reduction of ventricular arrhythmias by early intravenous atenolol in suspected acute myocardial infarction. *Br*

Med J 1983;**286**:506–10.

23 Yusuf S, Peto R, Lewis J, Collins R, Sleight P. Beta blockade during and after myocardial infarction: an overview of the randomized trials. *Progr Cardiovasc Dis* 1985;**27**:335–71.

24 Kirschenbaum HL, Rosenberg JM. Clinical experience with sotalol in the treatment of cardiac arrhythmias. *Clin Ther* 1994;**16**:346–64.

25 Prys-Roberts C, Foëx P, Biro GP, Roberts JG. Studies of anaesthesia in relation to hypertension V. Adrenergic beta-receptor blockade. *Br J Anaesth* 1973;**45**:671–81.

26 Prys-Roberts C. Interactions of anaesthesia and high pre-operative doses of beta-receptor antagonists. *Acta Anaesthesiol Scand* 1982(Suppl);**76**:47–53.

27 Roberts JG, Foëx P, Clarke TNS, Prys-Roberts C, Bennett MJ. Haemodynamic interactions of high-dose propranolol pre-treatment and anaesthesia in the dog. II. The effects of acute arterial hypoxaemia at increasing depths of halothane anaesthesia. *Br J Anaesth* 1976;**48**:403–10.

28 Roberts JG, Foëx P, Clarke TNS, Bennett MJ, Saner CA. Haemodynamic interactions of high-dose propranolol pre-treatment and anaesthesia in the dog. III. The effects of haemorrhage during halothane and trichloroethylene anaesthesia. *Br J Anaesth* 1976;**48**:411–18.

29 Foëx P, Ryder WA. Interaction of adrenergic beta-receptor blockade (oxprenolol) and PCO_2 levels in the anaesthetized dog. The influence of intrinsic beta-sympathomimetic activity. *Br J Anaesth* 1981;**53**:19–26.

30 Perel A, Krumholtz A, Kohn W, Shneider A. Equipotent doses of propranolol and esmolol reduce MAC of halothane in rats. *Anesthesiology* 1992;**77**:A406.

31 Jakobsen C-J, Blom L. Pre-operative assessment of anxiety and measurement of arterial plasma catecholamine concentrations. The effect of oral beta-adrenergic blockade with metoprolol. *Anaesthesia* 1989;**44**:249–53.

32 Deanfield JE, Selwyn AP, Chierchia S *et al.* Myocardial ischaemia during daily life in patients with stable angina: its relation to symptoms and heart rate changes. *Lancet* 1983;**2**:753–8.

33 Quyyumi AA, Wright CM, Mockus LJ, Fox KM. Effect of partial agonist activity in beta-blockers in severe angina pectoris: a double-blind comparison of pindolol and atenolol. *Br Med J* 1984;**289**:951–3.

34 Parodi O, Simonetti I, Michelassi C *et al.* Comparison of verapamil and propranolol therapy for angina pectoris at rest: a randomized, multiple cross-over, controlled trial in the coronary care unit. *Am J Cardiol* 1986;**57**:800–906.

35 Imperi GA, Lambert CR, Coy K, Lopez L, Pepine CJ. Effects of titrated beta-blockade (metoprolol) on silent myocardial ischemia in ambulatory patients with coronary disease. *Am J Cardiol* 1987;**60**:519–24.

36 Pepine CJ, Hill JA, Imperi GA, Norvell N. Beta-adrenergic blockers in silent myocardial ischemia. *Am J Cardiol* 1988;**61**:18B–21B.

37 Stone JG, Foëx P, Sear J, Johnson LL, Khambatta HJ, Triner L. Myocardial ischemia in untreated hypertensive patients: effect of a single small oral dose of a beta-blocker. *Anesthesiology* 1988;**68**:495–500.

38 Dodds TM, Torkelson AT, Fillinger MP, Tosteson A. Prophylactic beta-blockade reduces perioperative myocardial ischemia in high-risk patients undergoing noncardiac surgery. *Anesth Analg* 1994;**78**:S92.

39 Wallace A, Layung E, Browner W *et al.*, SPI Research Group. Randomized, double blind, placebo controlled trial of atenolol for the prevention of perioperative myocardial ischemia in high risk patients scheduled for non cardiac surgery. *Anesthesiology* 1994;**81**:A99.

40 Clarke TNS, Prys-Roberts C, Biro G *et al.* Aortic input impedance and left ventricular energetics in acute isovolumic anaemia. *Cardiovasc Res* 1978;**12**:49–55.

41 Clarke TNS, Foëx P, Roberts JG *et al.* Circulatory responses of the dog to acute isovolumic anaemia in the presence of high-grade adrenergic beta-receptor blockade. *Br J Anaesth* 1980;**52**:337–41.

42 Biro GP, Foëx P, Clarke TNS, Prys-Roberts C. Cardiac responsiveness to B-adrenergic stimulation in experimental anaemia. *Can J Physiol Pharmacol* 1976;**54**:675–82.

43 Crystal GJ, Ruiz JR, Rooney MW, Salem MR. Regional hemodynamic and oxygen supply during isovoluemic hemodilution in the absence and presence of high-grade beta-

adrenergic blockade. *J Cardiothorac Anesth* 1988;**2**:772–9.

44 Hagl S, Heimish W, Meisner H *et al.* The effect of hemodilution on regional myocardial function in the presence of coronary stenosis. *Basic Res Cardiol* 1977;**72**:344–64.

45 Zaroslinski J, Borgman RJ, O'Donnell JP *et al.* Ultra-short acting beta-blockers: a proposal for the treatment of the critically ill patient. *Life Sci* 1982;**31**:899–907.

46 Sum CY, Yacobi A, Kartzinel R *et al.* Kinetics of esmolol, an ultrashort-acting beta-blocker, and its major metabolite. *Clin Pharmacol Ther* 1983;**34**:427–34.

47 Lowenthal DT, Porter RS, Saris SD *et al.* The clinical pharmacology of an ultrashort-acting beta-blocker. In: Kaplan JA, ed. *Esmolol and the adrenergic response to adrenergic stimuli.* New York: BMI, 1985;31–5.

48 Reynolds RD, Gorczynski RJ, Quon CY. Pharmacology and pharmacokinetics of esmolol. *J Clin Pharmacol* 1986;**26**(Suppl A):A3–A14.

49 Gorczynski RJ, Shaffer JE, Lee RJ. Pharmacology of ASL-8052, a novel beta-adrenergic receptor antagonist with an ultrashort duration of action. *J Cardiovasc Pharmacol* 1983;**5**:668–77.

50 Sung JS, Blamski L, Kirshenbaum J *et al*, Esmolol Research Group. Clinical experience with esmolol, short-acting beta-adrenergic blocker in cardiac arrhythmias and myocardial ischemia. *J Clin Pharmacol* 1986;**26**:A15–A26.

51 Reilly CS, Wood M, Koshakji RP, Wood AJJ. Ultra-short acting beta-blockade: a comparison with conventional blockade. *Clin Pharmacol Ther* 1985;**38**:579–85.

52 Jacobs JR, Maier GW, Rankin JS, Reves JG. Esmolol and left ventricular function in the awake dog. *Anesthesiology* 1988;**68**:373–8.

53 Cucchiara RF, Benefiel DJ, Matteo RS *et al.* Evaluation of esmolol in controlling increases in heart rate and blood pressure during endotracheal intubation in patients undergoing carotid endarterectomy. *Anesthesiology* 1986;**65**:528–31.

54 Harrison L, Ralley FE, Wynands JE *et al.* The role of an ultrashort-acting adrenergic blocker (esmolol) in patients undergoing coronary artery bypass surgery. *Anesthesiology* 1987;**66**:413–18.

55 Gold MI, Sacks DJ, Grosnoff DB, Herrington C, Skillman CA. Use of esmolol during anesthesia to treat tachycardia and hypertension. *Anesth Analg* 1989;**68**:101–4.

56 Newsome LR, Roth JV, Hug CC, Nagle D. Esmolol attenuates hemodynamic responses during fentanyl-pancuronium anesthesia for aortocoronary bypass surgery. *Anesth Analg* 1986;**65**:451–6.

57 Gray RJ, Bateman TN, Czer LS, Coonklin CM, Matloff JM. Esmolol, a new ultrashort-acting beta-blocking agent for rapid control of heart rate in postoperative supraventricular tachycardias. *J Am Coll Cardiol* 1985;**5**:1451–6.

58 Kaplan JA. Dupont critical care lecture: role of ultrashort-acting beta-blockers in the perioperative period. *J Cardiothorac Anesth* 1988;**2**:683–91.

59 Byrd RC, Sung RJ, Marks J, Parmley WW. Safety and efficacy of esmolol (ASL-8052; an ultrashort-acting beta-adrenergic blocking agent) for control of ventricular rate in supraventricular tachycardias. *J Am Coll Cardiol* 1984;**3**:394–9.

60 Anderson S, Blanski L, Byrd R. Comparison of esmolol, a short-acting beta-blocker, with placebo in the treatment of supraventricular tachyarrhythmias. *Am Heart J* 1986;**111**:42–8.

61 Platia EV, Michelson EL, Porterfield JK, Das G. Esmolol versus verapamil in the acute treatment of atrial fibrillation and flutter. *Am J Cardiol* 1989;**63**:925–9.

62 Slogoff S, Keats AS. Does perioperative myocardial ischemia lead to postoperative myocardial infarction? *Anesthesiology* 1985;**62**:107–14.

63 Thomson IR, Putnis CL. Adverse effect of pancuronium during high-dose fentanyl anesthesia for coronary artery bypass grafting. *Anesthesiology* 1985;**62**:708–13.

64 Girard D, Shulman BJ, Thys DM, Mindich BP, Mikula SK, Kaplan JA. The safety and efficacy of esmolol during myocardial revascularization. *Anesthesiology* 1986;**65**:157–64.

65 Sanders DJ, Jewkes CF, Sear JW, Verhoeff F, Foëx P. Thoracic bioimpedance measurement of cardiac output and cardiovascular responses to the induction of anaesthesia and to laryngoscopy and intubation. *Anaesthesia* 1992;**47**:736–40.

66 Reves JG, Croughwell N, Hawkins E, Jacobs JR. Esmolol for treatment of intraoperative tachycardia and/or hypertension – bolus loading technique. *Anesthesiology*, 1983;**59**:A33.

67 Gibson BE, Black S, Maass L, Cucchiara RF. Esmolol for the control of hypertension

after neurologic surgery. *Clin Pharmacol Ther* 1988;**44**:650–3.

68 Kapur PA, Bochenek E. Esmolol as an adjunct to nitroprusside for controlled hypotension in anesthetized dogs. *Anesth Analg* 1988;**67**:S108.

69 Garson A, Gillette PC, McNamara DG. Propranolol: the preferred palliation for tetralogy of Fallot. *Am J Cardiol* 1981;**47**:1098–104.

70 Nussbaum J, Zane EA, Thys D. Esmolol for the treatment of hypercyanotic spells in infants with tetralogy of Fallot. *J Cardiothorac Anesth* 1989;**3**:200–2.

71 Zakowski M, Kaufman B, Berguson P, Tissot M, Yarmush L, Turndorf H. Esmolol during resection of pheochromocytoma: report of three cases. *Anesthesiology* 1989;**70**:875–7.

72 Trench AJ, Buckley FP, Drummond GB, Arthur GR, Scott DB. Propranolol in thyrotoxicosis. Cardiovascular changes during thyroidectomy in patients pre-treated with propranolol. *Anaesthesia* 1978;**33**:535–9.

73 Hamilton WF, Forrest AL, Gunn A, Peden NR, Feely J. Beta-adrenoceptor blockade and anaesthesia for thyroidectomy. *Anaesthesia* 1984;**39**:335–42.

74 Thorne AC, Bedford RF. Esmolol for perioperative management of thyrotoxic goiter. *Anesthesiology* 1989;**71**:291–4.

75 Leslie JB, Kalayjian RW, McLoughlin TM, Plachetka JR. Attenuation of the hemodynamic responses to endotracheal intubation with preinduction intravenous labetalol. *J Clin Anesth* 1989;**1**:194–200.

76 Bernstein JS, Ebert TJ, Stowe DF, Schmeling WT, Nelson MA, Woods MP. Partial attenuation of hemodynamic responses to rapid sequence induction and intubation with labetalol. *J Clin Anesth* 1989;**1**:444–51.

77 Inada E, Cullen DJ, Nemeskal AR, Teplick R. Effect of labetalol or lidocaine on the hemodynamic response to intubation: a controlled randomized double-blind study. *J Clin Anesth* **1**:207–13.

78 Chung KS, Sinatra RS, Chung JH. The effect of an intermediate dose of labetalol on heart rate and blood pressure responses to laryngoscopy and intubation. *J Clin Anesth* 1992;**4**:11–15.

79 Singh PP, Dimich I, Sampson I, Sonnenklar NA. A comparison of esmolol and labetalol for the treatment of perioperative hypertension in geriatric ambulatory surgical patients. *Can J Anaesth* 1992;**39**:559–62.

80 Le Bret F, Coriat P, Gosgnach M, Baron JF, Reiz S, Viars P. Transesophageal echocardiographic assessment of left ventricular function in response to labetalol for control of postoperative hypertension. *J Cardiothorac Vasc Anesth* 1992;**6**:433–7.

81 Toivonen J, Virtanen H, Kaukinen S. Deliberate hypotension induced by labetalol with halothane, enflurane or isoflurane for middle-ear surgery. *Acta Anaesth Scand* 1989;**33**:283–9.

82 Nuttall A, Snow HM. The cardiovascular effects of ICI 118587: a beta$_1$-adrenoceptor partial agonist. *Br J Pharmacol* 1982;**77**:381–8.

83 Harry JD, Marlow HF, Wardleworth AG, Young J. The action of ICI 118587 (a beta-adrenoceptor partial agonist) on heart response to exercise in man. *Br J Clin Pharmacol* 1981;**12**:266P–267P.

84 Sato H, Inoue M, Matsuyama T *et al.* Hemodynamic effects of the beta$_1$-adrenoceptor partial agonist xamoterol in relation to plasma norepinephrine levels during exercise in patients with left ventricular dysfunction. *Circulation* 1987; **75**:213–20.

85 Detry JM, Decoster PM, Buy JJ, Rousseau MF, Brasseur LA. Antianginal effects of Corwin, a new beta-adrenoceptor partial agonist. *Am J Cardiol* 1984;**53**:439–43.

86 Pouleur H, van Eyll C, Hanet C, Cheron P, Charlier AA, Rousseau MF. Long-term effects of xamoterol on left ventricular diastolic function and late remodeling: a study in patients with anterior myocardial infarction and single-vessel disease. *Circulation* 1988;**77**:1081–9.

87 Braunwald E, Kloner RA. The stunned myocardium: prolonged, postichemic ventricular dysfunction. Circulation 1982;**66**:1146–9.

88 The German and Austrian Xamoterol Study Group. Double-blind placebo-controlled comparison of digoxin and xamoterol in chronic heart failure. *Lancet* 1988;**1**:489–93.

89 Persson H, Rythe'n-Alder E, Melcher A, Erhardt L. Effects of beta receptor antagonists in patients with clinical evidence of heart failure after myocardial infarction: double blind comparison of metoprolol and xamoterol. *Br Heart J* 1995;**74**:140–8.

27

90 Lawson-Matthew PJ, McLean KA, Dent M, Austin CA, Channer KS. Xamoterol improves the control of chronic atrial fibrillation in elderly patients. *Age-Ageing* 1995;**24**:321–5.

91 Molajo AO, Bennett DH. Effect of xamoterol (ICI 118587) a new beta$_1$-adrenoceptor partial agonist, on resting haemodynamic variables and exercise tolerance in patients with left ventricular dysfunction. *Br Heart J* 1985;**54**:17–21.

92 Hitzenberger VG, Takacs F, Pittner H. Pharmacokinetics of the beta-adrenergic receptor blocking agent celiprolol after single intravenous and oral administrations to man. *Azneimittelforschung* 1983;**33**:50–2.

93 Frishman WH, Flamenbaum W, Schoenberger J *et al.* Celiprolol in systemic hypertension. *Am J Cardiol* 1989;**63**:839–42.

94 Dunn CJ, Spencer CM. Celiprolol. An evaluation of its pharmacological properties and clinical efficacy in the management of hypertension and angina pectoris. *Drugs Aging* 1995;**7**:394–411.

95 Saner H, Seiler A, Mahler F. Different hemodynamic effects of celiprolol and atenolol in patients with mild to moderate hypertension. *Arzneimittelforschung* 1995;**45**:790–5.

96 Sybertz EJ, Watkins RW. Preclinical pharmacologic properties of dilevalol, an anti-hypertensive agent possessing selective beta$_2$ agonist-mediated vasodilation and beta antagonism. *Am J Cardiol* 1989; **63**:3I–6I.

97 Kramer WG, Perentesis G, Affrime MB, Patrick JE. Pharmacokinetics of dilevalol in normotensive and hypertensive volunteers. *Am J Cardiol* 1989;**63**:7I–11I.

98 Bellissant E, Annane D, Thuillez C, Giudicelli JF. Comparison of the effects of dilevalol and propranolol on systemic and regional haemodynamics in healthy volunteers at rest and during exercise. *Eur J Clin Pharmacol* 1994;**47**:39–47.

99 Krum H, Sackner-Bernstein JD, Goldsmith RL *et al.* Double-blind, placebo-controlled study of the long-term efficacy of carvedilol in patients with severe chronic heart failure. *Circulation* 1995;**92**:1499–506.

100 Olsen SL, Gilbert EM, Renlund DG, Taylor DO, Yanowitz FD, Bristow MR. Carvedilol improves left ventricular function and symptoms in chronic heart failure: a double-blind randomized study. *J Am Coll Cardiol* 1995;**25**:1225–31.

101 Feuerstein GZ, Ruffolo RR jr. Carvedilol, a novel multiple action antihypertensive agent with antioxidant activity and the potential for myocardial and vascular protection. *Eur Heart J* 1995;**16**(Suppl F):38–42.

102 Lopez BL, Christopher TA, Yue TL, Ruffolo R, Feuerstein GZ, Ma XL. Carvedilol, a new beta-adrenoceptor blocker antihypertensive drug, protects against free-radical-induced endothelial dysfunction. *Pharmacology* 1995;**51**:165–73.

103 Ahlquist RP. A study of the adrenotropic receptors. *Am J Physiol* 1948;**153**:586–99.

2: Calcium-channel blockers

JEAN-JACQUES LEHOT, PIERRE-GEORGES DURAND, VINCENT PIRIOU

Verapamil and diltiazem were used first to treat tachycardia, angina pectoris or hypertension. Dihydropiridines (DHP) have been used to treat only the two last-named conditions. Calcium-channel blockers (CCBs) are now given to treat other disorders, such as cerebral artery spasm. As many anaesthetic drugs decrease intracellular calcium flux, they may interact with CCBs. Moreover, CCBs are increasingly administered intravenously (iv) during anaesthesia and in critical patients.

Comparative pharmacology of calcium-channel blockers

Classification and chemical characteristics

Spedding's classification[1] divides CCBs into three groups according to their mechanism of action: Group I is made up of DHPs which bind to a hydrophobic amino acid sequence at the external site of the cellular membrane; Group II (verapamil, diltiazem) is a heterogenous group made up of hydrophobic molecules acting through two different sites on the calcium channels; Group III (flunarizine, perhexiline, bepridil) possesses a structural homogeneity and is made up of lipophilic molecules which exhibit less selective mechanisms of action. 'Classic' CCBs inhibit the (long-lasting) L-channel; those include DHPs (for example, nifedipine), phenylalkylamines (for example, verapamil), and benzothiazepines (for example, diltiazem).

Mechanism of action

Calcium plays a fundamental role in the excitation–contraction coupling in myocardial cells and smooth muscle. Its penetration into the cell allows the Ca^{++} release from the sarcoplasmic reticulum which is responsible for muscle contraction. Contraction takes place in the myocardial cell because of the actin–myosin interaction facilitated by the troponin–Ca^{++} complex. In the vascular smooth muscle, calmodulin plays the same role as troponin in the cardiac muscle and allows the actin–myosin interaction.[2, 3]

Calcium enters into the cell through two types of channels: receptor operated channels (ROC) and voltage operated channels (VOC). Calcium-channel blockers decrease Ca^{++} entry through the VOC during phase 2 of the action potential of the fast response cells (ventricular contractile cells) and during phase 0 of the action potential of the slow response cells contained in the sinoatrial and atrioventricular nodes.

Voltage operated channels are made up of five protein subunits.[4] Some subunits allow the CCB to link to the channels,[5] others allow phosphorylation and activation of VOC through indirect stimulation by H_2-agonists and β-agonists[6] leading to Ca^{++} entry into the cell.

Calcium-channel blockers prevent activation of VOC, block Ca^{++} entry into the cell, and inhibit the excitation–contraction coupling. Verapamil decreases allosterically the fixation of DHPs to the cell whereas diltiazem increases this fixation.[7] Additionally, bepridil can attach to smooth muscle calmodulin.[8] The blockade of VOC takes place at rest with DHPs but is frequency-dependent with verapamil and diltiazem.[9, 10]

Pharmacokinetic parameters

Most calcium-channel blockers exhibit relatively similar pharmacokinetic properties (Table 2.1).[11–13] The bioavailability of diltiazem shows wide individual variations.[14] This has been shown also in diltiazem-treated patients undergoing coronary artery bypass graft (CABG) surgery.[15] Calcium channel-blocker metabolism is essentially hepatic through demethylation and dealkylation, leading to several biologically active metabolites. Thus hepatic failure or decreased hepatic blood flow due to cardiac failure slows CCB metabolism.[16] Elimination of inactivated compounds takes place mainly in the kidney. However, chronic treatment prolongs half-life because of saturation of the hepatic first-pass effect, for example verapamil elimination half-life is extended to 6–9 hours.[11] Van Harten et al.[17] suggested that sublingual absorption of nifedipine was negligible.

At the onset of cardiopulmonary bypass (CPB), plasma concentrations of diltiazem and of its two main active metabolites decrease due to haemodilution.[18] During CPB, these concentrations remain constant, suggesting that the rates of metabolism and excretion are altered during the bypass procedure.

Interactions

Interactions with other drugs have been reported frequently.[19, 20] Serum digoxin concentrations increase with CCB treatment, probably through diminution of renal clearance.[21] CCBs increase cyclosporin concentration by 49–110%, potentially leading to nephrotoxicity.[20] Verapamil increases

Table 2.1 Pharmacological properties of calcium-channel blockers

	Verapamil	Diltiazem	Bepridil	Nifedipine	Nicardipine	Nimodipine
Doses oral	80–160 mg 8 hourly	30–120 mg 8 hourly	200–300 mg/24 h	10–40 mg 8 hourly (intranasal 10 mg 4 hourly)	20 mg 8 hourly	240 mg/24 h
iv (bolus)	75–150 µg/kg	250 µg/kg	—	—	10–15 µg/kg	—
iv (maintenance)	15–45 mg/24 h	75–150 mg/24 h	4 mg/kg per 24 h	5–15 µg/kg	2–5 mg/h	2 mg/h
Oral absorption (%)	>90	>90	90	>90	99	>90
Onset of action (min)	<30	15	48–72 h	(intranasal 3, oral 20)	20–60	30–90
First-pass extraction by liver after oral administration (%)	75–90	70–80	30–40	40–60	20–40	90
Bioavailability (%)	20	25–50	60	50	30	5–10
Protein binding (%)	90	80	99	90	98	99
Elimination half-time (h)	4–10	2–6	33	3–5	3–5	2
Therapeutic plasma concentration (ng/ml)	50–250	100–250	300–1100	10–100	5–100	10–30
Excretion (%) renal	85	40	1	80	55	20
hepatic	15	60	99	20	45	80

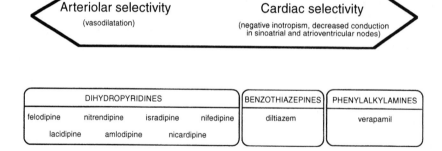

Fig 2.1   Cardiac and vascular selectivity of calcium-channel blockers

serum theophylline levels in some patients.[22] Conversely, cimetidine increases bioavailability and serum levels of verapamil, diltiazem, and DHP.[23]

Pharmacodynamic effects

Cardiovascular effects differ according to the CCB considered (Figure 2.1) and result from direct effects and effects elicited by stimulation of the baroreflex.[24]

Calcium-channel blockers act on nodal tissue. In rat isolated atrial cells, Kawai *et al.*[25] found a similar dose-dependent inhibitory effect of nifedipine, verapamil, and diltiazem characterised by increases in sinus recovery time, and effective and functional refractory periods of the atrioventricular node. In clinical studies, however, inhibitory effects were observed only with verapamil and diltiazem, while opposite effects were observed with nifedipine[25] and nicardipine.[26] All CCBs decreased mean arterial pressure and systemic vascular resistance (SVR) in a dose-dependent manner.[27] The baroreflex-induced increase in heart rate was greater with nifedipine than with verapamil or diltiazem,[24] due to a more potent vasodilatory effect of DHP.[28]

The effects of CCBs on cardiac performance are complex (Figure 2.2). All CCBs demonstrate potent negative inotropic effects *in vitro*,[29] but clinical studies have shown variations of heart rate and afterload.[27] However, verapamil seemed to be more,[28] and nicardipine less, cardiac depressant after intracoronary injection.[30]

Decreases in contractility, heart rate, and afterload reduce myocardial oxygen consumption (MVO_2). In normal and ischaemic myocardium intracoronary administration of CCB impairs left ventricular (LV) relaxation, but conversely, because of decreased afterload and sympathetic response, iv administration enhances ventricular relaxation.[28] Calcium-channel blockers have spasmolytic and vasodilatory properties on the coronary circulation. Spasmolytic effects have been demonstrated in pharmacologically induced spasm,[31] and clinical studies have confirmed functional improvement.[32] A dose-dependent increase in coronary blood flow (CBF) has been shown with all CCBs in normal and constricted coronary arteries.[33, 34]

Dihydropyridines have spasmolytic effects on the cerebral circulation and increase carotid blood flow.[35, 36] Calcium-channel blockers reverse the decrease in renal blood flow caused by angiotensin II.[37] Diltiazem and nicardipine may increase glomerular blood flow in patients with nephro-pathies.[37, 38] Calcium-channel blockers may also protect kidneys from ischaemia. In sheep, verapamil 50 µg/kg was injected into the renal artery prior to one hour of ischaemia and improved post-ischaemic creatinine excretion.[39] During infrarenal aortic cross-clamping, nicardipine prevented the decreases in glomerular filtration rate and effective renal plasma flow.[40] During abdominal surgery nicardipine increased urine flow, sodium, and phosphate excretion.[41] A continuous nifedipine infusion during CPB improved postoperative creatinine clearance and glomerular filtration rate.[42] Conversely, nifedipine may induce acute renal failure in a few situations,[43] particularly when systemic arterial pressure is decreased.

Calcium-channel blockers may dilate pulmonary arteries, especially in the presence of hypoxaemic vasoconstriction[44] or at an early stage of

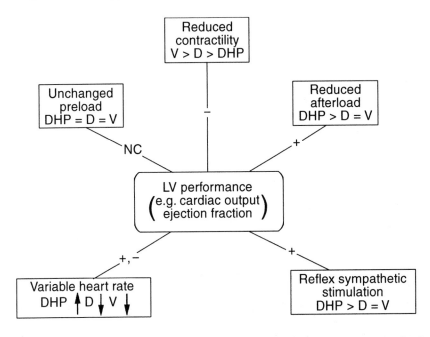

Fig 2.2 Effects of calcium-channel blockers on the major determinants of left ventricular function. V, verapamil; D, diltiazem; DHP, dihydropiridines; NC, no change

primary pulmonary hypertension.[45, 46] Rich *et al.*[47] showed in a 5-year follow-up study that patients responsive to high-dose nifedipine or diltiazem (26% of patients) had a higher survival rate (94 vs 55%). No increase in venous admixture has been found.[48] Antiatherogenic properties of CCBs such as isradipine have been demonstrated experimentally[49] but not confirmed in humans. Platelet aggregability was attenuated by verapamil.[50] CCBs increased plasma angiotensin II concentrations without change in plasma aldosterone concentration, or in renin activity.[51]

The L-type CCBs, including nifedipine, potentiate the analgesic effects of narcotics[52] by stimulating spinal $5HT_3$ receptor subtypes. This effect can be blocked by ondansetron.[53]

Indications not related to anaesthesia

Confirmed indications

The efficacy of CCBs has been confirmed in coronary artery disease (CAD),[54] especially coronary spasm,[32] in which most CCBs have demonstrated similar effects; CCBs reduced the number of episodes by 50% in more than 60% of patients. Diltiazem and nifedipine had additive effects but induced more untoward effects than when the drugs were administered separately.[55]

The action of CCBs in angina pectoris results from an increase in CBF in the ischaemic area,[56] and from a reduction in MVO_2. MVO_2 decreases due to: (1) a reduction in afterload, which is more pronounced with DHP, and (2) negative chronotropic and inotropic effects induced by verapamil and diltiazem. A dose-dependent improvement in performance during exercise, and a decrease in the incidence of angina crises, have been demonstrated.[57] In stable angina pectoris, diltiazem and nifedipine had additional effects.[58] In patients with moderately depressed LV function, the combination of diltiazem with propranolol increased LV ejection fraction during exercise compared with propranolol alone;[54] this might be attributed to afterload reduction caused by diltiazem. Dihydropyridines seem to be tolerated better than diltiazem or verapamil when LV failure is present.[59] Long-term vasodilatory therapy with nifedipine reduced or delayed the need for aortic valve replacement in asymptomatic patients with aortic regurgitation and normal LV systolic function.[60]

Acute hypertension can be treated by CCBs. Bauer *et al.*[61] observed a 10% decrease in systolic blood pressure in patients given diltiazem 0·3 mg/kg iv administered over 3 minutes. Oral nifedipine 5–30 mg or iv verapamil 5–10 mg have been used.[62]

Calcium-channel blockers are also utilised in chronic hypertension.[63] Oral verapamil 240 mg daily in adults was as efficient as atenolol or propranolol.[64] Dihydropyridines such as nicardipine or nitrendipine have also been utilised.[65] Hypotension may occur, however, leading to myocardial ischaemia, especially with nifedipine.[66–68]

Whilst DHPs do not possess antiarrhythmic properties, verapamil has been used for many years to treat paroxysmal supraventricular tachycardias.[69] The success rate of conversion to sinus rhythm was more than 80% after 10 mg iv in adults, and approached 100% when combined with carotid sinus massage.[70] Diltiazem 0·15 mg/kg or bepridil 24 mg/kg iv produced similar results.[70, 71] Calcium-channel blockers administered orally have been less successful.[72] Verapamil slowed the ventricular response in atrial fibrillation.[73] Verapamil, diltiazem or bepridil were used to treat ventricular arrhythmias during acute myocardial infarction (AMI) and idiopathic ventricular tachycardias with right bundle branch block and left axis deviation.[74, 75]

Cerebral artery spasms are associated with subarachnoid haemorrhage due to rupture of cerebral aneurysm. Nimodipine administered through a nasogastric tube every 4 hours for 3 weeks decreased the incidence of severe neurological deficits due to spasm,[76] and a recent meta-analysis confirmed the efficacy of prophylactic nimodipine in improving outcome after subarachnoid haemorrhage.[77] However, iv nimodipine therapy was associated with severe acute pulmonary hypertension.[78]

Possible indications

Due to the role of Ca^{++} in ischaemic myocardial cell injury,[79] CCBs have been proposed for use in AMI. Multicentre studies have shown no effect on mortality,[80, 81] but diltiazem decreased the incidence of cardiac events in AMI without Q wave,[82] and AMI without LV failure.[83] Diltiazem produced no significant overall effect in a postinfarction study.[83]

Verapamil brought a functional improvement in 50% of patients with obstructive cardiomyopathy.[84] This improvement occurred at rest and during exercise, was greater with verapamil than with nifedipine, and coincided with an improvement in LV diastolic function.[85] The LV intraventricular outflow pressure gradient decreased when the verapamil-induced cardiac depression was more pronounced than the fall in SVR.

In monkeys, nimodipine 10 µg/kg administered 5 minutes after cerebral ischaemia improved the outcome, and the histological score.[86] In humans after cardiac arrest, iv nimodipine decreased the coma duration but did not change the final outcome.[87] The administration of lidoflazine after cardiac arrest was not beneficial.[88]

Gelmers et al.[89] found a decrease in mortality when nimodipine was started orally within 24 hours of acute ischaemic stroke, possibly because this treatment decreased the incidence of cardiovascular complications. The beneficial effects of nimodipine could also be attributed to increased cerebral blood flow[90] without significant change in post-ischaemic cerebral metabolism,[91] but these effects are disputed.[92] Moreover, CCB therapy may be limited by cerebral vasodilatation and increased intracranial pressure.[93]

Pharmacological interactions during anaesthesia

Both volatile and iv anaesthetic agents depress the L-current in cardiac, and in neuronal, tissues.[94] As many anaesthetic agents depress sympathetic responses, the combination of CCBs and anaesthetics may have additional effects, particularly on the cardiovascular system.

Volatile anaesthetics

Experimental studies have determined the interactions between CCBs and volatile anaesthetics on the cardiovascular system. The negative inotropic effect of these combinations has been shown on isolated myocardial cells[95, 96] and in experimental studies with open[97, 98] or closed[99–101] chest. Enflurane combined with CCBs caused more myocardial depression than halothane or isoflurane. This has been demonstrated with verapamil in closed chest animals during acute[100, 101] and chronic[102] experiments, and with diltiazem on isolated myocardial cells.[95] Diltiazem or verapamil in combination with halothane decreased cardiac performance more than nifedipine[98] or nicardipine.[103] The combination of CCBs with volatile anaesthetics decreased mean arterial pressure.[97–100] At equianaesthetic potency, enflurane combined with verapamil decreased arterial pressure more than halothane or isoflurane.[100] This was accompanied by increased SVR and decreased cardiac output with both enflurane[100] and halothane.[104] Isoflurane in combination with CCBs either increased,[105] did not change[106] or decreased SVR. In swine anaesthetised with halothane, for a similar decrease in arterial pressure, SVR was reduced only by nifedipine.[98]

Calcium-channel blockers and volatile anaesthetics may modify CBF through two mechanisms: (1) decrease in coronary perfusion pressure, or (2) coronary artery vasodilatation. Most studies found no change in CBF despite a decrease in coronary perfusion pressure.[99, 101, 105, 106] A study in open chest sheep found a 66% decrease in CBF with halothane (inspired concentration = 1·2%) and after a verapamil cumulative dose of 0·16 mg/kg.[104] The combination of nicardipine and isoflurane (at one and two MAC), caused a substantial decrease in arterial pressure and an increase in CBF.[103] In open chest animals, asynchronism of LV wall motion was observed with[107] or without[104, 105, 108] critical coronary constriction. In this circumstance the mechanism of contraction asynchrony did not seem to be ischaemia but rather excitation–contraction uncoupling.[109, 110]

Verapamil and diltiazem slow AH conduction;[25] as halothane and enflurane similarly slow AH conduction, and halothane, enflurane and isoflurane slow HV conduction and intraventricular conduction,[111] CCBs and volatile anaesthetics may exert additive effects on the conduction system. Hantler et al.[112] reported episodes of sinus bradycardia in patients treated preoperatively with diltiazem and anaesthetised with enflurane and fentanyl.

In dogs anaesthetised with halothane, enflurane or isoflurane (1·2 and 1·5 MAC), verapamil increased AH interval more than did diltiazem.[111] Atlee et al.,[111] in an experimental study with verapamil or diltiazem, reported atrioventricular block with enflurane and complete heart block with halothane or isoflurane. Bepridil 5 mg/kg iv increased AH interval in dogs anaesthetised with enflurane but not with halothane or isoflurane.[113] However, nifedipine in combination with volatile anaesthetics did not modify atrioventricular conduction.[111] One patient described by Hantler et al.[112] presented with a Mobitz I atrioventricular block associated with sinus bradycardia.

Calcium-channel blockers did not increase the depressant effects of volatile anaesthetics on His–Purkinje and intraventricular conduction.[111] Verapamil and diltiazem exhibited protective effects against adrenaline-induced dysrhythmias in dogs anaesthetised with halothane.[114, 115]

Experimentally, CCBs enhanced the reduction of renal and carotid blood flows induced by volatile anaesthetics. This has been shown with several combinations: nicardipine and isoflurane;[103] and verapamil and either halothane, enflurane or isoflurane.[99, 101] In rats, verapamil and halothane or isoflurane inhibited hypoxaemic pulmonary vasoconstriction.[116]

Pharmacodynamic and pharmacokinetic reasons explain these interactions. Pharmacodynamic interactions occur at the cellular level and in the autonomic nervous system. Lynch et al.[117, 118] showed that halothane and enflurane had similar effects on the slow calcium channels in myocardial cells but the effects of isoflurane were different.[119] Wheeler et al.[120] showed that halothane decreased Ca^{++} release from the sarcoplasmic reticulum. Terrar and Victory[121] showed that isoflurane depressed the inward calcium current and the amplitude of contraction in myocytes isolated from guinea-pig ventricle. Thus volatile anaesthetics and CCBs have additive effects on myocytes. Nakao et al.[122] and Blanck et al.[123] observed that nitrendipine could be displaced from its membrane site by volatile anaesthetics in proportion to their anaesthetic potency. Maze et al.[124] showed that verapamil decreased the MAC of halothane.

Volatile anaesthetics impair the baroreflex responses[125] and therefore decrease the sympathetic response to CCB. In dogs anaesthetised with halothane 1% (inspired concentration), the administration of nifedipine 10 μg/kg iv was accompanied by reductions in arterial pressure and SVR together with increases in heart rate and cardiac output; with halothane 2%, nifedipine decreased arterial pressure to a greater extent but did not increase heart rate or cardiac output.[125]

Pharmacokinetic interactions have also been demonstrated. Serum

37

verapamil concentrations were increased by halothane, enflurane or isoflurane.[126] This increase was explained by a reduction of hepatic blood flow[127] or dysfunction of the autonomic nervous system.[126]

Calcium chloride reversed the negative inotropic effects but not the conduction defects induced by the combination of CCBs and volatile anaesthetics.[104]

Few clinical studies have assessed the effects of the combination of CCBs and volatile anaesthetics. Schulte–Sasse et al.[128] showed that verapamil 0·15 mg/kg iv was well tolerated during anaesthesia with low inspired concentrations of halothane (0·35%) in patients with coronary artery disease. Intravenous administration of verapamil may be hazardous in some circumstances. For example, Moller[129] reported a cardiac arrest during halothane anaesthesia when verapamil 5 mg was injected iv to reduce tachycardia in a 56-year-old patient who had presented with haemorrhagic shock. However, the combination of iv nicardipine and halothane seemed to be safe.[130] For Merin,[131] and in our experience, preoperative CCB treatment does not preclude the use of volatile anaesthetics. However, iv administration of verapamil or diltiazem is not recommended in patients anaesthetised with halothane or enflurane, especially when these patients present with cardiac failure or conduction disturbances.

Other anaesthetics

During high dose narcotic anaesthesia CCBs are usually well tolerated. In dogs given fentanyl 150 μg/kg,[132] 500 μg/kg[133] or alfentanil 160 μg/ kg,[134] CCB caused no deleterious effects but serum diltiazem levels greater than 1 mg/ml induced atrioventricular blocks. In dogs receiving fentanyl 150 μg/kg iv, nifedipine 20 μg/kg caused a decrease in arterial pressure and tachycardia which induced myocardial ischaemia.[135] In dogs with critical coronary constriction receiving similar fentanyl anaesthesia, verapamil decreased coronary perfusion pressure and increased heart rate, leading to a reduction in systolic function and to early diastolic dysfunction.[136] In patients with coronary artery disease with normal LV function during high-dose fentanyl anaesthesia, verapamil 75–150 μg/kg iv was well tolerated.[137] No pharmacokinetic interaction has been reported with narcotics.[133]

Barbiturates decrease calcium uptake from sarcoplasmic reticulum[138] and most general anaesthetics inhibit sodium–calcium exchange in the sarco-lemma.[139] However, Pierrot et al.[140] injected diltiazem 0·15 mg/kg iv in swine anaesthetised with thiopentone 100 mg/kg, and observed only a transient decrease in arterial pressure without any change in cardiac output. In patients receiving oral nimodipine, induction of anaesthesia with thiopentone produced only a slight decrease in arterial pressure.[141]

The combination of CCBs with local anaesthetics can enhance their cardiac toxicity. This was demonstrated in dogs with diltiazem or verapamil associated with lignocaine.[142]

Neuromuscular relaxants

Potentiation of suxamethonium or pancuronium muscle relaxation by CCBs has been observed in cats[143] and rats.[144] Calcium-channel blockers decreased the magnitude of the twitch or the vecuronium dosage necessary to obtain a 50% reduction of twitch.[145] In a rat phrenic nerve hemidiaphragm preparation, Salvador et al.[146] showed substantial potentiation of suxamethonium by diltiazem or verapamil, and a potentiation of pancuronium by nicardipine. In the same preparation nicardipine potentiated atracurium-induced neuromuscular block.[147] Neostigmine had no effect on this potentiation.[147] The interaction site may be the cholinergic postsynaptic membrane.[144] These interactions do not seem clinically relevant,[148] possibly because smaller concentrations are used.

Perioperative use

Myocardial ischaemia

While a number of studies reported the value of continuing β-blocker therapy before anaesthesia to prevent myocardial ischaemia,[149] the answer is still unclear for CCBs. However, the recurrence of angina pectoris 24 hours after discontinuing CCB has been reported.[150]

Cardiac surgery

The administration of nifedipine until the day of CABG surgery was accompanied by the need for more inotropic support but less vasodilatator therapy after CPB compared with patients who had received their last dose of nifedipine on the eve of surgery.[151] Conversely, the continuation of diltiazem until anaesthesia did not introduce haemodynamic differences compared with a control group.[15] In spite of continuing verapamil and nifedipine until surgery, tachycardia occurred during laryngoscopy in patients with coronary artery disease.[152] The pretreatment dose seems important; for example, pretreatment with nicardipine up to 25 μ/kg preserved ventricular function after hypothermic ischaemic arrest in rats but greater doses decreased cardiac performance.[153]

Two studies attempted to define the role of CCBs administered until surgery to prevent myocardial ischaemia during CABG surgery.[154, 155] Slogoff and Keats[154] in 444 patients observed significantly more ischaemic episodes in patients administered no treatment or only a CCB prior to surgery than in patients administered β-blockers with or without a CCB. Chung et al.[155] confirmed these findings in 92 patients. In these two studies, CCBs seemed to prevent ischaemia less than β-blockers.

However, these studies were not randomised. As tachycardia was correlated with ischaemic episodes,[154] the inclusion of patients administered different CCBs might have induced methodological bias.

Moreover, when diltiazem was chronically administered orally before cardiac surgery, only 25–33% of subjects had therapeutic levels of diltiazem before anaesthesia and all patients had subtherapeutic levels during and after CPB.[15, 156] Logically, Colson et al.[157] proposed continuous iv administration of diltiazem intraoperatively to reduce myocardial ischaemia. Seitelberger et al.[158] compared the effects of the iv administration of nifedipine and glyceryl trinitrate (GTN). Nifedipine reduced the incidence of myocardial ischaemia and necrosis. Finally, Henling et al.[159] showed that the preoperative concomitant administration of β-blockers and CCB was not accompanied by a greater incidence of conduction disturbances.

Bukowski et al.[160] administered diltiazem 0·3 mg/kg to prevent coronary graft spasm. Verapamil (50 mg) added to the priming solution was also preventive in patients with variant angina.[161] Intravenous bepridil or oral nifedipine resolved coronary artery spasm during CABG surgery[162] and sublingual nifedipine 10 mg reduced the vascular resistance of venous coronary grafts.[163]

A similar dose of verapamil caused more pronounced and longer cardiac depressant effects on the first postoperative day than on the eve of surgery.[164] This may be due to greater free plasma concentrations or postoperative cardiac depression. Calcium-channel blockers have been included in cold crystalloid cardioplegic solutions during cardiac surgery. Nifedipine 200 μg/l decreased myocardial ischaemia but brought difficulties for weaning from CPB.[165, 166] Diltiazem (150 μg/kg) improved myocardial protection but elicited myocardial depression and conduction disturbances.[167] More studies are needed to define the role of CCBs in cardioplegia.[166, 167]

Non-cardiac surgery

In two randomised studies[168, 169] diltiazem 0·15 mg/kg iv followed by a continuous infusion of 3–5 mg/kg per min initiated before induction of anaesthesia and continued up to 3–12 hours after tracheal extubation in patients with coronary artery disease was administered. Diltiazem infusion decreased the incidence of ischaemic episodes and was accompanied by few cardiovascular side effects.

Hypertension

The efficacy of CCB to prevent or to treat perioperative hypertensive episodes is widely recognised.

Intraoperative period

Verapamil 0·1 mg/kg iv[170] or sublingual nifedipine 10 mg[171, 172] prevented the pressor response to laryngoscopy without an effect on heart rate. Verapamil 0·1 mg/kg was more effective than nicardipine 30 μg/kg or diltiazem 0·2 mg/kg for controlling hypertension and tachycardia associated with intubation.[173] Similarly, diltiazem 0·3 mg/kg controlled the circulatory response to tracheal intubation in hypertensive patients.[174] Kishi et al.[175] administered nicardipine (1–2 mg iv) to control hypertensive episodes in vascular surgery and observed no change in right and left filling pressures or heart rate. Van Wezel et al.[176] compared iv verapamil, nifedipine, and GTN to maintain arterial pressure less than 20% of control in CABG surgery. Nifedipine and GTN were well tolerated but verapamil increased the PQ interval, and pulmonary artery and pulmonary artery occlusion pressures. Nicardipine 16 μg/kg decreased arterial pressure during normothermic CPB by decreasing SVR.[177] The absence of venodilatation prevented the decrease in the venous reservoir level.[178]

Intravenous nicardipine was used perioperatively to prevent and treat hypertension during surgery for removal of phaeochromocytoma.[179, 180] However, diltiazem as monotherapy did not prevent occasional hypertension in this setting.[181]

The cardiodepressant effect of anaesthetics, the depression of sympathetic activity, the cardiac status of the patient and the level of cardiac monitoring must be considered on an individual basis prior to administering iv CCBs. For example, nicardipine has been shown occasionally to induce transient left ventricular failure.[182]

Postoperative period

Mullen et al.[183] compared iv diltiazem, intranasal nifedipine and iv sodium nitroprusside (SNP) to treat hypertension after CABG surgery. The dosages necessary to obtain equivalent effects on arterial pressure were 150–300 μg/kg, 20–50 mg and 1 μg/kg/min respectively. Heart rate and MVO_2 decreased only with diltiazem. Indices of LV systolic function were reduced by diltiazem or nifedipine but not by SNP. Only SNP decreased myocardial lactate uptake, suggesting that myocardial ischaemia might occur. After myocardial revascularisation,[184] israpidine decreased systemic arterial pressure and SVR, and increased heart rate and cardiac index. Pulmonary artery and filling pressures did not change. In a study comparing isradipine and SNP,[185] both drugs reduced systemic arterial pressure and resistance. Isradipine infusion was associated with an increase in cardiac output but also increases in pulmonary artery and central venous pressures, whereas the last two parameters decreased with SNP. Heart rate and MVO_2 did not change with isradipine.

Finally, nicardipine or isradipine appear to be safe and effective alternatives to SNP in patients with normal or moderately altered ventricular function. In patients with poor ventricular function pure vasodilators such as SNP or urapidil may be safer.

Deliberate hypotension

Calcium-channel blockers have been used to induce hypotension during surgery. Zimpfer et al.[186] administered verapamil 0·7 mg/kg iv during neuroleptanalgesia; arterial pressure decreased by 10–20% during the first 10 minutes, due mainly to decreased SVR. During cerebral aneurysm surgery nicardipine (but not diltiazem) increased cerebral blood flow and blood flow velocity in the internal carotid artery.[187] Carbon dioxide reactivity did not change after nicardipine infusion.[188]

Arrhythmias

Intravenous verapamil or diltiazem have been used to treat supraventricular tachyarrhythmias during[189] or after[190] surgery, with few untoward cardiovascular effects.

Malignant hyperthermia

Experimental data suggested that CCBs could prevent malignant hyperthermia.[191, 192] Unfortunately, the combination of dantrolene with verapamil induced cardiovascular collapse in swine[193] and man.[194] However, a study in swine suggested that dantrolene may be administered safely with amlodipine.[195]

Summary and conclusions

Like β-blockers, CCBs were initially prescribed exclusively by cardiologists. They are now at the disposal of anaesthetists and intensive care physicians, especially since the development of iv preparations. As these drugs could have profound cardiovascular effects and potential neuronal effects, extensive knowledge of their pharmacology, including interactions with anaesthetic agents, should lead to more efficient and safer use.

Indications for iv calcium-channel blockers

- Verapamil — Supraventicular tachycardia except ventricular pre-excitation[196]
- Diltiazem — Coronary spasm
- Nicardipine — Systemic hypertension
  Isradipine
- Nitrendipine — Prevention and treatment of cerebral artery spasm in patients with subarachnoid haemorrhage

---

1 Spedding M. Activators and inactivators of Ca^{2+} channel: new perspectives. *J Pharmacol* 1985;**16**(4):319–43.
2 Braunwald E. Mechanism of action of calcium channel blocking agents. *N Engl J Med* 1982;**307**:1618–27.
3 McCall D. Excitation–contraction coupling in cardiac and vascular smooth muscle: modification by calcium entry blockade. *Circulation* 1987;**75**(Suppl V):V3–V14.

4 Arvieux CC, Lehot JJ. Calcium antagonists and anaesthesia. *Curr Opin Anaesthesiol* 1993;6:171-8.

5 Borsotto M, Barhanin J, Norman RI, Ladzunski M. Purification of the dihydropyridine receptor of the voltage dependent Ca^{2+} channel from skeletal muscle transverse tubules using (+) [^{3}H] PN 200- 110. *Biochem Biophys Res Commun* 1984;122:1357-66.

6 Bkaily G, Sperelakis N. Injection of protein kinase inhibitor into cultured heart cells blocks calcium slow channels. *Am J Physiol* 1984;246:630-4.

7 Murphy KMM, Gould RJ, Largent L, Snyder SH. A unitary mechanism of calcium antagonist drug action. *Proc Natl Acad Sci* 1983;80(12):860-4.

8 Itoh H, Ishikawa T, Hidaka H. Effects on calmodulin of bepridil, an antianginal agent. *J Pharmacol Exp Ther* 1984;230:737-41.

9 Lee KS, Tsien RW. Mechanism of calcium channel blockade by verapamil, D600, diltiazem and nitrendipine in single dialysed heart cells. *Nature* 1983;302:790-4.

10 Dupuis BA. Electropharmacologie des inhibiteurs du canal calcique lent. Les inhibiteurs du canal calcique lent en thérapeutique cardiovasculaire. *Geneva Excerpta Medica* 1985:69-84.

11 Thuillez C, Giudicelli JF. Pharmacologie clinique cardiovasculaire des inhibiteurs du canal calcique lent. Les inhibiteurs du canal calcique lent en thérapeutique cardiovasculaire. *Geneva Excerpta Medica* 1985:85-108.

12 Henry PD. Comparative pharmacology of calcium antagonists: nifedipine, verapamil and diltiazem. *Am J Cardiol* 1980;46:1047-58.

13 Kates RE. Calcium antagonists. Pharmacokinetics properties. *Drugs* 1983;25:113-24.

14 Kinney EL, Moskowitz RM, Zelis R. The pharmacokinetics and pharmacology of oral diltiazem in normal volunteers. *J Clin Pharmacol* 1981;21:337-42.

15 Larach DR, Hensley FA, Pae WE, Derr JA, Campbell DB. Diltiazem withdrawal before coronary artery bypass surgery. *J Cardiothorac Anesth* 1989;3:688-99.

16 Somogyi A, Albrecht M, Kliems G. Pharmacokinetics, bioavailability and ECG response of verapamil in patients with liver cirrhosis. *Br J Clin Pharmacol* 1981;12:51-60.

17 Van Harten J, Burggraaf K, Danhof M, Van Brummelen P, Breimer DD. Negligible sublingual absorption of nifedipine. *Lancet* 1987,ii:1363-5.

18 Boulieu R, Bonnefous JL, Lehot JJ, Durand PG, Chassignolle JF, Ferry S. Effect of cardiopulmonary bypass on plasma concentrations of diltiazem and its two active metabolites. *J Pharm Pharmacol* 1994;46:310-12.

19 Piepho RW, Culbertson VL, Rhodes RS. Drug interactions with the calcium entry blockers. *Circulation* 1987;75(Suppl V):V181-V194.

20 Hunt BA, Self TH, Lalonde RL, Bottorff MB. Calcium channel blockers as inhibitors of drug metabolism. *Chest* 1989;96:393-9.

21 De Vito JM, Friedman B. Evaluation of the pharmacokinetic interaction between calcium antagonists and digoxin. *Pharmacotherapy* 1986;6:73-82.

22 Burnakis TG, Seldon M, Czaplicki AD. Increased serum theophylline concentrations secondary to oral verapamil. *Clin Pharmacol* 1983;2:458-61.

23 Loi CM, Rollins DE, Dukes GE, Peat UA. Effect of cimetidine on verapamil disposition. *Clin Pharmacol Ther* 1985;37:65-7.

24 Nakaya H, Schwartz A, Millard RW. Reflex chronotropic and inotropic effects of calcium channel blocking agents in conscious dogs: diltiazem, verapamil and nifedipine compared. *Circ Res* 1983;52:302-12.

25 Kawai C, Konishi T, Matsuyama E, Okasaki H. Comparative effects of three calcium antagonists: diltiazem, verapamil and nifedipine, on the sino-atrial and atrioventricular nodes. Experimental and clinical studies. *Circulation* 1981;63(5):1035-12.

26 Matsui M, Mishiwaki H, Yoshino J *et al.* Effects of nicardipine hydrochloride on the conduction system of the heart in man. *Jpn Heart J* 1982;23(Suppl I):243-5.

27 Low RI, Takeda P, Mason DT, De Maria A. The effects of calcium channel blocking agents on cardiovascular function. *Am J Cardiol* 1982;49:547-53.

28 Walsh RA. The effects of calcium entry blockade on left ventricular systolic and diastolic function. *Circulation* 1987;75(Suppl V):V43-V55.

29 Nabata H. Effects of calcium antagonistic coronary vasodilatators on myocardial contractility and membrane potentials. *Jpn J Pharmacol* 1977;77:239-49.

30 Rousseau MF, Pouleur H. Calcium antagonism free of negative inotropic effects? A

comparison of intracoronary nifedipine and nicardipine. *Circulation* 1984;70(Suppl 11): 304:1217.

31 Theroux P, Waters DD, Affaki GS *et al*. Provocative testing with ergonovine to evaluate the efficacy of treatment with calcium antagonists in variant angina. *Circulation* 1979;**60**: 504–10.

32 Feldman RL. A review of medical therapy for coronary artery spasm. *Circulation* 1987;75(Suppl V):V96–V102.

33 Thuillez C, Maury M, Giudicelli J. Differential effects of verapamil and diltiazem on regional blood flow and function in the canine normal and ischemic myocardium. *J. Cardiovasc Pharmacol* 1983;5:19–27.

34 Pepine CJ, Lambert CR. Effects of nicardipine on coronary blood flow. *Am Heart J* 1988;**116**:248–54.

35 Tanaka K, Gatoh F, Maramatsu F. Effect of nimodipine, a calcium antagonist, on cerebral vasospasm after subarachnoid hemorrhage in cats. *Drug Res* 1982;**32**: 1529–34.

36 Payen D, Pinaud M, Lampron N, De Kersaint Gilly A, Nicolas F. Quantitative evaluation of hemodynamic and metabolic cerebral effects of acutely administered nifedipine in human subarachnoid hemorrhage. *Cardiovasc Res* 1984;**18**:626–31.

37 Bauer JH, Reams G. Short and long term effects of calcium entry blockers on the kidney. *Am J Cardiol* 1987;**59**:66A–71A.

38 Baba T, Boku A, Ishikazi T, Sone R, Takebe K. Renal effects of nicardipine in patients with mild to moderate essential hypertension. *Am Heart J* 1986;**111**:551–7.

39 Wooley JL, Barker GR, Jacobsen WK *et al*. Effect of the calcium entry blocker verapamil on renal ischemia. *Crit Care Med* 1988;**16**:48–51.

40 Colson P, Ribstein J, Seguin JR, Marty-Ane C, Roquefeuil B. Mechanisms of renal hemodynamic impairment during infrarenal aortic cross-clamping. *Anesth Analg* 1992;75:18–23.

41 Goto F, Sudo I. Treatment of intraoperative hypertension with enflurane, nicardipine or human atrial natriuretic peptide: haemodynamic and renal effects. *Can J Anaesth* 1992;**39**:932–7.

42 Bertolissi M, Antomucci F, De Monte A, Padovani R, Giordano F. Effects on renal function of a continuous infusion of nifedipine during cardiopulmonary bypass. *J. Cardiothorac Anesth* 1996;**10**:238–42.

43 Eicher JC, Morelon P, Chalopin JM, Tanter Y, Louis P, Rifle G. Acute renal failure during nifedipine therapy in a patient with congestive heart failure. *Crit Care Med* 1988;**16**:1163–4.

44 Simonneau G, Escourrou P, Duroux P, Lokhart A. Inhibition of hypoxic pulmonary vasoconstriction by nifedipine. *N Engl J Med* 1981;**304**:1582–5.

45 Camerini F, Alberti E, Klugmann S, Salvi A. Primary pulmonary hypertension: effects of nifedipine. *Br Heart J* 1980;**44**:352–6.

46 Landmark K, Refsum AM, Simonsen J, Storstein O. Verapamil and pulmonary hypertension. *Acta Med Scand* 1978;**204**:299–302.

47 Rich S, Kaufmann E, Levy PS. The effect of high doses of calcium channel blockers on survival in primary pulmonary hyertension. *N Engl J Med* 1992;**327**:76–81.

48 Boldt J, Bormann B, Kling D, Ratthey K, Hempelmann G. Influence of nimodipine and nifedipine on intrapulmonary shunting. A comparison to other vasoactive drugs. *Intens Care Med* 1987;**13**:52–6.

49 Weinstein DB, Heider JG. Antiatherogenic properties of calcium antagonists. *Am J Cardiol* 1987;**59**:163B–172B.

50 Wallen NH, Held C, Rehnguist N, Hjemdahl P. Platelet aggregability in vivo is attenuated by verapamil but not by metoprolol in patients with stable angina pectoris. *Am J Cardiol* 1995;75:1–6.

51 Haufe MC, Gerzer R, Weil J, Ernst JE, Theisen K. Verapamil impairs secretion of stimulated atrial natriuretic factor in humans. *J Am Coll Cardiol* 1988; 11:1199–203.

52 Carta F, Bianchi M, Argentons S *et al*. Effect of nifedipine on morphine induced analgesia. *Anesth Analg* 1990;**70**:493–8.

53 Hunt TE, Wu W, Zbuzek VK. Ondansetron blocks nifedipine induced analgesia in rats. *Anesth Analg* 1996;**82**:498–500.

54 Kostuk WJ, Pflugfelder P. Comparative effects of calcium entry-blocking drugs, beta

blocking drugs and their combination in patients with chronic stable angina. *Circulation* 1987;75(Suppl V):V114–V121.

55 Prida XE, Gelman JS, Feldman RL, Hill JA, Pepine CJ, Scott E. Comparison of diltiazem and nifedipine alone and in combination in patients with coronary artery spasm. *J Am Coll Cardiol* 1987;**9**:412–19.

56 Henry PD, Schuchleib R, Borda LJ. Effects of nifedipine on myocardial perfusion and ischemic injury in dogs. *Circ Res* 1978;**43**:372–80.

57 Low RI, Takeda P, Lee G. Effects of diltiazem-induced calcium blockade upon exercise capacity in effort angina due to chronic coronary artery disease. *Am Heart J* 1981;**101**:713–18.

58 Frishman W, Charlap S, Kimmel B *et al.* Diltiazem, nifedipine and their combination in patients with stable angina pectoris: effects on angina, exercise tolerance, and the ambulatory electrocardiographic ST segment. *Circulation* 1988;**77**(4):774–86.

59 Johnston DL, Lesoway R, Humen DP, Kostuk WJ. Clinical and hemodynamic evaluation of propanolol in combination with verapamil, nifedipine and diltiazem in exertional angina pectoris: a placebo controlled, double blind, randomized, cross-over study. *Am J Cardiol* 1985;**55**:680–7.

60 Scognamiglio R, Rahimtoola SH, Fasoli G, Nistri S, Dalla Volta S. Nifedipine in asymptomatic patients with severe aortic regurgitation and normal left ventricular function. *N Engl J Med* 1994;**331**:689–94.

61 Bauer JH, Reams GP. The role of calcium entry blockers in hypertensive emergencies *Circulation* 1987;75(Suppl V): V174–V180.

62 Fenakel K, Fenakel G, Appelman Z, Lurie S, Katz Z, Shoham Z. Nifedipine in the treatment of severe eclampsia. *Obstet Gynecol* 1991;**77**:331–7.

63 Massie BM, Tuban JF, Szlachcic J. Comparative studies of calcium channel blockers and beta-blockers in essential hyertension: clinical implications. *Circulation* 1987;75(Suppl V):V163–V169.

64 Dargie H, Cleland J, Findlay I, Murray G, McImes G. Combination of verapamil and beta-blockers in systemic hypertension. *Am J Cardiol* 1986;**57**:80D–82D.

65 De Divitiis O, Petitto M, Di Somma S *et al.* Nitrendipine and atenolol: comparison and combination in the treatment of arterial hypertension. *Arzneimittelforschung* 1985;**35**:727–9.

66 Wachter RM. Symptomatic hypotension induced by nifedipine in the acute treatment of severe hypertension. *Arch Intern Med* 1987;**147**:556–8.

67 O'Mailia JJ, Sander GE, Giles TD. Nifedipine associated myocardial ischemia or infarction in the treatment of hypertensive urgencies. *Ann Intern Med* 1987;**107**:185–6.

68 Casolo GC, Balli E, Poggesi L, Gensini F. Increase in number of myocardial ischemic episodes following nifedipine administration in two patients. Detection of silent episodes by holter monitoring. *Chest* 1989;**95**:541–3.

69 Krikler DM, Spurrell RA. Verapamil in the treatment of paroxysmal supraventricular tachycardia. *Postgrad Med J* 1974;**50**:447–53.

70 Singh BN, Nademanee K. Use of calcium antagonists for cardiac arrhythmias. *Am J Cardiol* 1987;**59**:153B–162B.

71 Bertin A, Chaitman BR, Bourassa MG *et al.* Beneficial effect of intravenous diltiazem in the acute management of supraventricular tachyarrhythmias. *Circulation* 1983;**67**:88–94.

72 Mauritson DR, Winniford MD, Walker WS, Rude RE, Cary JR, Hillis LD. Oral verapamil for paroxysmal supraventricular tachycardia. A long term double blind randomized trial. *Ann Intern Med* 1982;**96**:409–12.

73 Klein HO, Pauzner H, Di Segni E *et al.* The beneficial effects of verapamil in chronic atrial fibrillation. *Arch Intern Med* 1979;**139**:747–9.

74 Fazzini PF, Marchi F, Pucci P. Effects of verapamil on ventricular premature beats of acute myocardial infarction. *Acta Cardiol* 1978;**33**:25–9.

75 Lin FC, Finley D, Rahimtoola SH, Wu D. Idiopathic paroxysmal ventricular tachycardia with a QRS pattern of right bundle branch block and left axis deviation: a unique clinical entity with specific properties. *Am J Cardiol* 1983;**52**:95–100.

76 Allen GS, Ahn HS, Preziosi TJ *et al.* Cerebral arterial spasm. A controlled trial of nimodipine in patients with subarachnoid hemorrhage. *N Engl J Med* 1983;**308**:619–24.

77 Barker FG, Ogilvy CS. Efficacy of prophylactic nimodipine for delayed ischemic deficit

after subarachnoid hemorrahge: a meta analysis. *J Neurosurg* 1996;**84**:405–14.

78 Lovell AT, Smith M. Pulmonary vasoconstriction following intravenous nimodipine. *Anaesthesia* 1992;**47**:409–10.

79 Murphy JG, Marsh JD, Smith TW. The role of calcium in ischemic myocardial injury. *Circulation* 1987;**75**(Suppl V):V15–V24.

80 Moss AJ. Secondary prevention with calcium channel blocking drugs in patients after myocardial infarction: a critical review. *Circulation* 1987;**75**(Suppl V):V148–V153.

81 Roberts R. Recognition, diagnosis and prognosis of early reinfarction: the role of calcium channel blockers. *Circulation* 1987;**75**(Suppl V): V139–V147.

82 Gibson RS, Boden WE, Theroux P *et al.* The diltiazem reinfarction study group: diltiazem and reinfarction in patients with non-Q-wave myocardial infarction. *N Engl J Med* 1986;**315**:423–9.

83 The Multicenter Diltiazem Postinfarction Trial Research Group. The effect of diltiazem on mortality and reinfarction after myocardial infarction. *N Engl J Med* 1988;**319**:385–92.

84 Chatterjee K. Calcium antagonist agents in hypertrophic cardiomyopathy. *Am J Cardiol* 1987;**59**:146B–152B.

85 Rosing DR, Cannon RO, Watson RM, Kent KM, Lakatos E, Epstein SE. Comparison of verapamil and nifedipine effects on symptoms and exercise capacity in patients with hypertrophic cardiomyopathy. *Circulation* 1982;**66**(Suppl II):24:95.

86 Sten PA, Gisvold SE, Milde JH *et al.* Nimodipine improves outcome when given after complete cerebral ischemia in primates. *Anesthesiology* 1985;**62**:406–14.

87 Forsman M, Aarseth HP, Nordby HK, Skulberg A, Steen PA. Effects of nimodipine on cerebral blood flow and cerebrospinal fluid pressure after cardiac arrest: correlation with neurologic outcome. *Anesth Analg* 1989;**68**:436–43.

88 Brain Resuscitation Clinical Trial II Study Group. A randomized clinical study of a calcium-entry blocker (lidoflazine) in the treatment of comatose survivors of cardiac arrest. *N Engl J Med* 1991;**324**:325–31.

89 Gelmers HI, Gorter K, De Weerdt CJ, Wiezer HJA. A controlled trial of nimodipine in acute ischemic stroke. *N Engl J Med* 1988;**318**:203–7.

90 Prough DS, Furberg CD. Nimodipine and the 'No reflow phenomenon.' Experimenal triumph, clinical failure? *Anesth Analg* 1989;**68**:431–5.

91 Young WL, Josovitz K, Moralcs O, Chien S. The effect of nimodipine on post ischemic cerebral glucose utilization and blood flow in the rat. *Anesthesiology* 1987;**67**:54–9.

92 Trust Study Group. Randomised, double blind, placebo-controlled trial of nimodipine in acute stroke. *Lancet* 1990;**336**:1205–9.

93 Tietjen CS, Hurn PD, Vlatowski JA, Kirsch JR. Treatment modalities for hypertensive patients with intracranial pathology: options and risks. *Crit Care Med* 1996;**24**:311–22.

94 Hirota K, Lambert DG. Voltage-sensitive Ca^{2+} channels and anaesthesia. *Br J Anaesth* 1996;**76**:344–6.

95 Lynch CL. Combined depressant effects of diltiazem and volatile anesthetics on contractility in isolated ventricular myocardium. *Anesth Analg* 1988;**67**:1036–46.

96 Broadbent MP, Swan PC, Jones RM. Interactions between diltiazem and isoflurane. *Br J Anaesth* 1985;**57**:1018–21.

97 Kates RA, Kaplan JA, Guyton RA, Dorsey L, Hug CC, Hatcher CR. Hemodynamic interactions of verapamil and isoflurane. *Anesthesiology* 1983;**59**:132–8.

98 Kates RA, Zaggy AP, Norfleet EA, Heath KR. Comparative cardiovascular effects of verapamil, nifedipine and diltiazem during halothane anesthesia in swine. *Anesthesiology* 1984;**61**:10–18.

99 Chelly JE, Rogers K, Hysing ES, Taylor A, Hartley C, Merin RG. Cardiovascular effects of and interaction between calcium blocking drugs and anesthetics in the chronically instrumented dog. I. Verapamil and halothane. *Anesthesiology* 1986;**64**:560–7.

100 Kapur PA, Bloor BC, Flacke WE, Olewine SK. Comparison of cardiovascular responses to verapamil during enflurane, isoflurane or halothane anesthesia in the dog. *Anesthesiology* 1984;**61**:156–60.

101 Rogers K, Hysing ES, Merin RG, Taylor A, Hartley C, Chelly JE. Cardiovascular effects of and interaction between calcium blocking drugs and anesthetics in chronically instrumented dogs II. Verapamil, enflurane and isoflurane. *Anesthesiology*

1986;**64**:568–75.
102 Merin RG, Chelly JE, Hysing ES *et al.* Cardiovascular effects of and interaction between calcium blocking drugs and anesthetics in chronically instrumented dogs IV. Chronically administered oral verapamil and halothane, enflurane and isoflurane. *Anesthesiology* 1987;**66**:140–6.
103 Hysing ES, Chelly JE, Doursout MF, Hartley C, Merin RG. Cardiovascular effects of and interaction between calcium blocking drugs and anesthetics in chronically instrumented dogs III. Nicardipine and isoflurane. *Anesthesiology* 1986;**65**:385–91.
104 Lehot JJ, Leone BJ, Foëx P. Calcium reverses global and regional myocardial dysfunction caused by the combination of verapamil and halothane. *Acta Anaesthesiol Scand* 1987;**31**:441–7.
105 Videcoq M, Arvieux CC, Ramsay JG. The association isoflurane verapamil causes regional left ventricular dyssynchrony in the dog. *Anesthesiology* 1987;**67**:635–41.
106 Campos JH, Kapur PA. Combined effects of verapamil and isoflurane on coronary blood flow and myocardial metabolism in the dog. *Anesthesiology* 1986;**64**:778–84.
107 Leone BJ, Philbin DM, Lehot JJ, Wilkins M, Foëx P, Ryder WA. Intravenous diltiazem worsens regional function in compromised myocardium. *Anesth Analg* 1988;**67**:205–10.
108 Ramsay JG, Cutfield GR, Francis CM, Devlin WH, Foëx P. Halothane verapamil causes regional myocardial dysfunction in the dog. *Br J Anaesth* 1986;**58**:321–6.
109 Arvieux CC, Fagret D, Fargnoli JM *et al.* The association isoflurane–verapamil does not induce myocardial ischaemia. *Eur J Anaesthesiol* 1992;**9**:135–6.
110 Arvieux CC, Pernin Drouet N *et al.* Comparative effects of halothane associated with verapamil and ischaemia on myocardial metabolism in isolated perfused rat hearts. *Eur J Anaesthesiol* 1992;**9**:447–55.
111 Atlee JL, Hamann SR, Brownlee SW, Kreigh C. Conscious state comparisons of the effects of the inhalation anesthetics and diltiazem, nifedipine or verapamil on specialized atrioventricular conduction times in spontaneously beating dog hearts. *Anesthesiology* 1988;**69**:519–28.
112 Hantler CB, Wilton N, Learned DM, Hill AE, Knight PR. Impaired myocardial conduction in patients receiving diltiazem therapy during enflurane anesthesia. *Anesthesiology* 1987;**67**:94–6.
113 Larson LO, Hantler CB, Lynch JL *et al.* Cardiac electrophysiologic interactions of bepridil, a new calcium antagonist, with enflurane halothane and isoflurane. *J. Cardiothorac Anesth* 1988;**3**:346–55.
114 Kapur PA, Flacke WE. Epinephrine-induced arrhythmias and cardiovascular function after verapamil during halothane anesthesia in the dog. *Anesthesiology* 1981;**55**:218–25.
115 Iwatsuki N, Katoh M, Ono K, Amaha K. Antiarrhythmic effect of diltiazem during halothane anesthesia in dogs and in humans. *Anesth Analg* 1985;**64**:964–70.
116 Kjaewe J, Bjertnaes LJ. Interaction of verapamil and halogenated inhalation anaesthetics on hypoxic pulmonary vasoconstriction. *Acta Anaesthesiol Scand* 1989;**33**:193–8.
117 Lynch CL, Vogel S, Sperelakis N. Halothane depression of myocardial slow action potentials. *Anesthesiology* 1981;**55**:360–8.
118 Lynch CL, Vogel S, Pratila GM, Sperelakis N. Enflurane deression of myocardial slow action potentials. *J Pharmacol Exp Ther* 1982;**222**:405–9.
119 Lynch CL. Differential depression of myocardial contractility by halothane and isoflurane in vitro. *Anesthesiology* 1986;**64**:620–31.
120 Wheeler DM, Rice RT, Hansford RG, Lakatta EG. The effect of halothane on the free intra-cellular calcium concentration of isolated rat heart cells. *Anesthesiology* 1988;**69**:578–83.
121 Terrar DA, Victory JGG. Isoflurane depresses membrane currents associated with contraction in myocytes isolated from guinea-pig ventricle. *Anesthesiology* 1988;**69**:742–9.
122 Nakao S, Hirata H, Kagawa Y. Effects of volatile anaesthetics on cardiac calcium channels. *Acta Anaesthesiol Scand* 1989;**33**:326–30.
123 Blanck TJJ, Runge S, Stevenson RL. Halothane decreases calcium channel antagonist binding to cardiac membranes. *Anesth Analg* 1988;**67**:1032–5.
124 Maze M, Mason DM, Kates K. Verapamil decreases MAC for halothane in dogs. *Anesthesiology* 1983;**59**:327–9.

125 Tosone SR, Reves JG, Kissin I, Smith LR, Fournier SE. Hemodynamic responses to nifedipine in dogs anesthetized with halothane. *Anesth Analg* 1983;**62**:903–8.

126 Chelly JE, Hysing ES, Hill DC *et al.* Cardiovascular effects of and interaction between calcium blocking drugs and anesthetics in chronically instrumented dogs V. Role of pharmacokinetics and the autonomic nervous system in the interactions between verapamil and inhalational anesthetics. *Anesthesiology* 1987;**67**:320–5.

127 Gelman S, Fowler KC, Smith LR. Liver circulation and function during isoflurane and halothane anesthesia. *Anesthesiology* 1984;**61**:726–30.

128 Schulte-Sasse U, Hess W, Markschies-Hornung A, Tarnow L. Combined effects of halothane anaesthesia and verapamil on systemic hemodynamics and left ventricular myocardial contractility in patients with ischemic heart disease. *Anesth Analg* 1984;**63**:791–8.

129 Moller IW. Cardiac arrest following IV verapamil combined with halothane anaesthesia. *Br J Anaesth* 1987;**59**:522–6.

130 Ray DC, Drummond GB. Haemodynamic responses to nicardipine in humans anaesthetised with halothane. *Anaesthesia* 1989;**44**:382–5.

131 Merin RG. Calcium channel blocking drugs and anesthetics: is the drug interaction beneficial or detrimental? *Anesthesiology* 1987;**66**:111–13.

132 Griffin RM, Dimich I, Jurado R, Kaplan JA. Haemodynamic effects of diltiazem during fentanyl nitrous oxide anaesthesia. *Br J Anaesth* 1988;**60**:655–9.

133 Hill DC, Chelly JE, Delawati A, Abernethy DR, Doursout MF, Merin RG. Cardiovascular effects of and interaction between calcium blocking drugs and anesthetics in chronically instrumented dogs VI. Verapamil and fentanyl pancuronium. *Anesthesiology* 1988;**68**:874–9.

134 Lehd Pedersen J, Strom J, Berthelsen P, Eriksen J, Rasmussen JP. Haemodynamic effects of alfentanil in verapamil-treated dogs. *Acta Anaesthesiol Scand* 1985;**29**:354–7.

135 Griffin RM, Dimich I, Jurado R *et al.* Cardiovascular effects of a nifedipine infusion during fentanyl-nitrous oxide anesthesia in dogs. *J Cardiothorac Anesth* 1989;**3**:52–7.

136 Diedericks J, Leone BJ, Philbin DM, Foëx P. Effect of verapamil on canine left ventricular function in the presence of fentanyl when apical blood flow is critically limited. *Br J Anaesth* 1989;**63**:458–64.

137 Kapur PA, Norel EJ, Dajee H, Cohen G, Flacke W. Haemodynamic effects of verapamil administration after large doses of fentanyl in man. *Can Anaesth J* 1986;**33**:138–44.

138 Lain RF, Hess ML, Gertz EW, Briggs FN. Calcium uptake activity of canine myocardial sarcoplasmic reticulum in the presence of anesthetic agents. *Circ Res* 1968;**23**:597–604.

139 Hawortk RA, Goknur AB, Borkoff HA. Inhibition of Na–Ca exchange by general anesthetics. *Circ Res* 1989;**65**:1021–8.

140 Pierrot U, Blaise M, Hugon S, Bonnei F, Cupa M. Interférences hémodynamiques entre le diltiazem et le thiopental. Etude expérimentale chez le porc. *Can Anaesth J* 1984;**31**:166–72.

141 Stullken EH, Balestrieri F, Prough DS, McWhorther JM. The hemodynamic effects of nimodipine in patients anesthetized for cerebral aneurysm clipping. *Anesthesiology* 1985; **62**: 346–8.

142 Kapur PA, Grogan DL, Fournier DJ. Cardiovascular interactions of lidocaine with verapamil or diltiazem in the dog. *Anesthesiology* 1988;**68**:79–85.

143 Kraynack BJ, Lawson NW, Gintautas J. Neuromuscular blocking action of verapamil in cats. *Can Anaesth J* 1983;**30**:242–7.

144 Durant NN, Nguyen N, Katz RL. Potentiation of neuromuscular blockade by verapamil. *Anesthesiology* 1984;**60**:298–303.

145 Anderson KA, Marshall RJ. Interactions between calcium entry blockers and vecuronium bromide in anaesthetized cats. *Br J Anaesth* 1985;**57**:775–81.

146 Salvador A, Del Pozo E, Carlos R, Baeyens JM. Differential effects of calcium channel blocking agents on pancuronium and suxamethonium induced neuromuscular blockade. *Bt J Anaesth* 1988;**60**:495–9.

147 Sekerci S, Tulunay M. Interactions of calcium channel blockers with non-depolarising muscle relaxants *in vitro. Anaesthesia* 1996;**51**:140–4.

148 Bell PF, Mirakhur RK, Elliott P. Onset and duration of clinical relaxation of atracurium and vecuronium in patients on chronic nifedipine therapy. *Eur J Anaesthesiol*

1989;**6**:343–6.

149 Kaplan JA, Dunbar RW, Bland JW, Sumpter R, Jones EL. Propranolol and cardiac surgery: a problem for the anesthesiologist? *Anesth Analg* 1975;**54**:571–8.

150 Bala Subramanian V, Bowles MJ, Khurmi NS, Davies AB, O'Hara MJ, Raftery EB. Calcium antagonist withdrawal syndrome: objective demonstration with frequency modulated ambulatory SR-segment monitoring. *Br Med J* 1983;**286**:520–1.

151 Casson WR, Jones RM, Parsons RS. Nifedipine and cardiopulmonary bypass. Postbypass management after continuation or withdrawal of therapy. *Anaesthesia* 1984;**12**:1197–201.

152 Gorven AM, Cooper GM, Prys-Roberts C. Haemodynamic disturbances during anaesthesia in a patient receiving calcium channel blockers., *Br J Anaesth* 1986;**58**:357–60.

153 Brown PS, Parenteau GL, Holland FW, Clark RE. Pretreatment with nicardipine preserves ventricular function after hypothermic ischemic arrest. *Ann Thorac Surg* 1991;**51**:739–46.

154 Slogoff S, Keats AS. Does chronic treatment with calcium entry blocking drugs reduce perioperative myocardial ischemia? *Anesthesiology* 1988;**68**:676–80.

155 Chung F, Houston PL, Cheng DCH. Calcium channel blockade does not offer adequate protection from perioperative myocardial ischemia. *Anesthesiology* 1988;**69**:343–7.

156 Lehot JJ, Durand PG, Boulieu R *et al*. Concentrations plasmatiques du diltiazem et de ses métabolites en chirurgie coronarienne: relation avec le traitement préopératoire. *Ann Fr Anesth Réanim* 1993;**12**:452–6.

157 Colson P, Medioni P, Saussine M *et al*. Hemodynamic effect of calcium channel blockage during anesthesia for coronary artery surgery. *J. Cardiothorac Anesth* 1992;**6**:424–8.

158 Seitelberger R, Zwolfer W, Huber S *et al*. Nifedipine reduces the incidence of myocardial infarction and transient ischemia in patients undergoing coronary bypass grafting. *Circulation* 1991;**83**:460–8.

159 Henling CE, Slogoff S, Kodali SV, Arlund C. Heart block after coronary artery bypass. Effect of chronic administration of calcium entry blockers and beta blockers. *Anesth Analg* 1984;**63**:315–20.

160 Bukowski JG, Mattachione A, Moreau X, Corbeau JJ, Cottineau C, Jacob JP. Haemodynamic effects of intravenous diltiazem following aortocoronary bypass. *Cah Anesthesiol* 1995;**43**:195–8.

161 Katsumoto K, Niibori T. Prevention of coronary spasms during aorto-coronary bypass surgery for variant angina and effort angina wth ST elevation. *J Cardiovasc Surg* 1988;**29**:343–7.

162 Kapur PA. Calcium channel blockers and other vasodilating antianginal effects. In: Smith NT and Corbascio AN, eds. *Drug interactions in anesthesia*, 2nd edn. Philadelphia: Lea and Febiger, 1986:135–46.

163 Eide TR, Katz RI, Poppers PJ. The effect of sublingual nifedipine on coronary venous graft resistance immediately following cardiopulmonary bypass. *Anesth Analg* 1989;**68**:422–6.

164 Bjornstad PG, Storstein L, Semb BKH. Verapamil effects on left ventricular performance in patients with congestive heart failure studied with echochardiography before and after cardiac surgery. *Scand J Thorac Cardiovasc* 1986;**20**:61–6.

165 Flameng W, De Meyere R, Daenen W *et al*. Nifedipine as an adjunct to St Thomas' Hospital cardioplegia. *J Thorac Cardiovasc Surg* 1986;**91**:723–31.

166 Clark RE, Magovern GJ, Christlieb IY, Boe S. Nifedipine cardioplegia experience: results of a 3-year cooperative clinical study. *Ann Thorac Surg* 1983;**36**:654–63.

167 Christakis GT, Fremes SE, Weisel RD *et al*. Diltiazem cardioplegia. A balance of risk and benefit. *J Thorac Cardiovasc Surg* 1986;**91**:647–61.

168 Godet G, Coriat P, Baron JF *et al*. Prevention of intraoperative myocardial ischemia during non-cardiac surgery with intravenous diltiazem: a randomized trial versus placebo. *Anesthesiology* 1987;**66**:241–5.

169 Caramella JP, Goursot G, Carcone B. Prévention de l'ischémie myocardique per et postopératoire en chirurgie non cardiaque par le diltiazem intraveineux. *Ann Fr Anesth Réanim* 1988;**7**:245–50.

170 Nishikawa T, Namiki A. Attenuation of the pressor response to laryngoscopy and tracheal

intubation with intravenous verapamil. *Acta Anaesthesiol Scand* 1989;**33**:232–5.

171 Puri GD, Batra YK. Effect of nifedipine on cardiovascular responses to laryngoscopy and intubation. *Br J Anaesth* 1988;**60**:579–81.

172 Kale SC, Mahajan RP, Jayalakshami TA, Raghavan V, Das B. Nifedipine prevents the pressor response to laryngoscopy and tracheal intubation in patients with coronary artery disease. *Anaesthesia* 1988;**43**:495–7.

173 Mikawa K, Nishina K, Maekawa N and Obara H. Comparison of nicardipine, diltiazem and verapamil for controlling the cardiovascular responses to tracheal intubation. *Br J Anaesth* 1996;**76**:221–6.

174 Fuji Y, Tanaka H, Saitoh Y, Toyooka H. Effects of calcium channel blockers on circulatory response to tracheal intubation in hypertensive patients: nicardipine versus diltiazem. *Can J Anaesth* 1995;**42**:785–8.

175 Kishi Y, Okumura F, Furuya H. Haemodynamic effects of nicardipine hydrochloride. Studies during its use to control acute hypertension in anaesthetized patients. *Br J Anaesth* 1984;**56**:1003–6.

176 Van Wezel HB, Bovill JG, Schuller J, Gielen J, Hoeneveld MH. Comparison of nitroglycerine, verapamil and nifedipine in the management of arterial pressure during coronary artery surgery. *Br J Anaesth* 1986;**58**:267–73.

177 Delhumeau A, Granry JC, Cottineau C, Bukowski JG, Corbeau JJ, Moreau X. Comparaison des effets vasculaires du sulfate de magnésium et de la nicardipine pendant la circulation extracorporelle. *Ann Fr Anesth Réanim* 1995;**14**:149–53.

178 Lehot JJ, Durand PG, Villard J, Pelissier FT, Estanove S. Is nicardipine a venodilator during fentanyl-midazolam anaesthesia? *Eur J Anaesthesiol* 1992;**9**:154–5.

179 Arai T, Hatano Y, Ishida H, Mori K. Use of nicardipine in the anesthetic management of pheochromocytoma. *Anesth Analg* 1986;**65**:706–8.

180 Proye C, Thevenin D, Cecat P *et al.* Exclusive use of calcium channel blockers in preoperative and intraoperative control of pheochromocytomas: hemodynamics and free catecholamine assays in ten consecutive patients. *Surgery* 1989;**106**:1149–54.

181 Munro J, Hurlbert BJ, Hill GE. Calcium channel blockage and uncontrolled blood pressure during phacochromocytoma surgery. *Can J Anaesth* 1995;**42**:228–30.

182 Lehot JJ, Durand PG, Girard C. Nouveaux vasodilatateurs et bêta-bloqueurs. In SFAR, ed. *Congrès National d'Anesthésie et Réanimation.* Paris: Masson, 1991:117–29.

183 Mullen JC, Miller DR, Weisel RD *et al.* Postoperative hypertension: a comparison of diltiazem, nifedipine and nitroprusside. *J Thorac Cardiovasc Surg* 1988;**96**:122–32.

184 Brister NW, Barnette RE, Schartel SA, McClurken JB, Alpern J. Isradipine for treatment of acute hypertension after myocardial revascularisation. *Crit Care Med* 1991;**19**:334–8.

185 Underwood SM, Davies SW, Feneck RO, Lunnon MW, Wales RK. Comparison of isradipine with nitroprusside for control of blood pressure following myocardial revascularization: effects on hemodynamics, cardiac metabolism, and coronary blood flow. *J. Cardiothorac Anesth* 1991;**5**:348–56.

186 Zimpfer M, Fitzal S, Tonczar L. Verapamil as a hypotensive agent during neuro-leptanaesthesia. *Br J Anaesth* 1981;**53**:885–9.

187 Abe K, Iwanaga H, Inada E. Effect of nicardipine and diltiazem on internal carotid artery blood flow velocity and local cerebral blood flow during cerebral aneurysm surgery for subarachnoid hemorrhage. *J Clin Anesth* 1994;**6**:99–105.

188 Abe K, Iwanaga H, Shimada Y, Yoshiya I. The effect of nicardipine on carotid blood flow velocity, local cerebral blood flow and carbon dioxide reactivity during cerebral aneurysm surgery. *Anesth Analg* 1993;**76**:1227–33.

189 Brichard G, Zimmerman PE. Verapamil in cardiac dysrhythmias during anaesthesia. *Br J Anaesth* 1970;**42**:1005–12.

190 Iberti TJ, Benjamin E, Paluch TA, Gentili DR, Gabrielson GY. Use of constant infusion verapamil for the treatment of postoperative supraventricular tachycardia. *Crit Care Med* 1986;**14**(4):283–4.

191 Ilias WK, Williams CH, Fulfer RT, Dozier SE. Diltiazem inhibits halothane induced contractions in malignant hyperthermia susceptible muscles in vitro. *Br J Anaesth* 1985;**57**:994–6.

192 Adnet P J, Krivosic-Horber RM, Adamantidis MM, Reyford H, Cordonnier C, Handecoeur G. Effects of calcium-free solution, calcium antagonists, and the calcium

agonist BAY K8644 on mechanical responses of skeletal muscle from patients susceptible to malignant hyperthermia. *Anesthesiology* 1991;**75**:413–19.

193 Saltzman LS, Kates RA, Corke BC, Norfleet EA, Heath KR. Hyperkalemia and cardiovascular collapse after dantrolene and verapamil administration in swine. *Anesth Analg* 1984;**63**:473–8.

194 Robin AS, Zablocki AD. Hyperkalemia, verapamil and dantrolene. *Anesthesiology* 1987;**66**:246–9.

195 Freysz M, Timour Q, Bernaud C, Bertrix L, Faucon G. Cardiac implications of amodipine–dantrolene combinations. *Can J Anaesth* 1966;**43**:50–5.

196 Garratt C, Antoniou A, Ward D, Camm AD. Misuse of verapamil in pre-excited atrial fibrillation. *Lancet* 1987;**i**:367–9.

3: Angiotensin-converting enzyme inhibitors

PASCAL COLSON

Angiotensin-converting enzyme (ACE) inhibitors are increasingly used in the treatment of cardiovascular or other diseases.[1, 2, 3] The number of patients chronically treated with ACE inhibitors and scheduled for anaesthesia is increasing and the question arises as to whether renin–angiotensin system (RAS) blockade may affect haemodynamics during anaesthesia and surgery. In 1978, Miller *et al.* reported that the RAS is involved in the maintenance of normal blood presure during anaesthesia.[4] In contrast, anaesthesia is not invariably associated with deleterious haemodynamic events in ACE-blocked patients.[5-7] However, haemodynamic instability manifest as unexpected episodes of hypotension has been described in a few cases; most of these cases are not well documented but hypotension was always easily treated with volume loading.[8-10]

Acute responses of the unblocked RAS to haemodynamc stresses such as surgery or hypotension are also potentially deleterious. Angiotensin II induces vasoconstriction,[11] which may maintain blood pressure, but reduces blood flow to organs such as the kidneys and bowels. Accordingly, angiotensin II-induced reduction in blood flow may contribute to acute renal failure[12] and splanchnic ischaemia,[13] both of which are obvious contributors to postoperative morbidity.[14] RAS blockade with ACE inhibitors has been shown to decrease the haemodynamic consequences of the 'stress-response' on these regional circulations,[6, 15, 16] which, to some extent, are designed to contribute to body protection.

Nevertheless, recent advances in RAS physiology, ACE inhibitor pharmacology and ACE inhibitor use during anaesthesia and surgery may help to understand the haemodynamic risks of anaesthesia in ACE-blocked patients, to identify some predisposing factors, and to determine potential beneficial effects of ACE inhibitors during anaesthesia.

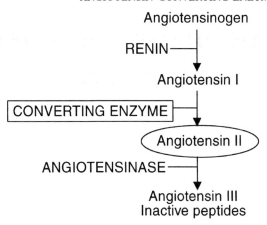

Fig 3.1   The renin–angiotensin biochemical cascade

Physiology of the renin–angiotensin system (RAS)

Biochemistry

The RAS is basically defined as a biochemical cascade[17] (Figure 3.1). A highly specific proteolytic enzyme, renin, cleaves an ineffective peptide precursor, angiotensinogen, to generate a decapeptide, angiotensin I. Angiotensin I is converted to an octapeptide, angiotensin II, by a non-specific carboxypeptidase, the angiotensin-converting enzyme. Angiotensin II is considered the effective final product of these enzymatic reactions.[17–19] The main biochemical controls of RAS activation are rapid metabolism of angiotensin II and feedback control of angiotensin II on renin release.[18]

The biochemical cascade originates from different organs: the kidneys produce renin, the liver generates angiotensinogen, and vascular endothelium synthesises angiotensin since almost all angiotensin I and angiotensin II (90 and 64%, respectively) have been shown to be generated within endothelium rather than in plasma.[19–21] Angiotensin II acts then on multiple target organs after binding on specific receptors. RAS was thus primarily described as a systemic, diffuse endocrine system. Using high performance liquid chromatography to measure angiotensins, immunohistological localisation of components of the RAS and hybridisation *in situ*, local formation of renin, angiotensinogen, and angiotensin have been suggested in various tissues (brain, kidney, heart, adrenal, testis, arterial wall).[18, 20] The implications of local angiotensin II production in cardiovascular physiology have been actively investigated,[21, 22] but claims for renin synthesis within cardiac and extrarenal vascular tissues have been refuted.[23] As a result of methodological shortcomings, evidence of *in situ* cardiac or vascular renin formation suggested by many studies of tissue RAS is now considered to be inadmissible. Regional formation of angiotensin II appears therefore to be subordinate to plasma renin. Interstitial fluids can bind or trap plasma renin and the angiotensin II formed may thus contribute either to the circulating angiotensin II (endocrine activity) or to the function of adjacent cells (paracrine activity) or cells to which the ACE is attached (autocrine activity).[21] The primary determinant of the rate of angiotensin II formation is the plasma concentration of renin created by the regulated secretion of renal renin.[23] However, the final activity of angiotensin II depends on the concentration of renin substrate and the availability of angiotensin-converting enzyme which both modulate local RAS activity. It is therefore more appropriate to consider diverse levels of regulation of angiotensin II formation, either systemic or local, rather than to distinguish endocrine or autocrine/paracrine functions of the RAS.

Mechanisms of RAS activation

The well-known primary mechanisms regulating renal renin secretion, that is renal baroreceptors, neurogenic stimulation, or macula densa-mediated RAS activation, have been confirmed at cellular as well as subcellular levels.[24] All these mechanisms regulate renin expression by Ca^{++}, adenosine $3',5'$-cyclic monophosphate, and chemiosmotic forces (K^+, Cl^-, and water flux coupled to H^+ movements). Under favourable conditions, prorenin is then processed to renin, which may be secreted by regulative degranulation or divergence translocation.[24]

Mechanisms of angiotensin II action

Angiotensin II binds at least to two specific receptors, angiotensin I receptor sybtypes AT1 and AT2. Although little is known about AT2 receptor-mediated effects, many actions of angiotensin II involved in blood pressure control (vasoconstriction, aldosterone secretion, stimulation of catecholamine release, central pressor and dipsogenic stimulations) are mediated through binding to AT1.[25] Angiotensin II-induced increases in noradrenaline release from guinea-pig atria have been shown recently to be mediated by AT1 receptors.[26] Besides direct actions of angiotensin II, a great body of evidence suggests a crossover potentiation between angiotensin II and other factors involved in blood pressure regulation. Vascular tone results therefore from interactions, either between vasoactive circulating peptides (angiotensin II, catecholamines)[27] or between angiotensin II and endothelial control of vasomotor tone,[28] e.g. by nitric oxide.[29] Regulation of vascular tone appears even more extraordinarily complex as angiotensin II can cause large significant reductions in blood pressure after losartan-induced AT1 receptor blockade. As shown experimentally in rats, this effect probably is mediated by AT2 receptors.[30] Similar interactions exist also with factors involved in angiotensin II-mediated body volume regulation; endothelin may increase angiotensin II-induced aldosterone

54

production,[31] and aldosterone may increase angiotensin II receptor numbers and enhance angiotensin II-stimulated protein synthesis.[32]

Role of angiotensin II

Local formation of angiotensin II seems to be involved in local regulation of vascular tone as well as angiogenesis[18, 19, 33, 34] that could be clinically relevant, particularly during anaesthesia.[6, 16] However, involvement of the RAS in blood pressure maintenance is of principal importance for clinical decision-making in the daily practice of anaesthesia.

The RAS and systemic haemodynamics

RAS endocrine activity is involved in blood pressure control. During hypovolaemia, RAS activation results first in angiotensin II-induced vasoconstriction. Then, angiotensin II stimulates fluid volume increases through stimulation of sodium and water reabsorption.[35]

RAS activation can be summarised as follows: (a) RAS is mainly dependent on body fluid volume; (b) effective blood volume (i.e. the blood volume that allows adequate cardiac output) is the regulating variable for RAS activation.[36] Blood pressure thus depends on RAS as a function of extracellular fluid volume and effective volaemia[36] (Figures 3.2, 3.3). While there is moderate RAS dependence in normovolaemia,[36, 37] and minimal effects with extracellular fluid volume expansion,[36, 38] the RAS contribution to blood pressure becomes crucial in hypovolaemia (Figure 3.2).[36, 37] The final purpose of RAS activation is to increase body fluid volume;[36–38]

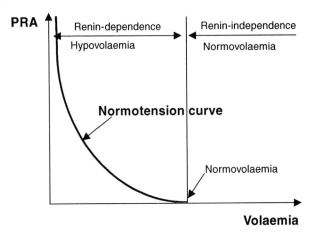

Fig 3.2 Plasma renin activity/effective volaemia relationship. In a physiological steady state, normotension is maintained without renin–angiotensin system activity or plasma renin activity (PRA). When (effective) volaemia is increased, blood pressure is renin-dependent. Inversely, blood pressure becomes renin-dependent when volaemia is decreased

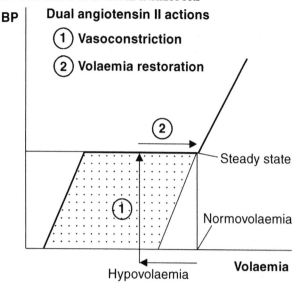

Fig 3.3 Dual action of angiotensin II. When (effective) volaemia decreases, angiotensin first induces (arterial and venous) vasoconstriction that sustains blood pressure (1), then volaemia is restored (2)

angiotensin II is the primary stimulus to aldosterone secretion,[36, 38] but contributes also to sodium regulation directly[39] as well as fluid volume regulation indirectly.[40] Any renin-dependent, volume-independent state tends therefore to be converted into a renin-independent, volume-dependent state by RAS action itself (Figure 3.3). For example, elevated blood pressure in experimental renovascular hypertension or coarctation hypertension[37, 41] is maintained initially by direct pressor actions of angiotensin II (renin-dependent state) and is thus sensitive to RAS blockade.[42] During a later chronic phase, hypertension is due to hyper-volaemia which is the result of angiotensin II activity,[37, 41] but then becomes insensitive to RAS blockade (renin-independent state).[42, 43]

Fluid volume regulation requires hours to days but angiotensin II-induced vasoconstriction is rapid so that acute changes in volume status, which are not uncommon during anaesthesia and surgery, result first in vasoconstriction. Angiotensin II-induced vasoconstriction is well known for arterioles and contributes to maintenance of blood pressure by increasing vascular resistance.[36-38] Angiotensin II also produces constriction of veins either directly[44-46] or through potentiation of the effect of the sympathetic nervous system,[44] which results in reduced vascular capacitance (a decrease in either unstressed vascular volume or compliance or both). Arterial angiotensin induced-vasoconstriction may also improve venous return because cardiac output is redistributed from long time-constant compartments to short time-constant compartments. An effective blood volume may therefore be maintained in spite of a decrease in absolute blood volume[47, 48] (Figure 3.3). Both arterial and venous actions of angiotensin II improve venous return to the heart, and cardiac output is then preserved[49] (Figure 3.3).

RAS and regional circulations

Angiotensin-induced vasoconstriction is one of the mechanisms of blood pressure control during renin-dependent states but results in cardiac output redistribution.

Renal circulation is the most extensively investigated regional circulation with regard to the role of RAS on regulation of regional vascular tone.[50–52] Moreover, the kidney was one of the first tissues where *in situ* formation of angiotensin II was demonstrated.[20, 53] Intrarenal RAS is involved in the homeostatic regulation of renal blood flow and glomerular filtration,[50] mainly by angiotensin II-induced vasoconstriction of the efferent arteriole of the glomerulus.[51] Many other tissues are probably affected by the role of the RAS on regulation of region circulation, but definitive evidence for such a role on local vasoregulation is still lacking.[20] The mesenteric circulation is also very sensitive to angiotensin II-induced vasoconstriction, so that both renal and mesenteric circulations are altered adversely during RAS activation.[13, 53]

Pharmacology of ACE inhibitors

Mechanisms of action and pharmacokinetics

Angiotensin-converting enzyme is a non-specific carboxypeptidase and is involved in conversion of angiotensin I to angiotensin II as well as inactivation of central opioids (enkephalins), and bradykinin, a potent vasodilator. Inactivation of angiotensin II formation is the accepted main mechanism of ACE inhibition.[1, 54]

From the earliest utilisation of the first orally administered specific ACE inhibitor, captopril, in man, reported in 1977,[55] many products with similar basic activity have been developed. Drug specificities have emerged from pharmacological modulations when related to pharmacokinetic profies.[2, 56, 57] Some are prodrugs that need to be converted by esterase activity in the liver to active moieties (e.g. alecepril, benazepril, cilazapril, enalapril, fisinopril etc.), resulting in a delay in peak activity. Most have longer terminal half-lives than captopril, permitting once-daily dosage, but this results also in delayed recovery of ACE activity after ACE inhibitor withdrawal. Nevertheless, inhibition of angiotensin II formation remains the key action of any ACE inhibitor.[58]

Pharmacology of ACE inhibitors

ACE inhibitor effects on systemic haemodynamics

ACE inhibitor effects depend on the underlying pathophysiological state and the degree of RAS activation. As stated above, blood pressure is not affected markedly by RAS blockade in normal subjects in sodium balance.[35-37, 55] However, the vasodilating effect of ACE inhibitors may exceed the complete blockade of angiotensin II formation as evidenced by decreased blood pressure in normotensive, sodium-replete subjects, i.e. subjects with low plasma renin activity.[35] A 10% decrease in blood pressure may occur after a single oral dose of enalapril in normotensive subjects receiving a normal sodium intake (150 mmol daily).[59] This effect is probably a result of additional hormonal effects of ACE inhibition such as interference with degradation of bradykinin or accumulation of prostaglandins.[35]

The decrease in blood pressure associated with ACE inhibition is basically the result of a decrease in systemic vascular resistance in both normal and hypertensive subjects.[36-38] In addition, ACE inhibitors can impair adaptation of cardiac output to ventricular loading changes. Niarchos and co-workers[38] have demonstraed that fainting occurring during tilting in patients treated with an intravenous ACE inhibitor (treprotide) was associated with a striking reduction in cardiac output. The decreased cardiac output was related to inhibition of the effects of angiotensin II on veins, inducing a decrease in venous return.[45-47] In addition, decreased blood pressure was not associated with reflex tachycardia, and this may have exaggerated the inability to maintain cardiac output; the absence of a reflex tachycardia suggests a blunting of the baroreflex mechanisms. However, several studies in animals[60, 61] and in man[62-64] to evaluate the relationship between pulse intervals and blood pressure during ACE inhibition, have demonstrated an increased sensitivity of the baroreflex response associated with resetting, rather than a blunting of the cardiac baroreflex. Although ACE inhibition tilts the balance of autonomic nervous system activity towards increased parasympatheric tone, the sympathetic response of the baroreflex is intact and remains capable of appropriate adjustment.[63, 65] Parasympathetic tone is basically increased,[62, 64, 65] but sympathetic activity may increase acutely during hypotension as assessed by the steep gradient of the slope of the pulse interval/blood pressure relationship.[63] This works quite well in awake normovolaemic subjects, and orthostatic hypotension does not occur in ACE-inhibitor-pretreated patients.[63] Moreover, vasopressin, which may be involved in blood pressure regulation, is also maintained during ACE inhibition.[63, 66, 67] Therefore, during hypovolaemia and ACE inhibition, both the sympathetic nervous system and vasopressin may act as overlapping vasopressor systems to maintain blood pressure.[68] Nevertheless, in spite of the dual control of blood pressure, blood pressure has been shown to be volume-dependent during ACE inhibition.[69]

ACE inhibitors and regional circulations

As expected from physiological considerations, renal and mesenteric circulations are the regional circulations that may benefit from ACE inhibition in renin-dependent states. In experimental studies, both circulations have been shown to be more sensitive to ACE inhibitor-induced vasodilatation than other regional circulations.[52, 53, 58, 70, 71] Recovery of impaired renal blood flow and glomerular filtration rate after administration of ACE inhibitors at doses that did not affect systemic blood pressure has been demonstrated early in sodium-restricted conscious dogs.[52] More recently, treatment with ACE inhibitors with different chemical structures has been found to improve both renal and splanchnic circulations in an experimental model of RAS activation (water-deprived Brattleboro-rats)[71] and in spontaneously hypertensive rats.[58] The potential benefit of RAS blockade on splanchnic perfusion has been shown in experimental haemorrhagic shock.[72–74] RAS blockade with either angiotensin II receptor antagonists[72] or the ACE inhibitors captopril and enalaprilat[73, 74] improved postoligaemic splanchnic perfusion and reduced significantly the subsequent formation of myocardial depressant factor (MDF) following haemorrhage in cats.[72–74]

ACE inhibitor therapy

Hypertension

Essential hypertension is related to increased vascular resistances. The main objective of antihypertensive treatment is to reduce vasoconstriction. The clinical use of ACE inhibitors was devoted initially to obvious physiopathological states associated with high plasma renin activity.[75] However, ACE inhibitors are presently considered effective in essential hypertension irrespective of the underlying plasma renin activity because vascular resistances can be reduced even when previous plasma renin activity is low.[1, 3] The suppression of endothelial angiotensin production has been advocated in non-renin hypertension.[18, 22] ACE inhibition is used increasingly in the treatment of hypertension[3] because of its good tolerance.[1]

Non-angiotensin II inhibition mechanisms are also involved in the pharmacological actions of ACE inhibitors. Direct effects of ACE inhibitors on vascular contraction and Ca^{++} influx in vascular smooth muscle cells are suggested mechanisms.[76] ACE inhibitors may increase the vasodilator effects of bradykinin by generating endothelium-derived relaxing factors such as nitric oxide.[77] The contribution of a prostaglandin-dependent component to the hypotensive action of ACE inhibitors remains controversial.[77, 78]

59

Reducing arterial blood pressure is not the sole criterion for success in the pharmacological management of essential hypertension. Associated metabolic and structural abnormalities may contribute to increase the risk of cardiovascular complications.[79] These factors must be taken into account when selecting the antihypertensive agent. Neither ACE inhibitors nor calcium blockers increase any risk factor of coronary artery disease and have characteristics close to those of the ideal antihypertensive drug.[79]

Heart failure

In congestive heart failure, stroke volume decreases because it is inversely related to changes in outflow resistances.[80] Vasodilator therapy can therefore improve stroke volume and cardiac output by decreasing afterload.[81] Increased release of neurohormones (plasma noradrenaline, plasma renin activity, atrial natriuretic peptide) correlates with decreased ejection fraction in congestive heart failure.[82] Besides sympathetic nervous system involvement and lysine vasopressin secretion, activation of the renin-angiotensin system increases systemic vascular resistance;[80] the more advanced is the stage of the disease, the more the RAS is activated.[83] ACE inhibitors improve left ventricular function in patients with chronic congestive heart failure[84-87] and have been shown to be beneficial in the treatment of congestive heart failure. However, similar improvements in haemodynamics (left ventricular ejection fraction) can be obtained with other vasodilators. Improved survival in severe heart failure associated with ACE inhibition is multifactorial and is related to haemodynamic effects as well as structural protection of the failing heart,[88] improvement of myocardial metabolism,[89] and prevention of ventricular arrhythmias.[90, 91]

The beneficial effect of ACE inhibition on mortality in chronic mild, moderate or severe heart failure is accepted.[92] This has encouraged the use of ACE inhibitors in earlier phases of heart disease, before overt heart failure develops. Administration of enalapril in patients with asymptotic left ventricular dysfunction reduced mortality and morbidity during an average follow-up of 37·4 months.[93] ACE inhibition has been evaluated also in the early phase following acute myocardial infarction. First results suggest that infarct expansion is attenuated and that the left ventricular remodelling is influenced favourably.[94, 95] Moreover, captopril given within 3–16 days after myocardial infarction to patients with ejection fractions of 40% or less improved mortality and reduced morbidity during a mean follow-up time of 42 months.[96] However, very early administration of enalapril following acute myocardial infarction (within 24 hours after the onset of chest pain) failed to improve mortality at 3 months.[97] This may be accounted for by the well-known deleterious effect of early administration of any potent vasodilator following infarction[98] and further studies are being required to identify the subgroup of patients who may benefit from early ACE inhibition.

Myocardial ischaemia

After myocardial infarction, ramipril given between the second and ninth day after myocardial infarction improved survival in patients with evidence of heart failure.[99] This effect has been attributed to prevention of ventricular remodelling,[100, 101] but ACE inhibitors may also reduce the incidence of recurrent myocardial infarction.[102] Cardioprotective effects of ACE inhibitors in acute myocardial ischaemia and infarction have been investigated intensively in recent years. Both experimental and clinical reports have revealed that coronary occlusion results in acute activation of the RAS.[103] Thus, ACE inhibitors could be expected to provide cardioprotection. Various mechanisms have been advocated on the basis of experimental studies. Angiotensin II may play a role as an independent arrhythmogen in ischaemic heart disease[104] and ACE inhibitor antiarrhythmic activity has been demonstrated through free radical scavenging, increased concentrations of bradykinin and prostaglandin, and attenuation of angiotensin II-related sympathetic facilitation.[105] Improvement of contractile function of the stunned myocardium is consistent with ACE inhibitor-induced potentiation of bradykinin or prostacyclin synthesis[106] or with SH-containing ACE inhibitors.[103] The clinical relevance of each mechanism remains under debate; for example, ACE inhibitors protect the myocardium against pathological structural remodelling created by reactive fibrosis[107] but have failed to prevent restenosis after coronary angioplasty.[107-109] Nevertheless, ACE inhibitors are recommended within the first week after infarction in patients with left ventricular dysfunction (ejection fraction less than 40%) because they reduce mortality and severe adverse cardiovascular events.[110] ACE inhibitors may also provide an anti-ischaemic effect on asymptomatic ischaemia during daily activity.[111]

Protection of regional circulation

In hypertension and heart failure, ACE inhibition is also associated with a redistribution of regional blood flow, especially in favour of the kidney[58, 71, 112, 113] provided that hypotensive episodes are avoided.[114] Evidence of improvement in renal function in diabetes and glomerulopathies[115, 116] has been demonstrated with ACE inhibitors.

ACE inhibitors and anaesthesia

Blood pressure regulation and anaesthesia

Blood pressure can be sustained by three vasopressor systems: the sympathetic nervous system, the RAS, and vasopressin. Anaesthesia decreases sympathetic contribution to blood pressure regulation and interferes with renin secretion. Some intravenous anaesthetics attenuate renal sympathetic nerve activity[117] and consequently induce a decrease in renin secretion. Similarly, epidural anaesthesia suppresses renin release in repsonse to arterial hypotension,[118] an effect mediated by the sympathetic nervous system because it is reversed by a β-agonist, adrenaline.[119] However, during anaesthesia and surgery, it is well established that blood pressure may become angiotensin-dependent.[4, 120, 121] In fact, the mechanism of RAS activation does not differ from awake conditions; decreased extracellular fluid volume activates RAS, as assessed by an increase in plasma renin activity.[120, 122] Blood pressure can therefore be maintained despite fluid volume changes.[120] RAS activation may also partly counterbalance the decrease in venous return associated with sympathetic blockade caused by anaesthesia.[123] Accordingly, blood pressure decreases markedly during general anaesthesia in renin-dependent states when angiotensin II action is impeded by an angiotensin II competitive inhibitor, saralasin.[120]

Besides the RAS and the sympathetic system, endogenous vasopressin may be involved in blood pressure regulation during anaesthesia. During epidural anaesthesia and enalaprilat-induced inhibition of the RAS, plasma vasopressin concentration increased significantly.[124] Conversely, as assessed by increased plasma renin activity, the RAS compensates for vasopressin blockade with vasopressin receptor (V1) antagonist.[124] Decreases in blood pressure induced by epidural anaesthesia are similar whether V1 receptors or the RAS are blocked. Each individual pressor system may act as a compensatory mechanism whenever other systems are depressed. The RAS contribution to blood pressure support is thus crucial when the sympathetic nervous system is blocked by epidural anaesthesia and endogenous vasopressin antagonised by a specific V1 receptor antagonist.[124] The greatest decrease in blood pressure occurred with the combination of enalaprilat with a V1 receptor antagonist and epidural blockade.[124]

ACE inhibitors and anaesthesia: risk or benefit?

The risk of hypotension

Preoperative ACE inhibition was used initially in order to prevent perioperative hypertension but was relatively ineffective.[5, 7, 125] In the studies in which preoperative ACE inhibition was associated with a significant reduction in the pressor response to intubation,[7, 126] the haemodynamic data were not sufficiently detailed to identify whether either cardiac ouput or vascular resistance or both were lowered when compared to control patients. It is noteworthy that most randomised clinical studies dealing with anaesthesia and preoperative ACE inhibition were not designed initially to evaluate the incidence and the magnitude of hypotension following induction of anaesthesia. Nevertheless, two of these studies reported severe, 'unexpected' deleterious haemodynamic events during anaesthesia.[8, 126] In Kataja and colleagues' study,[8] four out of 10 ACE-blocked patients (captopril 25 mg before and on the day of surgery) experienced marked decreases in blood pressure (systolic arterial blood pressure less than 70 mmHg) and heart rate (less than 40 b/min) just after induction of anaesthesia. However, mean pulmonary capillary wedge pressure was low (less than 6 mmHg) in the treated group, and the blood pressure decrease was corrected by fluid volume loading. Similarly, McCarthy et al.[126] reported three hypotensive episodes (systolic blood pressure less than 80 mmHg) following induction of anaesthesia in 22 normotensive patients undergoing gynaecological surgery following pretreatment with a single oral dose of captopril (12·5 or 25 mg, 25 minutes before tracheal intubation).[126] Although no data were given regarding filling pressures or cardiac output, hypotension was always treated successfully with volume loading. Two severe episodes of bradycardia which were not associated with hypotension also occurred, but in association with vagotonic stimuli.[126] These results further confirm the inability to adapt cardiac output to ventricular loading changes, the volume-dependence of blood pressure, and the increased vagal tone in anaesthetised ACE-blocked patients. Induction of anaesthesia impedes the sympathetic nervous system, one of the overlapping vasopressor systems which may contribute to maintain blood pressure in ACE-inhibited patients.[67, 127] In the presence of a combination of hypovolaemia, ACE inhibition and anaesthesia, vasopressin may therefore act as the only vasopressor system to maintain blood pressure.[127] However, vasopressin is less effective on systemic capacity than on arterial resistance,[44, 128] and the volume-dependence of blood pressure[69] is then amplified.

Results obtained after short-term preoperative ACE inhibition (1 to 2 days) in normotensive or mild hypertensive subjects may be inapplicable to chronically treated patients with moderate to severe hypertension, or with heart failure. First, chronic administration of ACE inhibitors may alter blood pressure regulation differently in comparison to short-term treatment; Raman, Waller and Warren[64] have shown that parasympathetic activity is further enhanced after chronic administration of ACE inhibitors when compared to acute administration. Second, in moderate and severe hyertension, chronic ACE inhibition is frequently associated with treatment with other antihypertensive agents that can also hinder adequate regulation of blood pressure. Moreover, the severity of hypertension correlates directly with the magnitude of potential haemodynamic changes.[129, 130] Acute sympathetic inhibition after induction of anaesthesia associated with preliminary RAS blockade may be expected to result in hypotensive episodes. The incidence of hypotension after induction of anaesthesia is therefore high in hypertensive patients when administration of ACE inhibitors is continued until the day of surgery.[131, 132] Haemodynamic effects of anaesthesia in hypertensive patients treated chronically with ACE inhibitors have been studied.[132] Hypotension (mean arterial blood pressure less than 70 mmHg) following induction of anaesthesia (flunitrazepam, fentanyl) occurred in 6 out of 8 ACE-blocked patients versus 3 out of 8 hypertensive patients not treated with an ACE inhibitor. In the ACE-blocked patients, decreased blood pressure was related mostly to decreases in cardiac output and pulmonary capillary wedge pressure. Mean pre-anaesthetic pulmonary capillary wedge pressure was higher in the ACE-blocked patients than in controls and hypotension was severe in patients who received a combination of three antihypertensive drugs. This is of interest and probably suggests that hypertension was more severe and associated with diastolic heart failure in the ACE-blocked patients. Diastolic dysfunction may thus have amplified the haemodynamic changes induced by anaesthesia in the presence of ACE inhibition since any decrease in venous return to the heart is tolerated poorly when ventricular compliance is reduced. However, episodes of hypotension are brief and corrected easily with volume infusion or sympathomimetic agents.[131, 132] Sudden changes in cardiac loading conditions may have affected haemodynamic stability drastically in patients with potential left ventricular diastolic dysfunction.[132] The decrease in blood pressure did not correlate with the decrease in plasma converting enzyme activity (PCEA).[131] However, PCEA was restored when ACE inhibitors were withdrawn before the day of anaesthesia,[131] and the incidence of hypotension after induction of anaesthesia was then reduced.[131]

Little is known about anaesthesia in patients suffering from heart failure and treated with ACE inhibitors. In an experimental model of doxorubicin-induced heart failure in rabbits, a combination of halothane and enalaprilat resulted in improvement of cardiac output and renal blood flow[133] but a higher halothane concentration (1·3 MAC) induced severe circulatory depression.[133] Cardiodepressant effects of a combination of halothane and an ACE inhibitor[134] may be deleterious in the presence of severe cardiomyopathy.[135] Because doxorubicin alters both diastolic and systolic functions and because enalaprilat was administered intravenously, it is difficult to draw any definite conclusions from these rabbit studies for the human situation of patients with pure systolic heart failure, such as regurgitant valvular diseases, chronically treated wih ACE inhibitors. Indeed, systolic heart dysfunction has been reported to be greatly improved by intravenous enalaprilat in one case.[136] The risk of hypotension following induction of anaesthesia seems to be less when ACE inhibitors are maintained until the day of surgery in patients with low left ventricular ejection fraction.[137]

Are there benefits?

Premedication with an ACE inhibitor attenuates sympathetic responses during surgery[138] and ACE inhibitors potentiate SNP-induced hypotension.[139] However, these effects are of limited clinical impact and whether

ACE inhibition during anaesthesia and surgery offers any true clinical benefits, remains an unresolved issue.

Experimental evidence suggests that ACE inhibitors may improve regional circulations, emphasising the importance of the interconnections between the RAS and endothelium-derived vasoactive substances.[29, 140] Some clinical evidence of a beneficial effect on regional circulation has been suggested in cardiac and vascular surgery (see below).

Systemic haemodynamics During cardiac surgery, ACE inhibitors were administered first to prevent hypertension. Hypertension following either noxious stimulation such as sternotomy[141] or coronary artery bypass graft surgery[5] does not seem to be mediated specifically by RAS activation. However, intravenous enalaprilat may reduce hypertension during cardiac surgery.[142] The RAS may be activated during cardiopulmonary bypass (CPB) as assessed by either increased plasma renin activity[6, 143, 144] or high plasma angiotensin II concentrations;[145] but the role of this RAS activation was more fully understood when ACE inhibition was used as a pharmacological tool to block the RAS. RAS inhibition with an ACE inhibitor is not usually associated with significant deleterious haemodynamic events during anaesthesia for coronary artry bypass grafting[6] or valvular surgery. In a double-blind placebo-controlled study, preoperative ACE inhibition in patients undergoing coronary artery bypass grafts did not alter the haemodynamic profile during anaesthesia and CPB when compared to control patients.[6] In contrast, preoperative chronic ACE inhibition before cardiac surgery contributes to increased vasoconstrictor requirements after moderate hypothermic CPB.[146] However, vasoconstrictors were required only for the first 4 hours in the ICU, and did not affect significantly the outcome. Two cases of very low systemic vascular resistance after hypothermic CPB in patients treated chronically with ACE inhibitor had been reported already.[147] In these two cases, anaesthesia and CBP before cooling were uneventful, but severe hypotension occurred during hypothermia and continued after rewarming. Weaning from CPB was possible only with an infusion of angiotensin II; α-adrenergic agonists were ineffective.[147] These two cases question the role of either hypothermia or inhibition of the RAS, or an association of both, on the dramatic α-adrenergic receptor desensitisation. These reports suggests also that the RAS may sometimes offset adrenergic system breakdown because an infusion of angiotensin II is successful in the management of such refractory low systemic vascular resistances.[147]

RAS activation is the accepted mechanism of the pathophysiology of hypertension in some vascular diseases such as renal artery stenosis or aortic coarctation[37, 41] which may require a surgical repair. However, ACE inhibition is restricted to unilateral renal artery stenosis when hypertension is severe. In fact, because of the potential risk of renal failure, ACE inhibition is usually contraindicated in unilateral as well as in bilateral renal artery stenosis.[3] In aortic coarctation, preoperative ACE inhibition is relatively ineffective in the treatment of hypertension because hypertension is mainly due to hypervolaemia during the chronic phase of the disease.[41] However, preoperative ACE inhibition does not impair blood pressure regulation or renal blood flow provided that volaemia is well maintained during anaesthesia and surgical repair (personal unpublished data).

Regional circulations   Impairment of renal haemodynamics during CPB is a model of decreased renal perfusion[6] and it has been suggested that the stimulated RAS during CPB may exert a deleterious effect.[145] Therefore, captopril was used as a pharmacological tool to block the RAS preoperatively in patients scheduled for coronary bypass.[6] Effective renal plasma flow and glomerular filtration rate as assessed by hippuran and DTPA clearances respectively, decreased during CPB in the control group but not in the ACE-blocked patients, although systemic haemodynamics were not significantly different between the groups.[6] Thus, the RAS does play a major role in modification of renal haemodynamics during CPB. Interestingly, this was a clinical demonstration of the exquisite sensitivity of the renal circulation to vasoconstriction induced by angiotensin II.[52]

RAS activation can be produced also by the surgical technique, mainly when thoracic aortic cross-clamping is used.[15] Joob *et al.* studied the effect of RAS blockade with enalapril on systemic and regional circulations using microspheres before, during and after thoracic clamping in a canine model.[15] In the control group, aortic clamping induced an increase in plasma renin activity, and decreases in renal and liver blood flows; both persisted after declamping. The ACE-blocked group experienced similar decreases in plasma flows during clamping but clamp release resulted in full recovery in renal and liver plasma flows. Although the small number of dogs studied precludes any definite conclusions, the apparent protective effect of ACE inhibition on organ blood flows in the treated group is noteworthy.

The decreased renal blood flow and increased plasma renin activity which occur during infrarenal aortic cross-clamping[148, 149] also suggest that the RAS is involved in renal haemodynamic impairment associated with infrarenal aortic surgery.[150] However, preoperative treatment with enalapril in patients scheduled for aortic reconstructive surgery failed to improve effective renal plasma flow and glomerular filtration rate during aortic cross-clamping.[151] The RAS is thus not an important determinant of the renal vasoconstriction associated with infrarenal aortic cross-clamping.[151] Although renal haemodynamics were not improved during clamping in the enalapril-treated group, it is of interest to consider that haemodynamic changes were less marked during surgery and that renal haemodynamics were well preserved before clamping in the enalapril-treated patients when compared to the controls.[151]

Conclusions

In addition to the long-term regulation of extracellular fluid volume, the RAS plays an important physiological role in maintaining venous return and blood pressure during acute haemodynamic stresses. ACE inhibitors may therefore alter venous return and cardiac output regulation during anaesthesia and surgery. This may be regarded as a disadvantage of ACE inhibition when other factors interfere with cardiovascular homeostasis; deleterious haemodynamic events may therefore occur when effective volaemia is decreased, which may be frequent during anaesthesia and surgery. However, the alternative solution should not be to stop ACE inhibitors preoperatively. This would allow recovery of RAS control on blood pressure but at the expense of some regional circulations. From this point of view, preliminary results from early studies during anaesthesia and surgery showing redistribution of regional blood flow with inhibition of ACE are encouraging; whether this might lead to improved postoperative outcome is a question which deserves further study. At this time, the evidence is that ACE inhibition does not allow the anaesthesiologist to be tolerant of hypovolaemia.

1 Breckenridge A. Angiotensin converting enzyme inhibitors. *Br Med J* 1988;**396**:618–20.
2 Kostis JB. Angiotensin converting enzyme inhibitors. I: Pharmacology. *Am Heeart J* 1988;**116**:1580–91.
3 Kostis JB. Angiotensin converting enzyme inhibitors. II: Clinical use. *Am Heart J* 1988;**116**:1591–506.
4 Miller ED, Ackerly JA, Peach MJ. Blood pressure support during general anaesthesia in renin-dependent state in the rat. *Anesthesiology* 1978;**48**:404–8.
5 Colson P, Grolleau D, Chaptal PA *et al.* Effect of preoperative renin–angiotensin system blockade on hypertension following coronary surgery. *Chest* 1988;**93**:1156–8.
6 Colson P, Ribstein J, Mimran M *et al.* Effect of angiotensin converting enzyme inhibition on blood pressure and renal function during open heart surgery. *Anesthesiology* 1990;**72**:23–7.
7 Yates AP, Hunter DN. Anaesthesia and angiotensin-converting enzyme inhibitors. *Anaesthesia* 1988;**43**:935–8.
8 Kataja JHK, Kaukinen S, Viinamäki OVK *et al.* Haemodynamic and hormonal changes in patients pretreated with captopril for surgery of the abdominal aorta. *J Cardiothorac Vasc Anesth* 1989;**3**:425–32.
9 McConachie I, Healy TEJ. ACE inhibitors and anaesthesia. *Postgrad Med J* 1988;**65**:273–4.
10 Selby DG, Richards JD, Marshman JM. ACE inhibitors (Letter). *Anaesth Intens Care* 1989;**17**:110–11.
11 Herd JA. Cardiovascular response to stress. *Physiol. Rev* 1991;**71**:305–30.
12 Moran SM, Myers BD. Pathophysiology of protracted acute renal failure in man. *J Clin Invest* 1985;**76**:1440–8.
13 Cohen MM, Sirar DS, McNeill JR, Grennway CV. Vasopressin and angiotensin on resistance vessels of spleen, intestine and liver. *Am. J Physiol* 1970;**218**:1704–6.
14 Björk M, Hedberg B. Early detection of major complications after abdominal aortic surgery: predictive value of sigmoid colon and gastric intramucosal pH monitoring. *Br J Surg* 1994;**81**:25–30.
15 Joob AW, Harman PK, Kaiser DL, Kron IL. The effect of renin-angiotensin system blockade on visceral blood flow during and after thoracic aortic cross-clamping. *J Thorac Cardiovasc Surg* 1986;**91**:411–18.

16 Mirenda JV, Grissom ThE. Anesthetic implications of the renin–angiotensin system and angiotensin-converting enzyme inhibitors. *Anesth Analg* 1991;72:667–83.

17 Oparil S, Haber E. The renin–angiotensin system. *N Engl J Med* 1974;291;:389–401.

18 Dzau V. Implications of local angiotensin production in cardiovascular physiology and pharmacology. *Am J Cardiol* 1987;59:59A–65A.

19 Campbell DJ. The site of angiotensin production. *J Hypertens* 1985;3:199–207.

20 Campbell DJ. Circulating and tissue angiotensin systems. *J Clin Invest* 1987;79:1–6.

21 Unger T, Gohlke P, Pal M, Retting R. Tissue renin–angiotensin systems: fact or fiction. *J Cardiovasc Pharmacol* 1991;18(Suppl 2):20–5.

22 Dzau VJ. Short and long term determinants of cardiovascular function and therapy: contributions of circulating and tissue renin angiotensin. *J Cardiovasc Pharmacol* 1989;14(Suppl 4):1–5.

23 Von Lutterotti N, Catanzaro DF, Sealey JE, Laragh JH. Renin is not synthesized by cardiac and extrarenal vascular tissues. *Circulation* 1994;89:458–70.

24 King JA, Lush DJ, Fray JCS. Regulation of renin processing and secretion: chemiosmotic control and novel secretory pathway. *Am J Physiol* 1993;265:C305–C320.

25 Greindling KK, Murphy TJ, Alexander RW. Molecular biology of the renin–angiotensin system. *Circulation* 1993;6:1817–28.

26 Brasch H, Sieroslawski L, Dominiak P. Angiotensin II increases norepinephrine release from atria by acting on angiotensin subtype 1 receptors. *Hypertension* 1993;22:699–704.

27 Dominiak P. Modulation of sympathetic control by ACE inhibitors. *Eur Heart J* 1993;14(Suppl 1):169–72.

28 Lüscher TF. Angiotensin, ACE-inhibitors and endothelial control of vasomotor tone. *Basic Res Cardiol* 1993;88(Suppl 1):15–24.

29 Sigmon DH, Beierwaltes WH. Angiotensin II. Nitric oxide interaction and the distribution of blood flow. *Am J Physiol* 1993;265:1276–83.

30 Scheuer DA, Perrone MH. Angiotensin type 2 receptors mediate depressor phase of biphasic pressure response to angiotensin. *Am J Physiol* 1993;28:E917–E923.

31 Cozza EN, Gomez-Sanchez CE. Mechanisms of ET-1 Potentiation of angiotensin II stimulation of aldosterone production. *Am J Physiol* 1993;28:E179–E183.

32 Ullian ME, Hutchison FN, Hazen-Martin DJ, Morinelli TA. Angiotensin II-aldosterone interactions on protein synthesis in vascular smooth muscle cells. *Am J Physiol* 1993;264:C1525–C1531.

33 Waeber B, Nussberger J, Juillierat L, Brunner H. Angiotensin converting enzyme inhibition: discrepancy between antihypertensive effect and inhibition of plasma enzyme activity. *J Cardiovasc Pharmacol* 1989;14(Suppl 4):57–63.

34 Campbell-Boswell M, Robertson AL jr. Effects of angiotensin II and vasopressin on human smooth muscle cells in vitro. *Exp Mol Pathol* 1981;35:265–76.

35 Kiowski W, Linder L, Kleinbloesem C, van Brummelen P, Bühler FR. Blood pressure control by the renin–angiotensin system in normotensive subjects. *Circulation* 1992;85:1–8.

36 Sancho J, Re R, Burton J et al. The role of the renin–angiotensin–aldosterone system in cardiovascular homeostasis in normal human subjects. *Circulation* 1976;53:400–5.

37 Haber E. The role of renin in normal and pathological cardiovascular homeostasis. *Circulation* 1976;54:849–61.

38 Niarchos AP, Pickering TG, Morganti A, Laragh JH. Plasma catecholamines and caradiovascular responses during converting enzyme inhibition in normotensive and hypertensive man. *Clin Exp Hypertens* 1982;A4:761–89.

39 Schuster VL, Kokko JP, Jacobson HR. Angiotensin II directly stimulates sodium transport in rabbit proximal convoluted tubules. *J Clin Invest* 1984;73:507–15.

40 Brooks VL, Keil LC, Reid IA. Role of the renin–angiotensin system in the control of vasopressin secretion in conscious dogs? *Circ Res* 1986;58:829–38.

41 Bagby SP, Mass RD. Abnormality of renin/body-fluid-volume relationship in serially studied inbred dogs with neonatally induced coarctation hypertension. *Hypertension* 1980;2:631–42.

42 Bagby SP. Acute responses of arterial pressure and plasma renin activity to converting enzyme inhibiton (SQ 20,881) in serially studied dogs with neonatally induced coarctation hypertension. *Hypertension* 1982;4:146–54.

43 Gavras H, Brunner HR, Vaughan ED, Laragh JH. Angiotensin-sodium interaction in blood pressure maintenance of renal hypertensive and normotensive rats. *Science* 1973;**180**:1369–74.

44 Benjamin N, Collier JG, Webb DJ. Angiotensin II augments sympathetically induced vasoconstriction in man. *Clin Sci* 1988;**75**:337–40.

45 Hernandez I, Ingles AC, Pinilla JM *et al.* Cardiocirculatory responses to angiotensin II and AVP in conscious rats. *J Cardiovasc Pharmacol* 1991;**17**:916–22.

46 Lee RW, Standeart S, Lancaster LD *et al.* Cardiac and peripheral circulatory responses to angiotensin and vasopressin in dogs. *J Clin Invest* 1988;**82**:413–19.

47 Drees JA, Rothe CF. Reflex venoconstriction and capacity vessel pressure-volume relationships in dogs. *Circ Res* 1974;**34**:360–73.

48 Shoukas AA, Sagawa K. Total systemic vascular compliance measured as incremental volume-pressure ratio. *Circ Res* 1971;**28**:277–91.

49 Hainsworth R. The importance of vasculature capacitance in cardiovascular control. *TIPS* 1990;**5**:250–4.

50 Freeman RH, Davis JO, Vitale SJ, Johnson JA. Intrarenal role of angiotensin II. Homeostatic regulation of renal blood flow in the dog. *Circ Res* 1973;**32**:692–8.

51 Hall JE, Guyton AC, Jackson ThE *et al.* Control of glomerular filtration rate by the renin-angiotensin system. *Am J Physiol* 1977;**233**:F366–F372.

52 Kimbrough HM, Vaughan ED, Carey RM, Ayers CR. Effect of intrarenal angiotensin II on renal function in conscious dogs. *Circ Res* 1977;**40**:174–8.

53 Levens NR, Peach MJ, Carey RM. Role of the intrarenal renin-angiotensin system in the control of the renal function. *Circ Res* 1981;**48**:157–67.

54 Hall JE, Granger JP. Mechanism of blood pressure and renal haemodynamic effects of captopril. *Am J Cardiol* 1982;**49**:1527–9.

55 Ferguson RK, Turini GA, Brunner HR, Gavras H. A specific orally active inhibitor of angiotensin-converting enzyme in man. *Lancet* 1977;**1**:775–8.

56 Becker RHA, Scholkens B. Ramipril: review of pharmacology. *Am J Cardiol* 1987;**59**:3D–11D.

57 Ulm EH, Hichens M, Gomez HJ *et al.* Enalapril maleate and a lysine analog (MK-521): disposition in man. *Br J Clin Pharmacol* 1982;**14**:357–62.

58 Richer C, Doussau MP, Guidicelli JF. Systemic and regional haemodynamic profile of five angiotensin I converting enzyme inhibitors in the spontaneously hypertensive rat. *Am J Cardiol* 1987;**59**:12D–17D.

59 MacGregor GA, Markandu ND, Bayliss J *et al.* Non-sulfhydryl-containing angiotensin-converting enzyme inhibitor (MK-421): evidence for role of the renin system in normotensive subjects. *Br Med J* 1981;**283**:401–3.

60 Garner MG, Phippard AF, Fletcher PJ *et al.* Effect of angiotensin II on baroreflex control of heart rate in conscious baboons. *Hypertension* 1987;**10**:628–34.

61 Petty MA, Reid JL. Captopril and baroreceptor reflex responses to pressor and depressor stimuli in the rabbit? *J Auton Pharmacol* 1981;**1**:211–15.

62 Ajayi AA, Campbell BC, Meredith A *et al.* The effect of captopril on the reflex control of heart rate: possible mechanisms. *Br J Pharmacol* 1985;**20**:17–25.

63 Mancia G, Parati G, Pomidossi G *et al.* Modification of arterial baroreflexes by captopril in essential hypertension. *Am J Cardiol* 1982;**49**:1415–19.

64 Raman GV, Waller DG, Warren DJ. The effect of captopril on autonomic reflexes in human hypertension. *J Hypertension* 1985;**3**(Suppl 2):111–15.

65 Cody RJ, Bravo EL, Fouad FM, Tarazi RC. Cardiovascular reflexes during long-term converting enzyme inhibiton and sodium depletion. The responses to tilt in hypertensive patients. *Am J Med* 1981;**71**:422–6.

66 Yamashita M, Oyama T, Kudo T. Effect of the inhibitor of angiotensin I converting enzyme on endocrine function and renal perfusion in haemorrhagic shock. *Can Anaesth Soc J* 1977;**24**:695–701.

67 Zierbe RL, Feuerstein G, Kopin IJ. Effect of captopril on cardiovascular, sympathetic and vasopressin responses to haemorrhage. *Eur J Pharmacol* 1981;**72**:391–5.

68 Courneya CA, Korner PI. Neurohumoral mechanisms and the role of arterial baroreceptors in the reno-vascular response to haemorrhage in rabbits. *J Physiol* 1991;**437**:393–407.

69 Mimran A, Ribstein J. Effect of converting enzyme inhibition on the systemic and renal response to acute isotonic volume expansion in normal man. *Clin Sci* 1981;**61**:285-7.
70 Gavras H, Liang CS, Brunner HR. Redistributon of regional blood flow after inhibiton of the angiotensin-converting enzyme. *Circ Res* 1978;3(Suppl I):59-63.
71 Muller AF, Gardiner SM, Compton AM, Bennett T. Regional haemodynamic effects of captopril, enalaprilat and lisinopril in conscious water-replete and water-deprived brattlebroro rats. *Clin Sci* 1990;**79**:393-401.
72 Trachte GJ, Lefer AM. Effect of angiotensin II receptor blockade by [Sar¹-Ala⁸]-angiotensin II in haemorrhagic shock. *Am J Physiol* 1979;**236**(2):H280–H285.
73 Rosenfeld LM, Cooper HS. Captopril and the intestinal response to haemorrhagic shock. *Arch Int Pharmacol Ther* 1982;**259**:144-52.
74 Freeman JG, Hock CE, Edmonds JS, Lefer AM. Anti-shock actions of a new converting enzyme inhibitor, enalaprilic acid, in haemorrhagic shock in cats. *J Pharmacol Exp Ther* 1984;**231**:610-15.
75 Oparil S, Haber E. The renin-angiotensin system (second of two parts). *N Engl J Med* 1974;**391**:446-57.
76 Zhu Z, Tepel M, Neusser M, Mehring N, Zidek W. Effect of captopril on vasoconstriction and Ca++ influx in aortic smooth muslce. *Hypertension* 1993;**22**:806-11.
77 Gräfe M, Bossaller C, Graf K et al. Effect of angiotensin-converting enzyme inhibition on bradykinin metabolism by vascular endothelial cells. *Am J Physiol* 1993;**264**:H1493–H1497.
78 Gerber JG, Franca G, Byyny RL, LoVerde M, Nies AS. The hypotensive action of captopril and enalapril is not prostaglandin dependent. *Clin Pharmacol Ther* 1993;**54**:523-32.
79 Houston MC. The management of hypertension and associated risk factors for the prevention of long-term cardiac complications. *J Cardiovasc Pharmacol* 1993;**21**(Suppl 2):S2-S13.
80 Levine TB, Francis GS, Goldsmith SR et al. Activity of the sympathetic nervous system and renin-angiotensin system assessed by plasma hormone levels and their relationship to haemodynamic abnormalities in congestive heart failure. *Am J Cardiol* 1982;**49**:1659-66.
81 Cohn JN, Franciosa JA. Vasodilator therapy of cardiac failure. *N Engl J Med* 1977;**297**:27-31.
82 Benedict CR, Weiner DH, Johnstone DE et al. Comparative neurohormonal responses in patients with preserved and impaired left ventricular ejection fraction: results of studies of left ventricular dysfuncton (SOLVD) registry. *J Am Coll Cardiol* 1993;**22**(Suppl A):146A-153A.
83 Schunkert H, Tang SS, Litwin SE et al. Regulation of intrarenal and circulating renin-angiotensin systems in severe heart failure in the rat. *Cardiovasc Res* 1993;**27**:731-5.
84 Dzau VJ, Colucci WS, Williams GH et al. Sustained effectiveness of converting-enzyme inhibition in patients with severe congestive heart failure. *N Engl J Med* 1980;**302**:1373-9.
85 Davis R, Ribner HS, Keung E et al. Treatment of chronic congestive heart failure with captopril; an oral inhibitor of converting enzyme. *N Engl J Med* 1979;**301**:117-21.
86 Ader R, Chatterjee K, Ports T et al. Immediate and sustained haemodynamic and clinical improvement in chronic heart failure by an oral angiotensin-converting enzyme inhibitor. *Circulation* 1980;**61**:931-7.
87 Powers ER, Chiaramida A, Demaria AN et al. A double-blind comparison of lisinopril with captopril in patients with symptomatic congestive heart failure. *J Cardiovasc Pharmacol* 1987;**9**(Suppl 3):82-8.
88 Kjekshus J, Sweldberg K, Snapinn S. Effects of enalapril on long-term mortality in severe congestive heart failure. *Am J Cardiol* 1992;**69**:103-7.
89 Kiowski W, Zuber M, Elsasser S et al. Coronary vasodilatation and improved myocardial lactate metabolism after angiotensin converting enzyme inhibition with cilazapril in patients with congestive heart failure. *Am Heart J* 1991;**122**:1382-8.
90 Fonarow GC, Chelimsky-Fallick C, Warner Stevenson L et al. Effect of direct vasodilation with hydralazine versus angiotensin-converting enzyme inhibition with captopril on mortality in advanced heart failure: the Hy-C Trial. *J Am Coll Cardiol* 1992;**19**:842-50.

91 Flapan AD, Nolan JN, Neilson JMM, Ewing DJ. Effect of captopril on cardiac parasympathetic activity in chronic failure secondary to coronary artery disease. *Am J Cardiol* 1992;**69**:532–5.

92 Braunwald E: ACE Inhibitors – a cornerstone of the treatment of heart failure. *N Engl J Med* 1991;**325**:351–3.

93 The SOLVD Investigators. Effect of enalapril on mortality and the development of heart failure in asymptomatic patients with reduced left ventricular ejection fractions. *N Engl J Med* 1992;**327**:685–91.

94 Oldroyd KG, Pye MP, Ray SG *et al*. Effects of early captopril administration on infarct expansion, left ventricular remodeling and exercise capacity after acute myocardial infarction. *Am J Cardiol* 1991;**68**:713–18.

95 Bonaduce D, Petretta M, Arrichiello P *et al*. Effects of captopril treatment on left ventricular remodeling and function after anterior myocardial infarction: comparison with digitalis. *J Am Coll Cardiol* 1992;**19**:858–63.

96 Pfeffer MA, Braunwald E, Moyé LA *et al*. Effect of captopril on mortality and morbidity in patients with left ventricular dysfunction after myocardial infarction. Results of the Survival and Ventricular Enlargement Trial. *N Engl J Med* 1992;**327**:669–77.

97 Sweberg K, Held P, Kjekshus J *et al*. Effects of the early administration of enalapril on the mortality in patients with acute myocardial infarction. Results of the Cooperative New Scandinavian Enalapril Survival Study II. *N Engl J Med* 1992;**327**:678–84.

98 Cohn JN. The prevention of heart failure – a new agenda. *N Engl J Med* 1992;**327**:725–7.

99 Ball SG and The Acute Infarction Ramipril Efficacy (AIRE) Study Investigators. Effect of ramipril on mortality and morbidity of survivors of acute myocardial infarction with clinical evidence of heart failure. *Lancet* 1993;**342**:821–8.

100 Bonarjee VVS, Carstensen S, Caidahl K, Nilsen DWT, Edner M, Berning J, Concensus II Multi-Echo Study Group. Attenuation of left ventricular dilatation after acute myocardial infarction by early initiation of enalapril therapy. *Am J Cardiol* 1993;**72**:1004–9.

101 Pouleur H, Rousseau MF, van Eyll C *et al*. Effects of long-term enalapril therapy on left ventricular diastolic properties in patients with depressed ejection fraction. *Circulation* 1993;**88**:481–91.

102 Ertl G. Angiotensin converting enzyme inhibitors in angina and myocardial infarction. What role will they play in the 1990s? *Drugs* 1993;**46**:209–18.

103 Przyklend K, Kloner RA. 'Cardioprotection' by ACE-inhibitors in acute myocardial ischaemia and infarction? *Basic Res Cardiol* 1993;**88**(Suppl 1):139–54.

104 Curtis MJ, Pugsley MK, Walker MJA. Endogenous chemical mediators of ventricular arrhythmias in ischaemic heart disease. *Cardiovasc Res* 1993;**27**:703–19.

105 Vogt M, Motz W, Strauer BE. ACE-inhibitors in coronary artery disease? *Basis Res Cardiol* 1993;**88**(Suppl 1):43–64.

106 Zughaib ME, Sun JZ, Boli R. Effect of angiotensin-converting enzyme inhibitors on myocardial ischaemia/reperfuson injury: an overview. *Basic Res Cardiol* 1993;**88**(Suppl 1):155–67.

107 Weber KT, Brilla CG, Campbell SE, Guarda E, Zhou G, Sriram K. Myocardial fibrosis: role of angiotensin II and aldosterone. *Basic Res Cardiol* 1993;**88**(Suppl 1):107–21.

108 Desmet W, Vrolix M, De Scheerder I, Van Lierde J, Willems JL, Piessens J. Angiotensin-converting enzyme inhibition with fosinopril sodium in the prevention of restenosis after coronary angioplasty. *Circulation* 1994;**89**:385–92.

109 Heyndrickx GR, MERCATOR Study Group. Angiotensin-converting enzyme inhibitor in a human model of restenosis. *Basic Res Cardiol* 1993;**88**(Suppl 1):169–82.

110 Sutton M St J. Should angiotensin converting enzyme (ACE) inhibitors be used routinely after infarction? Perspectives from the survival and ventricular enlargement (SAVE) Trial. *Br Heart J* 1994;**71**:115–18.

111 Ikram H, Low CJS, Shirlaw TM *et al*. Angiotensin converting enzyme inhibition in chronic stable angina: effects on myocardial ischaemia and comparison with nifedipine. *Br Heart J* 1994;**71**:30–3.

112 Hollenberg NK, Swartz SL, Passan DR, Williams GH. Increased glomerular filtration rate after converting-enzyme inhibition in essential hypertension. *N Engl J Med*

1979;**301**:9–12.
113 Ichikawa I, Pfeffer JM, Pfeffer MA *et al.* Role of angiotensin II in the altered renal function of congestive heart failure. *Circ Res* 1984;**55**:669–75.
114 Packer M, Huang Lee W, Yushak M, Medina N. Comparison of captopril and enalapril in patients with severe chronic heart failure. *N Engl J Med* 1986;**315**:847–53.
115 Fernandez-Repollet E, Tapia E, Martinez-Maldonado M. Effects of angiotensin-converting enzyme inhibition on altered renal haemodynamics induced by low protein diet in the rat. *J Clin Invest* 1987;**80**:1045–9.
116 Taguma Y, Kitamoto Y, Futaki G *et al.* Effect of captopril on heavy proteinuria in azotemic diabetics. *N Engl J Med* 1985;**313**:1617–20.
117 Matsukawa K, Ninomiya I, Nishiura N. Effects of anaesthesia on cardiac and renal sympathetic nerve activities and plasma catecholamines. *Am J Physiol* 1993;**265**:R793–R797.
118 Hopf HB, Schlaghecke R, Peters J. Sympathetic neural blockade by epidural anaesthesia suppresses renin release in response to arterial hypotension. *Anesthesiology* 1994;**80**:992–9.
119 Zayas VM, Blumenfeld JD, Bading B *et al.* Adrenergic regulation of renin secretion and renal haemodynamics during deliberate hypotension in humans. *Am J Physiol* 1993;**265**:F686–F692.
120 Miller ED, Longnecker DE, Peach MJ. The regulatory function of the renin-angiotensin system during general anaesthesia. *Anesthesiology* 1978;**48**:399–403.
121 Pettinger WA. Anesthetics and the renin–angiotensin aldosterone axis. *Anesthesiology* 1978;**48**:393–6.
122 Robertson D, Michelakis AM. Effect of anaesthesia and surgery on plasma renin activity in man. *J Clin Endocrinol* 1972;**34**:831–6.
123 Ecoffey C, Edouard A, Pruszczynnski W *et al.* Effects of epidural anaesthesia on catecholamines, renin activity and vasopressin changes induced by tilt in elderly men. *Anesthesiology* 1985;**62**:294–7.
124 Carp H, Vadhera R, Jayaram A, Garvey D. Endogenous vasopressin and renin–angiotensin systems support blood pressure after epidural block in humans. *Anesthesiology* 1994;**80**:1000–7.
125 Murphy JD, Vaughan RS, Rosen M. Intravenous enalaprilat and autonomic reflexes. *Anaesthesia* 1989;**44**:816–21.
126 McCarthy GJ, Hainsworth M, Lindsay K *et al.* Pressor responses to tracheal intubation after sublingual captopril. *Anaesthesia* 1990;**45**:243–5.
127 Ullman JE, Hjelmqvist H, Rundgren M, Leksell LG. Anaesthesia effects of vasopressin antagonism and angiotensin I converting enzyme inhibition during halothane anaesthesia in sheep. *Acta Anaesthesiol Scand* 1992;**36**:132–7.
128 Frederick G, Welt P, Rutlen DL. Effect of vasopressin on systemic capacity. *Am J Physiol* 1991;**261**:H1494–H1498.
129 Dagnino J, Prys-Roberts C. Studies of anaesthesia in relation to hypertension. VI: cardiovascular responses to extradural blockade of treated and untreated hypertensive patients. *Br J Anaesth* 1984;**56**:1065–73.
130 Folkow B. Physiological aspects of primary hypertension. *Physiol. Rev* 1982;**62**:347–504.
131 Coriat P, Richer C, Douraki T *et al.* Influence of chronic angiotensin-converting enzyme inhibition on anaesthetic induction. *Anesthesiology* 1994;**81**:299–307.
132 Colson P, Saussine M, Séguin JR *et al.* Haemodynamic effects of anaesthesia in patients chronically teated with angiotensin-converting enzyme inhibitors. *Anesth Analg* 1992;**74**:805–8.
133 Blake DW, Way D, Trigg L *et al.* Cardiovascular effects of volatile anaesthesia in rabbits: influence of chronic heart failure and enalaprilat treatment. *Anesth Analg* 1991;**73**:441–8.
134 Doherty NE, Seelos KC, Suzuki JI *et al.* Application of cine nuclear magnetic resonance imaging for sequential evaluation of response to angiotensin-converting enzyme inhibitor therapy in dilated cardiomyopathy. *J Am Coll Cardiol* 1992;**19**:1294–302.
135 Wisenbaugh T, Essop R, Rothlisberger C, Sareli P. Effects of a single oral dose of captopril on left ventricular performance in severe mitral regurgitation. *Am J Cardiol*

1992;**69**:348–53.

136 Acampora GA, Melendez JA, Keefe DL *et al.* Intraoperative administration of the intravenous angiotensin-converting enzyme inhibitor, enalaprilat, in a patient with congestive heart failure. *Anaesth Analg* 1989;**69**:833–9.

137 Colson P, Ryckwaert F, Calvet B, Raison D, Valat J, Roquefeuil B. Haemodynamic effect of anaesthesia in patients with congestive heart failure treated with ACE inhibitors (abstract). *Anesthesiology* 1993;**79**:A88.

138 Böttcher M, Behrens K, Moller EA, Christensen JH, Andreasen E. ACE inhibitor premedication attenuates sympathetic responses during surgery. *Br J Anaesth* 1994;**72**:633–7.

139 Woodside J, Garner L, Bedford RF *et al.* Captopril reduces the dose requirement of sodium nitroprusside inducted hypotension. *Anesthesiology* 1984;**60**:413–17.

140 Baker CH, Sutton ET, Dietz JR. Endotoxin alteration of muscle microvascular renin-angiotensin responses. *Circ Shock* 1992;**36**:224–30.

141 Cashman JN, Jones RM, Thompson MA. Renin–angiotensin activation is not primarily responsible for the changes in mean arterial pressure during sternotomy in patients undergoing cardiac surgery. *Eur J Anaesthesiol* 1984;**1**:299–303.

142 Boldt J, Schindler E, Härter K, Görlach G, Hempelmann G. Influence of intravenous administration of angiotensin-converting enzyme inhibitor enalaprilat on cardiovascular mediators in cardiac surgery patients. *Anesth Analg* 1995;**80**:480–5.

143 Bailey DR, Miller ED, Kaplan JA, Rogers PW. The renin-angiotensin-aldosterone system during cardiac surgery with morphine-nitrous oxide anaesthesia. *Anesthesiolgoy* 1975;**42**:538–44.

144 Lehot JJ, Villard J, Piriz H *et al.* Haemodynamic and hormonal responses to hypothermic and normothermic cardiopulmonary bypass. *J Cardiothorac Vasc Anesth* 1992;**6**:132–9.

145 Taylor KM, Morton IJ, Brown JJ *et al.* Hypertension and the renin-angiotensin system following open-heart surgery. *J Thorac Cardiovasc Surg* 1977;**74**:840–5.

146 Tuman KJ, McCarthy RJ, O'Connor CJ, Holm WE, Ivankovitch AD. Angiotensin-converting enzyme inhibitors increase vasoconstrictor requirements after cardiopulmonary bypass. *Anesth Analg* 1995;**80**:473–9.

147 Thaker U, Geary V, Chalmers P, Sheikh F. Low systemic vascular resistance during cardiac surgery: case reports, brief review, and management with angiotensin II. *J Cardiothorac Vasc Anesth* 1990;**4**:360–3.

148 Berkowitz HD, Shetty S. Renin release and renal cortical ischemia following aortic cross clamping. *Arch Surg* 1974;**109**:612–17.

149 Gal TJ, Cooperman LH, Berkowitz HD. Plasma renin activity in patients undergoing surgery of the abdominal aorta. *Ann Surg* 1973;**179**:65–9.

150 Gamulin Z, Forster A, Morel D *et al.* Effects of infrarenal aortic cross-clamping on renal haemodynamics in humans. *Anesthesiology* 1984;**61**:394–9.

151 Colson P, Ribstein J, Séguin JR *et al.* Mechanisms of renal haemodynamic impairment during infrarenal aortic cross-clamping. *Anesth Analg* 1992;**75**:18–23.

4: Antiarrhythmic agents

JEAN EMMANUEL de la COUSSAYE,
JEAN-JACQUES ELEDJAM

Several problems have been identified in the perioperative management of patients receiving antiarrhythmic treatment. All antiarrhythmic drugs induce a decrease in myocardial contractility.[1-3] Moreover, the margin of safety between their levels of efficacy and toxicity is often narrowed.[4] It is therefore essential that their pharmacology is understood. On the other hand, drugs used in anaesthetic practice also have electrophysiological effects and these have to be taken into account in evaluating possible interactions between anaesthetic and antiarrhythmic agents. Such interactions could induce or worsen conduction defects, arrhythmias and/or haemodynamic disturbances. Thus, when a patient presenting for operation is receiving antiarrhythmic treatment, the anaesthesiologist must determine why this medication has been given and whether there is a non-cardiac cause facilitating the occurrence of rhythm and/or conduction disturbances. Cardiac function should be evaluated and cardiac disease sought.[5-10] Any such concurrent heart disease will itself require management during the perioperative period.

Pharmacology of antiarrhythmic drugs

Many agents, such as digitalis, magnesium, or adenosine, can suppress arrhythmias by correcting electolyte or acid–base disorders, and/or by relieving cardiac failure or the effects of coronary artery disease.[11, 12] However, the term 'antiarrhythmic' is reserved for drugs that induce changes in the ionic currents responsible for the cardiac action potential.[13, 14] The *in vivo* antiarrhythmic property of these drugs comes from their additive effects on cardiac electrophysiology, myocardial vascularisation, and the autonomic nervous system.[15, 16] This could explain why two antiarrhythmic drugs may have similar electrophysiological effects but one drug will act preferentially on atrial arrhythmias while another will act on ventricular arrhythmias.[17]

The Vaughan Williams classification of antiarrhythmic effects[18-20] has been debated because it focuses only on cellular electrophysiological mechanisms. Moreover, one drug can act in several classes. Other

74

classifications based on electrophysiological and/or clinical data have therefore been proposed.[21-27] More recently, the working group on arrhythmias of the European Society of Cardiology proposed a new classification (the 'Sicilian Gambit'),[28] including electrophysiological effects, effects on the autonomic nervous system, and actions on arrhythmogenic mechanisms. Nevertheless, the classification of Vaughan Williams remains commonly used and will therefore be featured in this chapter (Tables 4.1 and 4.2). Finally, not all antiarrhythmic drugs are available in all countries, and the list offered here will not be exhaustive.

Table 4.1   Effects of Class 1 antiarrhythmic drugs

Class 1	Local anaesthetic effect=inhibition of fast inward sodium current (decrease in $\dot{V}_{max}$ of phase 0 of fast AP)=decrease in conduction velocity, excitability and automaticity
Sub-class 1a (quinidine, procainamide, disopyramide)	Moderated decrease in $\dot{V}_{max}$ APD prolongation ERP prolongation Lengthening of ERP/APD →QRS widening and jT lengthening
Sub-class 1b (lignocaine, mexiletine, diphenylhydantoin)	Mild decrease in $\dot{V}_{max}$ Shortening of APD and ERP Decrease in ERP/APD QRS and QT unchanged
Sub-class 1c (flecainide, propafenone, cibenzoline)	Marked decrease in $\dot{V}_{max}$ APD and ERP not or slightly modified QRS widening, jT not modified

AP, action potential; APD, action potential duration; ERP, effective refractory period.

Table 4.2   Vaughan Williams classification: classes 2, 3, and 4

Class 2 beta-blocking agents	Decrease in automaticity (SN and AVN) due to decrease in slope of spontaneous diastolic depolarisation Shortening of APD (ventricles) ERP slightly or not modified (atria and ventricles), or lengthened (AVN) QRS unchanged, QT unchanged or shortened, PR lengthened
Class 3 possible interaction with Na–Ca exchange, decrease in potassium channel current i_K (phase 3)	APD and ERP prolongation, increase in ERP/APD QRS unchanged, QT lengthened
Class 4 calcium-channel blocking drugs	Decrease in $\dot{V}_{max}$ of slow action potential Decrease in spontaneous diastolic depolarisation (SN and AVN) Increase in ERP (AVN) APD shortening (decrease in phase 2 of fast AP)

SN, sinus node; AVN, atrioventricular node; AP, action potential.

Class 1 antiarrhythmic drugs

The main effect of class 1 antiarrhythmic drugs is to inhibit the fast inward sodium current i_{Na}.[29] The maximum upstroke velocity, which is represented by the peak of the first derivative of phase 0 of atrial and ventricular action potentials (V_{max}), is therefore decreased. As the V_{max} is correlated to the conduction velocities, class 1 antiarrhythmic drugs therefore slow conduction velocities and widen the QRS complex. This is the main antiarrhythmic effect of propafenone and flecainide, while quinidine and disopyramide have other effects, such as inducing an increase in the duration of the action potential.[30–32] The efficacy of class 1 antiarrhythmic drugs also depends on their in-, out- kinetic on the sodium channel receptors (fast or slow block and recovery), on the state of the channel, and therefore on the heart rate. Quinidine and flecainide act mainly in the activated state of the cardiac sodium channel, while lignocaine interacts mainly in the inactivated state.[33–37] Moreover, the kinetic of block and recovery is different in the three subclasses,[38, 39] being fast in class 1B antiarrhythmic drugs, slow in class 1C and intermediate in class 1A.[40, 41] Thus, the faster the heart rate or the more depolarised the cardiac cells, the more inhibited the V_{max} owing to a greater receptor saturation induced by antiarrhythmic drugs. Moreover, the V_{max} is further decreased when this is a class 1C agent.

Class 1A antiarrhythmic drugs[42]

Quinidine and hydroquinidine

Electrophysiological effects (see Table 4.1) Quinidine decreases the slope of spontaneous diastolic depolarisation at low concentration and increases the threshold potential at high concentration.[43] It suppresses the normal automaticity of Purkinje fibres and ectopic pacemakers.[44] However, quinidine is not effective in arrhythmias caused by abnormal automaticity and after-depolarisations.[45]

These drugs have a vagolytic effect and induce sympathetic stimulation; they therefore increase the heart rate. They lengthen conduction times of the atrioventricular node (AVN, AH interval) and of the His–Purkinje system (HV interval) by direct effect. However, the AH interval is often shortened due to the vagolytic effect, so that the PR interval – consequent upon the AH and HV intervals – is not always altered. QRS widening and QT lengthening ($QT = QRS + jT$) are dependent on the plasma concentration and are useful for monitoring ($QT < 500$ ms).

Haemodynamic effects Quinidine depresses myocardial contractility and induces vasodilatation by blocking the α-adrenoceptors.[46] A decrease in blood pressure can thus be observed.

Indications Quinidine and its derivatives can be used to terminate ventricular or atrial arrhythmias. However, during an atrial tachycardial (flutter, or other variant), they can paradoxically accelerate the ventricular rate. This is due to slowing of the atrial rate and acceleration of conduction in the AVN.[44] The main indication for this group of drugs is prevention of atrial tachycardias. They are also used in supraventricular dysrhythmias in patients with Wolff–Parkinson–White syndrome because they slow conduction and lengthen the refractory period of accessory pathways.[47] Quinidine and its derivatives are particularly indicated in the prevention of recurrence of atrial arrhythmias.[48]

The oral dose of quinidine is 200–600 mg every 6 hours. There is effective digestive absorption and peak plasma concentration is obtained in 2 hours. First-pass hepatic metabolism occurs. The elimination half-life is 6 hours. Elimination is renal, with active and inactive metabolites after hepatic metabolisation. In renal, cardiac or hepatic failure dosage has to be reduced. Urine alkalinisation decreases renal excretion by more than 50%.[44] Therapeutic plasma levels are in the range 2–6 µg/ml, with toxic levels higher than 8 µg/ml.

Adverse effects Quinidine and its derivatives can induce conduction defects, depending on the dose and the cardiac state. In contrast, the occurrence of quinidine syncope does not seem to be related to dosage. It is due rather to torsades de pointes induced by lengthening of the QT interval.[49] Quinidine and its derivatives can also induce diarrhoea, vomiting, nausea, dizziness, visual disorders, hypoacousy, worsening of myasthenia gravis, a reaction of hypersensibility with fever, cutaneous disorders, thrombocytopena, and pancytopenia.

Quinidine increases plasma concentrations of digoxin. In contrast, hepatic enzyme inducers accelerate its metabolism. Combined with oral anticoagulants, it can induce haemorrhagic disorders whose mechanisms are not fully understood. Quinidine potentiates the effects of non-depolarising muscle relaxants.

Disopyramide
Electrophysiological effects Effects are similar to those of quinidine, although the vagolytic effect is more marked and the atrial and ventricular effective refractory periods are more lengthened. In contrast, disopyramide has a less significant action on the His–Purkinje system.[42] ECG modifications are similar to those induced by quinidine.

Haemodynamic effects Disopyramide can markedly impair myocardial contractility and precipitate latent cardiac failure.[50]

Indications Indications are similar to those of quinidine.[51, 52] The oral dose is 400–800 mg in three or four divided doses per day. In a slow-release form administration is two times per day. Digestive absorption is almost complete, with a peak plasma concentration reached at between 30 and 120 minutes. The half-life is 5–8 hours. Plasma protein binding is variable and non-linear; low protein binding may result in toxic plasma levels of free disopyramide.[42] Partially metabolised by the liver, elimination is 80% renal and 20% faecal; dosage has therefore to be reduced in renal failure. Therapeutic plasma levels range between 1·7 and 4 μg/ml, with the toxic level >7 μg/ml.[42]

Adverse effects Disopyramide has the same disadvantages as quinidine but induces a more marked impairment of myocardial contractility. These anticholinergic effects can induce urinary retention, constipation, and severe hypoglycaemia. Disopyramide prolongs the action of non-depolarising muscle relaxants and increases the plasma level of free lignocaine.

Procainamide

Electrophysiological effects These are similar to those of quinidine, but with a more marked local anaesthetic effect and with a less vagolytic action. ECG modifications induced by procainamide are similar to quinidine, but the PR interval is more likely to be lengthened.

Haemodynamic effects Procainamide depresses myocardial contractility and provokes vasodilatation via a ganglioplegic effect. Hypotension can therefore occur. It has no α-blocking effect.[44]

Indications Procainamide is especially used by the intravenous route in the termination of ventricular arrhythmias.[53, 54] Indeed, it has a marked action on the circular movement of re-entrant ventricular tachycardias.[55]

The oral dose is 500–1000 mg every 4 hours. Digestive absorption is almost complete, with a peak plasma concentration at 1 hour with no effect of first-pass hepatic metabolism.[43] It is metabolised in the liver by acetylation with inactive and active metabolites (N-procainamide or NAPA).

Procainamide has a short half-life (3–4 hours). It is eliminated by the kidney. NAPA has a longer half-life (7 hours) but is less potent than procainamide, with class 3 effects[56] (therapeutic levels of NAPA: 2–22 μg/ml). Doses of procainamide should be reduced in patients with slow hepatic acetylation, impairment of renal function or severe cardiac failure. Intravenous injection must never be rapid because it can induce cardiovascular collapse or cardiac arrest. Dosage is from 1 to 1·5 mg/kg over 2–4 minutes repeated every 5 minutes until termination of tachycardia, without exceeding 1 g. The ECG and blood pressure must be monitored during injection.[44] Infusion doses are from 20 to 80 μg/kg/min. Therapeutic plasma levels are in the range 4–10 μg/ml (toxicity >12–15 μg/ml).[43]

Adverse effects Adverse effects are dose-dependent and are similar to quinidine, although torsades de pointes is seen less often. Procainamide can also induce a lupus syndrome during chronic administration. Indeed, 50–70% of patients treated for 12 months have positive antinuclear antibodies, and 30% show cerebral, renal, and pericardial clinical manifestations. This lupic syndrome is reversible after stopping procainamide treatment.[44]

Class 1B antiarrhythmic drugs[57]

Lignocaine

Electrophysiological effects[58–60] (see Table 4.1)   Lignocaine has no marked effect on the autonomic nervous system. Its properties are enhanced by hyperkalaemia, acidosis, and hypoxia.[61–67] It decreases abnormal and normal automaticity[68] and raises the threshold of ventricular fibrillation.[69, 70] Lignocaine is especially effective on ischaemic cells because they become unexcitable. This explains its efficacy on arrhythmias due to ischaemia reperfusion.[71]

Haemodynamic effects   Lignocaine at therapeutic levels has no haemodynamic effects.

Indications   Lignocaine has an immediate antiarrhythmic action but it is effective only on ventricular arrhythmias, especially during the acute phase of myocardial infarction, in cardiac surgery, and during digitalis intoxication.[72] It is effective in suppression of ventricular premature contractions, and in ventricular tachycardias, and can avoid the occurrence of ventricular fibrillation.[48, 69, 70]

The usual iv dose is 1–1·5 mg/kg. One repeated dose of 0·5–1 mg/kg can be added. The recommended infusion rate is 15–50 μg/kg/min so as to obtain plasma levels of 1·5–5 μg/ml. By the intramuscular route, the dose is 4–5 mg/kg. The therapeutic rate is obtained in 15 minutes, for a duration of 90 minutes.[72, 73] Nevertheless its prophylactic use in the acute phase of mycardial infarction is not recommended because of the proarrhythmic effects of class 1B antiarrhythmic drugs.[74]

The half-life is short (100 minutes). Seventy per cent of lignocaine is bound to plasma proteins and is metabolised by the liver. Thus, any decline of the hepatic blood flow decreases its clearance, and in this case dosage must be reduced by 50%.[44]

Adverse effects   Side effects are dose-dependent, and tremor, confusion, a metallic taste in the mouth, convulsions, and coma are seen. Carciotoxicity is rarer; it occurs especially in cases of cardiac disease with myocardial depression, sometimes associated with serious conduction defects.[75–82]

Mexiletine

Electrophysiological, ECG, and haemodynamic effects and indications of mexiletine are similar to those of lignocaine.[83] Additionally, mexiletine is effective by the oral route. The dose is 200 mg every 6–8 hours which promotes a therapeutic plasma level in 1–3 days (0.75–2 μg/ml).[84] Absorption by the oral route is 75%, with no first-pass hepatic metabolism. Peak plasma concentration is obtained in 2–4 hours. The half-life of mexiletine is 10–15 hours, with some hepatic metabolism but mainly renal elimination. Hepatic, renal or cardiac failure necessitates a reduction in dosage. Similarly, combination with digitalis necessitates a reduction in dosage of both.[85]

Class 1C antiarrhythmic drugs

Flecainide

Electrophysiological effects (see Table 4.1) Flecainide acts on both atrial and ventricular arrhythmias and can depress the sinus function.[86, 87] It is effective for reperfusion arrhythmias but does not act on early after-depolarisations induced by barium.[88] It induces PR lengthening and QRS widening without major alteration of ventricular repolarisation represented on ECG by the jT interval. Flecainide provokes a prolonged sodium channel blockade.[89] This marked use-dependent effect is responsible for a QRS widening proportional to heart rate.[90, 91] Finally, flecainide raises the pacing threshold of implanted pacemakers, which may necessitate reprogramming.

Haemodynamic effects Flecainide does not induce dramatic haemodynamic depression in the healthy patient. In contrast, the ejection fraction can be decreased by more than 20% in congestive cardiac failure.[2]

Indications Flecainide is highly effective in terminating and preventing ventricular and atrial arrhythmias in a healthy heart.[92–97] It is also effective on junctional tachycardias with or without accessory pathway.

Flecainide given by the oral route has good bioavailability. Peak plasma concentration is reached at 2–4 hours with a prolonged elimination half-life of 12 hours in the healthy subject and 30 hours in the presence of congestive cardiac failure.[84, 98] Elimination is hepatic and renal. Renal elimination is decreased by alkaline pH[99] and the dose has therefore to be reduced in renal failure. Dosage is in the range 100–300 mg/day by mouth in two divided doses. In case of cardiac failure or conduction defects an initial total of 100 mg/day given in two doses is recommended. Therapeutic plasma levels are in the range 0.2–1 μg/ml. During treatment, close monitoring of widening of the QRS complex is required; a widening greater than 40 msec demands dose reduction.[100]

Adverse effects As with all potent antiarrhythmic drugs, flecainide can induce serious side effects. Proarrhythmic efffects,[97, 101–103] conduction defects at rest and during exercise[90, 104] and atrioventricular blocks can be seen. It can also precipitate cardiac failure.[2] Although a cardioprotective effect of class 1 antiarrhythmic drugs has been demonstrated experimentally on ischaemic myocardium,[88, 105] flecainide is ineffective in the prevention of sudden death after myocardial infarction. Indeed, in these patients, the CAST study reported a higher mortality in the group treated with flecainide or encainide than in placebo-treated controls.[106] Flecainide can be responsible for digestive disorders, dizziness, tremors, and visual disorders. Finally, flecainide increases the plasma level of digoxin and, in combination with propranolol, there is a resultant elevation of plasma levels of both propranolol and flecainide.

Propafenone[107]

Electrophysiological effects (see Table 4.1) Propafenone produces slight class 2 and 4 antiarrhythmic effects. It slows conduction velocity in accessory pathways and can increase the pacing threshold of stimulation of implanted pacemakers. Moreover, it induces sinus bradycardia, lengthens the PR interval (AH and HV) and widens the QRS complex in a frequency-dependent manner.[108–111] However, the jT interval is not modified.[112]

Haemodynamic effects Propafenone has slight haemodynamic effects on the healthy heart. It produces a moderate decrease of contractility,[43] blood pressure, and cardiac output.[113] These effects are more marked where there is pre-existing congestive cardiac failure.[114–116]

Indications Propafenone is used for terminating and preventing supraventricular and ventricular arrhythmias and in Wolff–Parkinson–White syndrome.[114, 117–124] After oral administration there is first-pass hepatic metabolism with significant inter-individual variations, so that a slight dose increase can induce a marked elevation of plasma level. Peak plasma concentration is reached at 2–3 hours. Elimination half-life is 7–8 hours and the liver is responsible for metabolism. Dosage must be decreased in hepatic, renal or cardiac failure. Similarly, dosage of digitalis,[85, 125] warfarin, metoprolol, quinidine, and theophylline[107, 126] must be reduced in combination with propafenone. Total daily dose by the oral route varies from 450 to 1200 mg; 900 mg given in three divided doses is usual (therapeutic plasma level: 0·5–1·5 μ/ml).

Adverse effects Propafenone has the same adverse effects as other class 1C antiarrhythmic drugs.

Cibenzoline[127]

Electrophysiological effects Cibenzoline, although classified as a 1C drug, mimics both *in vitro*[128, 129] and *in vivo*[130] effects produced by class 1A and also has class 4 antiarrhythmic effects. Moreover, it inhibits the ATP-dependent potassium current.[131] It is slightly vagolytic. It slows conduction velocity in the His–Purkinje system and in the ventricular myocardium, and lengthens ventricular effective refractory periods. Atrial and AV node conducion is slightly modified.[132] Cibenzoline also slows conduction in accessory pathways and sometimes induces a slight increase in heart rate.[133] Finally, it widens the QRS complex and slightly lengthens the QT interval.

Haemodynamic effects By the intravenous route, cibenzoline induces a slight decrease of myocardial contractility in the healthy patient. This effect is more marked in the presence of cardiac failure. Oral administration is usually well tolerated.

Indications Cibenzoline is indicated in the prevention and termination of supraventricular or ventricular arrhythmias and in Wolff–Parkinson–White syndrome.[134–136] Bioavailability is good when given by the oral route, with no first-pass hepatic metabolism. Peak plasma concentration is reached at 90 minutes; elimination half-life is about 4–5 hours but can be longer than 7 hours in congestive cardiac failure and during the acute phase of myocardial infarction.[43] Elimination is mainly renal. Dosage must be reduced in renal or cardiac failure. Administration is usually oral, with a dose of 4–6 mg/kg per day given in three divided doses (therapeutic plasma level: 0·3–0·4 μg/ml).

Adverse effects Cibenzoline can induce both conduction defects and proarrhythmic effects, and precipitate cardiac failure.[137] Like all class 1 antiarrhythmic drugs, it is also responsible for minor neurological and digestive disorders.

Class 2 antiarrhythmic drugs

Class 2 antiarrhythmic drugs are represented by the β-blocking agents, which are discussed in Chapter 1.

Class 3 antiarrhythmic drugs

Amiodarone[138, 139]

Electrophysiological effects (see Table 4.2) These are complex and imperfectly understood. The class 3 effect seems to be mainly due to the inhibition of i_k current.[140] The action of amiodarone differs according to the mode of administration.[141] By the intravenous route it slightly modifies atrial, His–Purkinje system, and ventricular effective refractory periods but amiodarone markedly lengthens AV node and accessory pathway effective refractory periods.[32] Moreover, it decreases sinus rate[142] and AV node conduction. In chronic administration, in addition to its class 3 action, amiodarone induces a class 4 effect proportional to the frequency of stimulation,[143-145] and class 1 effect.[146-149] The class 1 effect is also use-dependent.[150] It therefore slows ventricular conduction velocity by altering longitudinal rather than transverse conduction velocities.[151] It also has α- and β-adrenergic non-competititve antagonistic actions,[152-153] and blocks conversion of T4 to T3.[56] The mechanism is a down-regulation of β-adrenoceptors.[154] These effects, which appear from the second day and increase with the duration of treatment,[155, 156] are due to an antagonism between amiodarone and T3.[157, 158] Finally, amiodarone inhibits the microsomal Na-K-ATP-ase activity.[159]

Haemodynamic effects   The intravenous administration of amiodarone induces a drop in blood pressure and depresses left ventricular end-diastolic pressure and arterial resistance. This action is in part due to the solvent.[160] Moreover, there is an increase in coronary blood flow and a decrease in myocardial oxygen consumption, also partly due to the solvent.[161] In cardiac failure, cardiac output increases but blood pressure can fall in a significant but unpredictable manner through reduced contractility and arterial vasodilatation.[162, 163] Slow administration, by infusion or by the oral route, induces few haemodynamic side effects at rest.[164] However, prolonged administration produces a summation of class 1, 2, 3 and 4 effects that can be potentially deleterious to haemodynamic status and to conduction during anaesthesia.[165]

Indications   Amiodarone is used for the termination or prevention of all arrhythmias.[166-174] Although it has been proposed in the treatment of torsades de pointes during lengthening of the QT interval, it remains contraindicated in this condition.[175] Preliminary study results suggests that amiodarone is effective in prevention of post-infarction sudden death.[176, 177] However, it appears that small dosage regimes are more effective and less toxic than larger doses,[1, 178] even in the case of congestive cardiac failure.[178-182] By the oral route, the first dose is between 600 and 2000 mg/24 h (30 mg/kg) followed by 200–400 mg once daily. Digestive absorption is slow and incomplete, with peak plasma concentration reached in 4–7 hours and the steady state obtained in 3–5 weeks during chronic treatment;[156] this period can be shortened to one week by giving a large first dose.[166] Amiodarone is metabolised by the liver with an active metabolite, N-desethylamiodarone (NDA). The half-life is 14–20 hours after a single dose and 20–60 days in long-term administration. Amiodarone is widely distributed throughout the tissues. Iodides bind especially in the thyroid gland and are eliminated by the kidney. Therapeutic levels are $0.5–3$ μg/ml with great individual variation. Lengthening of the QT interval is closely correlated to the myocardial concentration of amiodarone.

Adverse effects   Torsades de pointes has been described following amiodarone but a direct causation has not been completely proven and is even controversial.[175] It can also induce AV block and sinus dysfunction.[183] During prolonged treatment, it can cause hypo- or hyperthyroidism,[184] hepatitis, corneal microdeposits, cutaneous pigmentation and photosensitivity. Pulmonary fibrosis[185] may also occur but regress on cessation of amiodarone, with treatment by corticosteroids or after plasmapheresis.[186] Side effects necessitate the discontinuation of treatment in more than 30% of patients.[143, 168, 187] These adverse effects are facilitated by long-term treatment using large doses.[185, 188] Finally, amiodarone can increase the concentration of digitalis[185] and DPH, and potentiate the effects of heparin and oral anticoagulants.

Class 4 antiarrhythmic drugs

Class 4 antiarrhythmic drugs are represented by the calcium-channel blocking agents. Three agents are used as antiarrhythmic drugs: verapamil, diltiazem, and bepridil.[189] These are discussed in Chapter 2.

Electrophysiological effects of anaesthetic agents and their possible interactions with antiarrhythmic drugs

Agents used for anaesthesia have electrophysiological and haemodynamic effects. The choice of anaesthetic technique has therefore to take into account the specific antiarrhythmic treatment of an individual patient and the underlying cardiac disorder. Failure to observe these precautions risks the induction of an increased antiarrhythmic effect, giving rise to or worsening conduction defects, and promoting haemodynamic depression and/or the occurrence of an arrhythmogenic effect.

Halogenated volatile anaesthetics

Halogenated volatile anaesthetics produce antiarrhythmic effects but can also facilitate the occurrence of arrhythmias.[190-196] In concentrations greater than 0·5%, they act in a dose-dependent manner at all levels of the heart by altering, in a non-uniform manner, the different electrophysiological structures.[190, 194, 197-200]

On the sinus node and atrioventricular node, halogenated volatile anaesthetics induce bradycardia and lengthening of the PR inteval. They decrease the $\dot{V}_{max}$ of phase 0 of slow action potentials and lengthen refractory periods of the atrioventricular node.[201-203] These actions are more marked with halothane and enflurane than with isoflurane. The effects of these agents are similar to those of calcium-channel blockers; indeed, they decrease the calcium entry through the slow calcium channel.[204-209] This suggests potentiation of effects with the calcium-channel blockers.[208, 210-212] Beta-blocking agents also act at the same level, and can theoretically worsen bradycardia and/or induce AV block. The potentiation of electrophysio-logical and haemodynamic effects of halogenated volatile anaesthetics with verapamil is clinically relevant, while it is less marked with diltiazem. Intravenous administration of diltiazem in dogs anaesthetised with halo-thane slightly lengthens the PR interval, decreases pulmonary and systemic vascular resistances, and slightly increases cardiac output.[213] Moreover, diltiazem decreases the impact of arrhythmias induced by adrenaline.[213] In humans anaesthetised with halogenated volatile anaesthetics, intravenous injection of diltiazem also decreases the rate of ventricular premature contractions and slows the ventricular rate of atrial fibrillations.[213]

In the atria and ventricles, halogenated volatile anaesthetics have a direct action by slowing conduction velocities.[214] Ozaki et al.[215] confirmed that slowing of conduction velocity induced by lignocaine was proportional to the decrease in $\dot{V}_{max}$. These authors also demonstrated that the slowing of ventricular conduction velocities induced by halothane and enflurane was not associated with as marked a decrease in $\dot{V}_{max}$. This fact calls into question the classic theory on the direct relationship between the maximum upstroke velocity ($\dot{V}_{max}$) and the conduction velocity.[36] This means that halogenated volatile anaesthetics slow the conduction velocity by decreas-ing the fast inward sodium current,[216] but also, and mainly, by altering gap-junction conduction (intercellular communications).[217, 218] Moreover, it was demonstrated that the mechanism of alteration of conduction velocity induced by halogenated volatile anaesthetics varies with tissue function. In Purkinje fibres, halogenated volatile anaesthetics notably decrease $\dot{V}_{max}$, in the manner of a class 1 antiarrhythmic drug. By contrast, they markedly slow conduction at the Purkinje–muscle junction by acting on both the $\dot{V}_{max}$ and on gap-junctions.[219] Thus, particular care is required in administering anaesthesia using halogenated volatile anaesthetics in patients treated with class 1 antiarrhythmic drugs. Indeed, as these two types of molecule slow conduction by two different mechanisms, this exposes the patient to a potentiation of effects and to the appearance of conduction block. This risk was demonstrated in vitro using a combination of quinidine and halothane.[220] However, using a high resolution epicardial mapping study in rabbit hearts, the present authors observed no marked alterations of longitudinal and transverse conduction velocities, nor the occurrence of ventricular effective refractory periods induced by halothane or enflurane.[221]

The class 1 and 4 action of halogenated volatile anaesthetics might suggest a possible potentiation of effects with amiodarone. This was demonstrated in vitro by Gallagher, and by Rooney et al.[222, 223] The combination of halothane and amiodarone enhances bradycardia and atrioventricular conduction time. Moreover, in vivo, the action of pro-longed administration of amiodarone on β-adronoceptors risks potentiation of all these effects.

More is known about the antiarrhythmic and/or arrhythmogenic effects of halogenated volatile anaesthetics.[191] *In vitro* they suppress or decrease late after-depolarisations induced by catecholamines,[224-226] demonstrating an antiarrhythmic action. In contrast, halogenated volatile anaesthetics, and especially enflurane, have demonstrable proarrhythmic action because they increase abnormal automaticity induced by catecholamines on Purkinje fibres, although this is controversial.[227, 228] On ischaemic myocardium *in vitro*, halogenated volatile anaesthetics do not increase abnormal automaticity. Moreover halothane and enflurane, in contrast to isoflurane, suppress late after-depolarisations.[229] Similarly, the slowing of conduction velocity associated with functional block and shortening of refractory periods increase the potential for re-entry arrhythmias.[191] However, this has never been shown to be a clinical reality. Moreover, in isolated rabbit heart, the present authors were not able to induce re-entry arrhythmias because halogenated volatile anaesthetics did not markedly modify either ventricular conduction velocity (whatever the pacing rate) or ventricular effective refractory period. Consequently, no conduction block could be created.[221] In contrast, in ischaemic myocardium re-entry arrhythmias might be facilitated by halogenated volatile anaesthetics. Finally, *in vivo*, Gallagher and McClernam[230] reported in dogs that halothane suppresses arrhythmias in the acute phase of experimental myocardial infarction and has variable effects on arrhythmias in the late phase. Moreover, halothane terminates tachycardias induced by ouabain, but has no effect on tachycardias induced by cesium. These authors suggest therefore that, *in vivo*, halothane can suppress abnormal automaticity due to ischaemia, terminate or, on the contrary, facilitate re-entries and terminate arrhythmias due to late after-depolarisations but cannot suppress arrhythmias induced by early after-depolarisations.[230] In conclusion therefore, halogenated volatile anaesthetics have membrane properties causing either antiarrhythmic or arrhythmogenic action, but these actions occur at high concentrations only and are completely reversible.

Opiates

Opiates, and especially fentanyl, are used classically as a major component of anaesthesia in patients with cardiovascular risk.[231-235] They are often responsible for bradycardia, the mechanism for which remains controversial. Royster et al.[236] demonstrated in dogs that fentanyl induces a dose-dependent bradycardia but also a lengthening of conduction of the atrioventricular node and an increase in atrioventricular node and ventricular effective refractory periods. Romero et al.[237] reported that, in isolated rat atria, the negative chronotropic effect of morphine is not modified by naloxone or by atropine, even after reserpine pretreatment. Blair et al.[238, 239] described an increase in action potential duration of

Purkinje fibres with fentanyl and sufentanil. Saini *et al.*[240] demonstrated in anaesthetised dogs with haemorrhagic shock that fentanyl increases the fibrillation threshold. Rabkin[241] reported in guinea-pigs that morphine and dynorphine (an endogenous opiate) decrease the severity of arrhythmias induced by digoxin. All these studies suggest that opiates have actions on the cardiac membrane.[242] However, while the implication of opiate receptors is controversial,[242-244] the autonomic nervous system seems to participate in producing antiarrhythmic effects. In the opinion of some authors, this action is due more to the depression of the sympathetic system than the activation of the parasympathetic system.[240] In contrast, the study of Rabkin[241] suggests that the antiarrhythmic effect of opiates is mediated by the activation of the central cholinergic system.

The antiarrhythmic action of opiates is therefore similar to a class 3 antiarrhythmic effect. Opiates can increase the effects of calcium-channel blocking agents and of β-blocking agents.[245, 246] However, effects described in experimental models only appear with large doses.

Muscle relaxants

The action of muscle relaxants on cardiac electrophysiology is variable. Pancuronium bromide corrects bradycardia induced by fentanyl as well as the depression that fentanyl induces on the atrioventricular node.[236] This action does not seem to be solely mediated by the autonomic nervous system.[30] Indeed, while pancuronium bromide antagonises the bradycardia induced by acetylcholine, it also antagonises the bradycardia induced by large doses of opiates, which are very often insensitive to the administration of atropine.[236, 247] It would seem therefore that a direct membrane action of pancuronium bromide might explain this effect. However, pancuronium bromide has arrhythmogenic properties; indeed, it induces oscillations of the resting potential with increased occurrence of after-depolarisations in response to adrenaline.[248] This arrhythmogenicity is reversed by calcium-channel blocking agents.[248]

Vecuronium bromide is known to have little cardiovascular impact.[249, 250] *In vitro*, it slightly increases heart rate and myocardial contractility.[251] However, *in vivo*, combined with opiates, it can worsen opiate-induced bradycardia and/or can facilitate the occurrence of junctional rhythm or atrioventricular block.[252, 253] This effect is increased by the administration of calcium-channel or β-blocking agents.[246] The administration of physostigmine or edrophonium to reverse muscle relaxant action classically precipitates bradycardia or atrioventricular block. These disorders are more frequent during anaesthesia using fentanyl and vecuronium bromide,[254] and necessitate the administration of large doses of atropine. It is our opinion that this combination should be avoided in patients with sinus dysfunction and/or pre-existing conduction defect and/or treatment with a class 1C antiarrhythmic drug. Finally, class 1 and 4 antiarrhythmic drugs can potentiate the action of muscle relaxants.[255, 256]

Intravenous anaesthetics and the adjuvants of general anaesthesia

Barbiturates have no or few arrythmogenic effects *in vivo*. However, they prolong ventricular action potential duration and refractory periods.[257] They also facilitate late after-depolarisations at high concentration and at rapid pacing rate on the rabbit papillary muscle.[258] Propofol seems to have a mild calcium-channel inhibitory effect and M_2-muscarinic receptor competitive actions.[209, 259] This only partially explains propofol-induced bradycardia. Benzodiazepines are not reputed to be arrhythmogenic. They decrease experimental arrhythmias of reperfusion.[260] Among neuroleptic agents, promethazine has antiarrhythmic properties similar to class 1 antiarrhythmic drugs.[261] Haloperidol increases the threshold of ventricular fibrillation in pigs.[262] Droperidol has quinidine-like effects:[197] it increases anterograde and retrograde refractory periods in accessory pathways in patients with Wolff–Parkinson–White syndrome.[263] Large dose of droperidol, however, can induce torsades de pointes, probably by creating triggered activity induced by early after-depolarisations. Nitrous oxide facilitates arrhythmias induced by catecholamines in dogs anesthetised with halothane.[264] Finally, high nitrous oxide concentrations can facilitate the occurrence of junctional rhythm.[265]

Local anaesthetic drugs

Local anaesthetic drugs have a direct action on conduction due to their class 1 antiarrhythmic property. These effects on the infranodal conduction are clinically relevant only in the case of overdosage.[14] Lignocaine and mepivacaine have been shown to have good safety margins,[75, 266] but bupivacaine and etidocaine are more cardiotoxic. Indeed, although bupivacaine has been shown not to worsen a pre-existing conduction defect at anaesthetic concentrations during lumbar epidural anaesthesia,[267, 268] its use for these patients remains debatable.[14] Indeed, the inhibitory effect induced by bupivacaine on the fast inward sodium current is more potent than that of lignocaine.[40, 59] Moreover, bupivacaine also inhibits the potassium[269, 270] and calcium[271] currents. Lignocaine and mepivacaine are therefore to be preferred in patients taking antiarrhythmic medication. Worsening of haemodynamic status and of conduction velocities has been demonstrated in anaesthetised dogs receiving bupivacaine combined with β-blocking agents,[272] calcium-channel inhibitors[273] or class 1 antiarrhythmic drugs.[274] Finally, verapamil, more than diltiazem, potentiates ECG and haemodynamic effects in conscious dogs receiving 'anaesthetic' doses of bupivacaine or lignocaine.[275]

Complications induced by antiarrhythmic drugs: implications for anaesthsia

Despite their therapeutic effects, antiarrhythmic drugs have an impact on haemodynamic status, on the occurrence of conduction defect and/or on proarrhythmic effects. Thus, the indication for antiarrhythmic drug treatment has to be discussed in the case of minor arrhythmias detected preoperatively or during the perioperative period.[276] Furthermore, the initiation of antiarrhythmic treatment imposes the need for clinical and ECG supervision. Finally, it must be remembered that the best antiarrhythmic treatment in congestive cardiac failure remains the improvement of haemodynamic status.[277-281]

Haemodynamic impact of antiarrhythmic drugs

Most antiarrhythmic drugs depress myocardial contractility.[282, 283] Myocardial depression is more marked when the antiarrhythmic drug is administered intravenously, and/or when cardiac function is previously impaired.[3] Moreover, their indirect or direct action, mediated by the autonomic nervous system, on arterial and venous tone and their efficacy or otherwise on the arrhythmia also influence the haemodynamic state.[3]

For class 1 antiarrhythmic drugs, myocardial depression seems to depend on the slowing of ventricular conduction and the duration of sodium channel blockade.[284] The reduced intracellular pool of calcium also decreases myocardial function.[59, 128, 129, 285-287] Myocardial impairment will depend, however, on the drug and on the type of autonomic nervous system response. Indeed, lignocaine and mexiletine induce little alteration in cardiovascular status,[35, 83] while effects of quinidine are counterbalanced by the vasodilatation that it induces.[46] In contrast, disopyramide, by its vasoconstrictor effect, can induce severe cardiac failure.[50, 288] Finally, class 1C antiarrhythmic drugs are reputed to cause cardiovascular depression, to the extent that cardiac failure may occur.[289] However, the occurrence of acute cardiac failure is unpredictable.[108, 110, 116, 290]

Haemodynamic effects of β-blocking agents are due mainly to the decrease in heart rate and in calcium entry into the cell by reduction of phosphorylation of calcium channels.[291] Moreover, β-blockers induce an increase in systemic vascular resistances and therefore modify the capacity of adaptation and can precipitate cardiac failure. Among class 3 antiarrhythmic drugs, amiodarone produces little modification of haemodynamic parameters when it is injected slowly by the intravenous route.[173] In chronic administration, it does not alter the ejection fraction even in patients whose initial ejection fraction is low.[164] However, these effects on the α- and β-adrenoceptors can dramatically modify the response to stress and may result in severe collapse or bradycardia during induction of anaesthesia.[165]

89

Serious conduction defects

Serious conduction defects induced by antiarrhythmic drugs include severe bradycardia, sinoatrial block or AV block. These conduction defects usually occur following absolute or relative overdosage in patients with pre-existing conduction defects. The type of conduction defect depends on the class of antiarrhythmic drug.[78] Class 1 drugs are usually responsible for AV blocks rather sinoatrial blocks. Widening of the QRS complex testifies directly to slowing of intraventricular conduction, and constitutes a basic element of monitoring.[292] In contrast, class 1B drugs do not widen the QRS complex.[9, 75, 77, 80–82, 293] Beta- and calcium-channel blocking agents may cause AV blocks, sinoatrial blocks or low atrial rhythm by alteration of sinus impulse.[294, 295] Finally, amiodarone can induce marked sinus bradycardia, sometimes AV block, and sinoatrial blocks in the case of overdosage.[165] In conclusion, these conduction defects are often poorly tolerated, and may necessitate the emergency use of catecholamines and/or cardiac pacing.[294]

Arrhythmogenic effects

Proarrhythmic effects of antiarrhythmic drugs may be defined as the occurrence of more serious arrhythmias than those motivating their prescription. Although possibly overestimated,[295] the frequency of these accidents has been estimated at 8% during treatment to prevent ventricular tachycardia or fibrillation.[103, 296] Virtually all antiarrhythmic drugs are susceptible to be arrhythmogenic through a variety of mechanisms.[56, 103, 296] An increase or decrease in the plasma level an idiosyncratic reaction, abnormalities of serum potassium or magnesium concentrations,[297] an interaction between the antiarrhythmic drug and the autonomic nervous system, or alterations of cardiac performance and/or vasomotor activity may all be implicated. These accidents mainly concern class 1C antiarrhythmic drugs (encainide, flecainide), and possible mechanisms may be sustained re-entries induced by an excessive slowing of conduction velocity around functional blocks,[101, 298–300] and/or non-uniform refractoriness.[301, 302] These mechanisms are suggested in the CAST 1 study, which demonstrated that mortality was higher in patients taking encainide or flecainide, more particularly when they had non-Q wave myocardial infarction, heart rate greater than 74 beats/min or frequent ventricular premature contractions.[303]

Amiodarone, class 1B[74] and 1A[103, 304] antiarrhythmic drugs may also be implicated. The proarrhythmic effect of class 1B antiarrhythmic drugs would be due to a marked elevation of their plasma level inducing slowing of ventricular conduction associated with non-uniform ventricular activation.[293] Moreover, in the CAST 2 study their combination with diuretics increased mortality.[303] Although torsades de pointes has been described with bepridil, sotalol and amiodarone,[305–307] these arrhythmias occur

90

especially in association with treatment with class 1A antiarrhythmic drugs, and particularly with quinidine and its derivatives. They seem to be due to a triggered activity induced by early after-depolarisations,[308-313] facilitated by bradycardia,[311-313] hypokalaemia and hypomagnaesemia,[313, 314] and low plasma concentration.[315] The lengthening of the QT interval corrected for the resting heart rate,[316] or its insufficient shortening during exercise,[317] testifies to the potential risk of occurrence of this complication.

In case of a proarrhythmic accident, the first move is to discontinue the incriminated drug immediately and to ensure symptomatic treatment.[103] Propranolol has been shown to be effective in reversing flecainide- or encainide-induced arrhythmogenic effects. This confirms the hypothesis of their interaction with the autonomic nervous system.[318]

In conclusion, the margin of safety between efficacy and toxicity is often narrow and unpredictable, especially with class 1 antiarrhythmic drugs. Indeed, cardiac arrests have been reported in children with normal cardiac function treated for non-lethal arrhythmias by encainide or flecainide,[319] while a meta-analysis of 808 patients treated with quinidine and its derivatives to maintain sinus rhythm after cardioversion for atrial tachy-cardias has confirmed the efficacy of the antiarrhythmic drug versus placebo. Despite controversy concerning the meta-analysis, this study suggests that quinidine and its derivatives have a tendency to increase the mortality over 1 year.[320] A study of 406 elderly patients allocated to treatment by quinidine or procainamide or no antiarrhythmic drug for complex ventricular premature contractions, confirmed that antiarrhyth-mic treatment showed no benefit in preventing the occurrence of sudden death.[321] Thus prescription of chronic antiarrhythmic treatment must be considered carefully, and the reasons documented. Treatment with antiar-rhythmics should never constitute a 'comfort therapy' in the case of non-documented palpitations.[304, 314] Finally, it must be remembered that some arrhythmias can be treated by non-pharmacological means (cardio-verter-defibrillators, radiofrequency ablation).[322-326] Radiofrequency ablation has even been proposed to manage symptomatic ectopic activ-ity.[327]

Implications for anaesthesia

Antiarrhythmic treatment is instigated, *a priori*, to prevent potentially serious arrhythmias. It follows, therefore, that antiarrhythmic drugs should be maintained during the perioperative period and, equally, that they should be effective. The choice of anaesthetic technique must therefore take into account the impact of anaesthetic agents on the antiarrhythmic drug and, *a fortiori*, on the underlying cardiac disease. When administration by the digestive route is not possible, antiarrhythmic drugs must be given by the i.v. route.

Nevertheless, except in the case of β-blocking agents and of amiodarone, one could make a case for the temporary discontinuation of antiarrhythmic treatment. Indeed, several facts have to be taken into account. No antiarrhythmic drug is ever 100% effective[328] and the occurrence of these drugs' adverse efects is facilitated during the perioperative perod.[329]Moreover, in patients with high risk of coronary artery disease and undergoing non-cardiac surgery, increased occurrence of arrhythmias was reported in 12%, this complication arising during the postoperative period in 10%. This study also found that preoperative antiarrhythmic treatment induced an increase in both peroperative and especially postoperative arrhythmias. Finally, this same study did not demonstrate a requirement for aggressive antiarrhythmic therapy during the postoperative course.[201] Finally, another argument is that the main goal of prescription by a cardiologist of antiarrhythmic treatment is the avoidance of sudden death in a patient suffering serious arrhythmias.[314] Such an event seems unlikely during the perioperative course if aggressive monitoring is employed.

Taking into account all the possible interactions induced by antiarrhythmic drugs, one may propose the temporary discontinuation of treatment, especially when an antiarrhythmic drug has been prescribed for a minor, non-sustained arrhythmia. This, however, is not possible with amiodarone because its prolonged half-life would require withdrawal of treatment for several weeks. Beta-blocking agents are also an exception because their abrupt withdrawal should always be avoided.[330]

1 Julian DG, Cowan JC. Successes and limitations of antiarrhythmic drug therapy. In: Vaughan Williams EM (ed). *Antiarrhythmic drugs.* Berlin: Sprnger-Verlag, 1989:105–20.
2 Ravid S, Podrid PJ, Lampert S, Lown B. Congestive heart failure induced by six of the newer antiarrhythmic drugs. *J Am Coll Cardiol* 1989;14:1326–30.
3 Schlepper M. Cardiodepressive effects of antiarrhythmic drugs. *Eur Heart J* (Suppl E) 1989;10:73–80.
4 Campbell RWF, Nimkhedar K. Risk-benefit profiles of antiarrhythmic therapy. *Am J Cardiol* 1989;64:50J–2J.
5 Akhtar M, Tchou PJ, Jazayeri M. Mechanisms of clinical tachycardias. *Am J Cardiol* 1988;61:9A–19A.
6 Allessie MA, Schalij MJ, Krichhof CJHJ, Boersma L, Huybers M, Hollen J. Experimental electrophysiology and arrhythmogenicity. Anisotropy and ventricular tachycardia. *Eur Heart J* (Suppl E) 1989;10:2–8.
7 Arnsdorf MF, Bup TE. Management of arrhythmias in heart failure. *Cardiol Clin* 1989;7:145–69.
8 Breithardt G, Borggrefe M, Martinez-Rubio A, Budde T. Pathophysiological mechanisms of ventricular tachyarrhythmias. *Eur Heart J* (Suppl E) 1989;10:9–18.
9 Dennis AR, Ross DL, Richards DA *et al.* Effect of antiarrhythmic therapy on delayed potentials detected by the signal-averaged electrocardiogram in patients with ventricular tachycardia after acute mycardial infarction. *Am J Cardiol* 1986;58:261–5.
10 Lazzara R, Scherlag BJ. Generation of arrhythmias in myocardial ischemia and infarction. *Am J Cardiol* 1988;61:20A–6A.
11 Gang ES, Lew AS, Hong MA, Wang FZ, Siebert CA, Peter T. Decreased-incidence of ventricular late potentials after successful thrombolytic therapy for acute myocardial infarction. *New Engl J Med* 1989;321:712–16.
12 Rosen MR. Mechanisms for arrhythmias. *Am J Cardiol* 1988;61:2A–8A.

13 Dupuis B. Antiarythmiques. *Sem Hôp Paris* 1985;**61**:109–29.
14 Eledjam JJ, Bruelle P, de La Coussaye JE, Brugada J. Bupivacaine toxicity: pathophysiology and treatment. In: Van Zundert A (ed). *Highlights in regional anaesthesia and pain therpy. III.* Barcelona: Publicidad Permanyer, 1994:95–108.
15 de La Coussaye JE, Eledjam JJ, Bruelle P *et al.* Mechanisms of the putative cardioprotective effect of hexamethonium in anesthetized dogs given a large dose of bupivacaine. *Anesthesiology* 1994;**80**:595–605.
16 Huikuri H, Zaman L, Castellanos A *et al.* Changes in spontaneous sinus node rate as an estimate of cardiac autonomic tone during stable and unstable ventricular tachycardia. *J Am Coll Cardiol* 1989;**13**:646–52.
17 Zipes DP. A consideration of antiarrhythmic therapy. *Circulation* 1985;**72**:949–56.
18 Vaughan Williams EM. Classification of antiarrhythmic actions. In: Vaughan Williams EM (ed). *Antiarrhythmic drugs.* Berlin: Springer-Verlag, 1989:45–68.
19 Vaughan Williams EM. Classification of antiarrhythmic drugs. In: Sandoe E, Flensted Janasene, Olesen KH (eds). *Symposium of cardiac arrhythmias.* Sodertalje: AB Astra, 1970:449–72.
20 Vaughan Williams EM. Subgroups of class 1 antiarrhythmic drugs. *Eur J Heart* 1984;**5**:96–8.
21 Arnsdorf MF. Basic understanding of the electrophysiologic actions of antiarrhythmic drugs. Sources, sinks, and matrices of information. *Med Clin North Am* 1984;**68**:1247–80.
22 Borchard V, Berger F, Haffner D. Classification and action of antiarrhythmic drugs. *Eur Heart J* (Suppl E) 1989;**10**:31–40.
23 Campbell TJ. Kinetics of onset of rate-dependent effects of class I antiarrhythmic drugs are important in determining their effects on refractoriness in guinea pig ventricle and provide a theoretical basis for their subclassification. *Cardiovasc Res* 1983;**17**:344–52.
24 Harrison DC. Antiarrhythmic drug classification: new science and practical applications. *Am J Cardiol* 1985;**56**:185–7.
25 Harumi K, Tsutsumi T, Sato T, Sekiya S. Classification of antiarrhythmic drugs based on ventricular fibrillation threshold. *Am J Cardiol* 1989;**64**:10J–14J.
26 Nattel S. Antiarrhythmic drug classifications. A critical appraisal of their history, present status, and clinical relevance. *Drugs* 1991;**41**:672–701.
27 Touboul P, Attalah G, Gressard A, Michelon G, Chatelain MT, Delahaye JP. Effets electrophysiologiques des agents antiarythmiques chez l'homme. Tentative de classification. *Arch Mal Coeur* 1978;**72**:72–81.
28 Task Force of the Working Group on Arrhythmias of the European Society of Cardiology. The Sicilian Gambit. A new approach to the classification of antiarrhythmic drugs based on their actions on arrhythmogenic mechanisms. *Circulation* 1991;**84**:1831–51.
29 Kohlhardt M, Fichtner H, Froebe U, Herzig J W. On the mechanism of drug-induced blockage of Na$^+$ currents: interaction of antiarrhythmic compounds with DPI-modified single cardiac Na$^+$ channels. *Circ Res* 1989;**64**:867–81.
30 Echt DS, Black JN, Barbey JT, Coxe DR, Cato E. Evaluation of antiarrhythmic drugs on defibrillation energy requirements in dogs. Sodium channel block and action potential prolongation. *Circulation* 1989;**79**:1106–17.
31 Roden DM, Bennett PB, Snyders DJ, Balser JR, Hondeghem LM. Quinidine delays Ik activation in guinea pig ventricular myocytes. *Circ Res* 1988;**62**:1055–8.
32 Spinelli W, Hoffman BF. Mechanisms of termination of reentrant atrial arrhythmias by class I and class III antiarrhythmic agents. *Circ Res* 1989;**65**:1565–79.
33 Anno T, Hondeghem LM. Interactions of flecainide with guinea pig cardiac sodium channels. Importance of activation unblocking to the voltage dependence of recovery. *Circ Res* 1990;**66**:789–803.
34 Clarkson CW, Follmer CH, Ten Eick RE, Hondeghem LM, Yeh JZ. Evidence for two components of sodium channel block by lidocaine in isolated cardiac myocytes. *Circ Res* 1988;**63**:869–78.
35 Clarkson CW, Hondeghem LM. Evidence for a specific receptor site for lidocaine, quinidine, and bupivacaine associated with cardiac sodium channels in guinea pig ventricular myocardium. *Circ Res* 1985;**56**:496–506.
36 Hondeghem LM, Katzung BG. Test of model of antiarrhythmic action. Effects of

93

quinidine and lidocaine on myocardial conduction. *Circulation* 1980;**61**:1217–26.
37 Nitta JI, Sunami A, Marumo F, Hiaraoka M. States and sites of actions of flecainide on guinea-pig cardiac sodium channels. *Eur J Pharmacol* 1992;**214**:191–7.
38 Hoffmann BF. Modification of the electrophysiologic matrix by antiarrhythmic drugs. *J Am Coll Cardiol* 1985;**5**:28B–30B.
39 Hondeghem LM, Katzung BG. Antiarrhythmic agents: the modulated receptor mechanism of action of sodium and calcium channel-blocking drugs. *Ann Rev Pharmacol Toxicol* 1984;**24**:387–423.
40 Clarkson CW, Hondeghem LM. Mechanism for bupivacaine depression of cardiac conduction: fast block of sodium channels during the action potential with slow recovery from block during diastole. *Anesthesiology* 1985;**62**:396–405.
41 Hondeghem LM, Katzung BG. Time and voltage dependent interaction of antiarrhythmic drugs with cardiac sodium channels. *Biochim Biophys Acta* 1977;**472**:373–98.
42 Campbell TJ. Clinical use of class Ia antiarrhythmic drugs. In: Vaughan Williams EM (ed). *Antiarrhythmic drugs*. Berlin: Springer-Verlag, 1989:175–99.
43 Dupuis B. Antiarythmiques II. Les divers anti-arythmiques. *Sem Hôp Paris* 1985;**61**:625–54.
44 Davies LK, Davis RF. Pharmacologic treatment of arrhythmias. *Anesth Clin North Am* 1989;**7**:421–58.
45 Wit AL. The effects of quinidine on the cellular electrophysiology of the heart: a brief review. *J Electrophysiol* 1989;**3**:316–22.
46 Crawford M, White D, O'Rourke R. Effects of oral quinidine on left ventricular performance in normal subjects and patients with congestive cardiomyopathy. *Am J Cardiol* 1979;**44**:714–18.
47 Fauchier JP, Cosnay P, Rouesnel Ph, Moquet B, Huguet RG. Effects of hydroquinidine hydrochlorate on the atrioventricular accessory pathways with or without paroxysmal arrhythmias. *J Electrophysiol* 1989;**3**:370–7.
48 Nakaya Y, Nii H, Nomura M, Fuajino K, Mori H. Effects of lidocaine and quinidine on post-repolarization refractoriness after the basic and premature action potentials: consideration of aim of antiarrhythmic drug therapy. *Am Heart J* 1989;**118**:907–12.
49 Hohnloser SH, Van de Loo A, Baedeker F. Efficacy and proarrhythmic hazards of pharmacologic cardioversion of atrial fibrillation: prospective comparison of sotalol versus quinidine. *J Am Coll Cardiol* 1995;**26**:852–8.
50 Podrid PJ, Schoenenberger A, Lown B. Congestive heart failure caused by oral disopyramide. *N Engl J Med* 1980;**302**:614–16.
51 Della Bella P, Marenzi G, Tondo C *et al*. Effects of disopyramide on cycle length, effective refractory period and excitable gap of atrial flutter, and relation to arrhythmia termination by overdrive pacing. *Am J Cardiol* 1989;**63**:812–16.
52 Fujimura O, Klein GJ, Sharma AD, Yee R, Szabo T. Acute effect of disopyramide on atrial fibrillation in the Wolff–Parkinson–White syndrome. *J Am Coll Cardiol* 1989;**13**:1133–7.
53 Marchlinski FE, Buxton AE Vassalo JA *et al*. Comparative electrophysiologic effects of intravenous and oral procainamide in patients with sustained ventricular arrhythmias. *J Am Coll Cardiol* 1984;**4**:1247–54.
54 Stamato NJ, Frame LH, Rosenthal ME, Almendral JM, Gottlieb CD, Josephson ME. Procainamide-induced slowing of ventricular tachycardia with insights from analysis of resetting response patterns. *Am J Cardiol* 1989;**63**:1455–61.
55 Kay GN Epstein AE, Plumb VJ. Preferential effect of procainamide on the reentrant circuit of ventricuar tachycardia. *J Am Coll Cardiol* 1989;**14**:382–90,
56 Zipes DP. Management of cardiac arrhythmias: pharmacological, electrical and surgical techniques. In: Braunwald E (ed). *Heart disease*. Saunders: Philadelphia, 1988:621–57.
57 Harron DWG, Shanks R. Clinical use of class Ib antiarrhythmic drugs. In: Vaughan Williams EM (ed). *Antiarrhythmc drugs*. Berlin: Springer-Verlag, 1989:201–33.
58 Collinsworth KA, Kalman SM, Harrison DC. The clinical pharmacology of lidocaine as an antiarrhythmic drug. *Circulation* 1974;**50**:1217–30.
59 Josephson IR. Lidocaine blocks NA, Ca and K currents of chick ventricular myocytes. *J Mol Cell Cardiol* 1988;**20**:593–604.
60 Rosen MR, Merker C, Pippenger CE. The effects of lidocaine on the canine ECG and electrophysiologic properties of Purkinje fibers. *Am Heart J* 1976;**91**:191–202.

61 Avery P, Redon D, Schaenzer G, Rusy BF. The influence of serum potassium on the cerebral and cardiac toxicity of bupivacaine and lidocaine. *Anesthesiology* 1984;**61**:134–8.

62 Bosjnak ZJ, Stowe DF, Kampine JP. Comparison of lidocaine and bupivacaine depression of sinoatrial nodal activity during hypoxia and acidosis in adult and neonatal guinea pigs. *Anaesth Analg* 1986;**65**:911–17.

63 Campbell TJ, Wyse KR, Hemsworth PD. Effects of hyperkalemia, acidosis, and hypoxia on the depression of maximum rate of depolarization by class I antiarrhythmic drugs in guinea pig myocardium: differential actions of class Ib and Ic agents. *J Cardiovasc Pharmacol* 1991;**18**:51–9.

64 Evans J, Gilmour RF, Zipes DP. The effects of lidocaine and quinidine on impulse propagation across the canine Purkinje-muscle junction during combined hyperkalemia, hypoxia, and acidosis. *Circ Res* 1984;**55**:185–96.

65 Komai H, Rusy BF. Effects of bupivacaine and lidocaine on A-V conduction in the isolated rat heart: modification by hyperkalaemia. *Anesthesiology* 1981;**55**:281–5.

66 Sage DJ, Feldman HS, Richard S, Arthur G. Influence of lidocaine and bupivacaine on isolated guinea pig atria in the presence of acidosis and hypoxia. *Anesth Analg* 1984;**63**:1–7.

67 Wyse KR, Ye V, Campbell TJ. Effects of hyperkalaemia on the depression of maximum rate of depolarization by class I antiarrhythmic agents in guinea-pig myocardium. *Br J Pharmacol* 1993;**108**:255–61.

68 Abete P, Ferrara N, Rengo F, Vassalle M. Mechanisms of lidocaine actions on normal and abnormal rhythms in canine cardiac tissues *in vivo* and *in vitro*. *Clin Exp Pharmacol Physiol* 1991;**18**:179–91.

69 Chow MSS, Kluger J, Dipersio DM, Lawrence R, Fielman A. Antifibrillatory effects of lidocaine and bretylium immediately post cardiopulmonary resuscitation. *Am Heart J* 1985;**110**:938–43.

70 Sugimoto T, Murakawa Y, Toda I. Evaluation of antifibrillatory effects of drugs. *Am J Cardiol* 1989;**64**:33J–36J.

71 Li G-R, Ferrier GR. Effects of lidocaine on reperfusion arrhythmias and electrophysiological properties in an isolated ventricular muscle model of ischemia and reperfusion. *J Pharmacol Exp Ther* 1991;**257**:997–1004.

72 Koster RW, Dunnings AJ. Intramuscular lidocaine for prevention of lethal arrhythmias in the prehospitalization phase of acute myocardial infarction. *N Engl J Med* 1985;**313**:1105–10.

73 Lie KI, Liem KL, Louridtz WJ *et al.* Efficacy of lidocaine in preventing primary ventricular fibrillation within 1 hour after a 300 mg intramuscular injection. *Am J Cardiol* 1978;**42**:486–91.

74 The Cardiac Arrhythmia Suppression Trial Investigators. Effect of antiarrhythmic agent moricizine on survival after myocardial infarction. *N Engl J Med* 1991;**327**:227–33.

75 Bruelle P, Lefrant J-Y, de La Coussaye JE *et al.* Comparative electrophysiologic and hemodynamic effects of several amide local anesthetic drugs in anesthetized dogs. *Anesth Analg* 1996;**82**:648–56.

76 de La Coussaye JE, Brugada J, Eledjam JJ. Cardiac complications of local anesthetic agents. In: Vincent JL (ed). *Yearbook of Intensive Care and Emergency Medicine*. Berlin: Springer-Verlag, 1992:129–36.

77 Demczuk RJ. Significant sinus bradycardia following intravenous lidocaine injection. *Anesthesiology* 1984;**60**:69–70.

78 Dhingra RC, Deedwania PC, Cummings JM *et al.* Electrophysiologic effects of lidocaine on sinus node and atrium in patients with and without sinoatrial dysfunction. *Circulation* 1978;**57**:448–54.

79 Gupta PK, Lichstein E, Chadda KD. Lidocaine induced heart block in patients with bundle branch block. *Am J Cardiol* 1974;**33**:487–92.

80 Keidar S, Grenadier E, Palant A. Sino-atrial arrest due to lidocaine injection in sick sinus syndrome during amiodarone administration. *Am Heart J* 1982;**104**:1384–5.

81 Lichstein E, Chadda KD, Gupta PK. Atrioventricular block with lidocaine therapy. *Am J Cardiol* 1973;**31**:277–81.

82 Roos TC, Dunning AJ. Effects of lidocaine on impulse formation and conduction defects

in man. *Am Heart J* 1975;**89**:686–99.
83 Campbell NPS, Zaidi SA, Adgey AAJ, Patterson GC, Pantridge JF. Observations on haemodynamic effects of mexiletine. *Br Heart J* 1979;**41**:182–6.
84 Woosley RL, Funck-Brentano C. Overview of the clinical pharmacology of antiarrhythmic drugs. *Am J Cardiol* 1988;**61**:61A–69A.
85 Sphakianaki E, Tsouderos I, Morali A *et al.* Interactions between digitoxin and some antiarrhythmic drugs. *Meth Find Exp Clin Pharmacol* 1992;**14**:355–60.
86 Kodama I, Honjo H, Kamiya K, Toyama J. Two types of sodium channel block by class-I antiarrhythmic drugs by using V max of action potential in single ventricular myocytes. *J Mol Cell Cardiol* 1990;**22**:1–12.
87 Le Grand B, Le Heuzey JY, Perier P *et al.* Cellular electrophysiological effects of flecainide on human atrial fibres. *Cardiovasc Res* 1990;**24**:232–8.
88 Ferrara N, Abete P, Leosco D *et al.* Effect of flecainide acetate on reperfusion and barium-induced ventricular tachyarrhythmias in the isolated perfused rat heart. *Arch Int Pharmacodyn* 1990;**308**:104–14.
89 Wang Z, Pelletier LC, Talajic M, Nattel S. Effects of flecainide and quinidine on human atrial action potentials. Role of rate-dependence and comparison with guinea pig, rabbit, and dog tissues. *Circulation* 1990;**82**:274–83.
90 Ranger S, Talajic M, Lemery R, Roy D, Nattel S. Amplification of flecainide-induced ventricular slowing by exercise. A potentially significant consequence of use-dependent sodium channel blockade. *Circulation* 1989;**79**:1000–6.
91 Ranger S, Talajic M, Lemery R, Roy D, Villemaire C, Nattel S. Kinetics of use-dependent ventricular conduction slowing by antiarrhythmic drugs in humans. *Circulation* 1991;**83**:1987–94.
92 Pritchett EL, Datorre SD, Platt ML, McCarville SE, Hougham AJ. The flecainide supraventricular tachycardia study group. Flecainide acetate treatment of paroxysmal supraventricular tachycardia and paroxysmal atrial fibrillation: dose–response studies. *J Am Coll Cardiol* 1991;**17**:297–303.
93 Suttorp MJ, Kingma JH, Jessurun ER, Lie-A-Huen L, Van Hemel NM, Lie KI. The value of class IC antiarrhythmic drugs for acute conversion of paroxysmal atrial fibrillation or flutter to sinus rhythm. *J Am Coll Cardiol* 1990;**16**:1722–7.
94 Suttorp MJ, Kingma JH, Lie-A-Huen L, Mast EG. Intravenous flecainide versus verapamil for acute conversion of paroxysmal atrial fibrillation or flutter to sinus rhythm. *Am J Cardiol* 1989;**63**:693–6.
95 Van Wijk LM, Crijns HJ, Kingma HJ *et al.* Flecainide: long-term effects in patients with sustained ventricular tachycardia or ventricular fibrillation. *J Cardiovasc Pharmacol* 1990;**15**:884–91.
96 Van Wijk LM, Crijns HJ, Van Gilst WH, Wesseling H, Lie KI. Flecainide acetate in the treatment of supraventricular tachycardias: value of programmed electrical stimulation for long term prognosis. *Am Heart J* 1989;**117**:365–9.
97 Van Gelder IC, Crijns HJGM, Van Gilst WH, Van Wijk LM, Hamer HPM, Lie KI. Efficacy and safety of flecainide acetate in the maintenance of sinus rhythm after electrical cardioversion of chronic atrial fibrillation or atrial flutter. *Am J Cardiol* 1989;**64**:1317–21.
98 Boriani G, Stocchi E, Capucci A *et al.* Flecainide: evidence of non-linear kinetics. *Eur J Clin Pharmacol* 1991;**41**:57–9.
99 Hertrampf R, Gunder-Remy U, Beckmann J, Hoppe U, Elsaesser W, Stein H. Elimination of flecainide as a function of urinary flow rate and pH. *Eur J Clin Pharmacol* 1991;**41**:61–3.
100 Padrini R, Piovan D, Busa M, Al-Bunni M, Maiolino P, Ferrari M. Pharmacodynamic variability of flecainide assessed by QRS changes. *Clin Pharmacol Ther* 1993;**53**:59–64.
101 Levine JH, Morganroth J, Kadish AH. Mechanisms and risk factors for proarrhythmia with type IA compared with IC antiarrhythmic drug therapy. *Circulation* 1989;**80**:1063–9.
102 Podrid PJ. Aggravation of arrhythmia: a complication of antiarrhythmic drug therapy. *Eur Heart J* (Suppl E) 1989;**10**:66–72.
103 Zipes DP. Proarrhythmic events. *Am J Cardiol* 1988;**61**:70A–76A.
104 Vik-Mo H, Ohm OJ, Lund-Johansen P. Electrophysiological effects of flecainide acetate

in patients with sinus nodal dysfunction. *Am J Cardiol* 1982;**50**:1090–4.

105 HanakiY, Sugihama S, Hieda N,Taki K, Hayashi H, OzaWA. Cardioprotective effects of various class I antiarrhythmic drugs in canine hearts. *J Am Coll Cardiol* 1989;**14**:219–24.

106 The Cardiac Arrhythmia Suppression Trial (CAST) Investigators. Preliminary report of encainide and flecainide on mortality in a randomized trial of arrhythmia suppression after myocardial infarction. *N Engl J Med* 1989;**321**:406–12.

107 Funck-Brentano C, Kroemer HK, Lee JT, Roden DM. Propafenone. *N Engl J Med* 1990;**322**:518–25.

108 Dukes ID, Vaughan Williams EM. The multiple modes of action of propafenone. *Eur Heart J* 1984;**5**:115–21.

109 Groschner K, LindnerW, Schneld H, KukovetzWR. The effects of the stereoisomers of propafenone and diprafenone in guinea-pig heart. *Br J Pharmacol* 1991;**102**:669–74.

110 McLeod AA, Stiles GL, Shand DG. Demonstration of beta-adrenoreceptor blockade by propafenone hydrochloride; clinical pharmacologic, radioligand bending and adenylate cyclase activation studies. *J Pharmacol Exp Ther* 1984;**228**:461–6.

111 Stoschitzky K, Klein W, Stark G *et al.* Different stereoselective effects of (R)- and (S)-propafenone: clinical pharmacologic, electrophysiologic, and radioligand binding studies. *Clin Pharmacol Ther* 1990;**47**:740–6.

112 Coumel P, Leclerq J, Assayag P. European experience with the antiarrhythmic efficacy of propafenone for supraventricular and ventricular arrhythmias. *Am J Cardiol* 1984;**54**:60D–66D.

113 Karagueuzian HR, Katoh T, McCullen A, Mandel WJ, Peter T. Electrophysiologic and hemodynamic effects of propafenone, a new antiarrhythmic agent, on the anesthetized, closed-chest dog; comparative study with lidocaine. *Am Heart J* 1984;**107**:418–24.

114 Bianconi L, Boccadamo R, Pappalardo A, Gentili C, Pistolese M. Effectiveness of intravenous propafenone for conversion of atrial fibrillation and flutter of recent onset. *Am J Cardiol* 1989;**64**:335–8.

115 Lange H, Lampert S, Sutton MSJ, Lown B. Changes in cardiac output determined by continuous-wave Doppler echocardiography during propafenone or mexiletine drug testing. *Am J Cardiol* 1990;**65**:458–62.

116 Podrid PJ, Lown B. Propafenone, a new agent for ventricular arrhythmias. *J Am Coll Cardiol* 1984;**4**:117–25.

117 Antman EM, Beamer AD, Cantillon C, McGowan N, Friedman PL. Therapy of refractory symptomatic atrial fibrillation and atrial flutter: a staged care approach with new antiarrhythmic drugs. *J Am Coll Cardiol* 1990;**15**:688–707.

118 Boahene KA, Klein GJ, Yee R, Sharma AD, Fujimura O. Termination of acute atrial fibrillation in the Wolff–Parkinson–White syndrome by procainamide and propafenone: importance of atrial fibrillatory cycle length. *J Am Coll Cardiol* 1990;**16**:1408–14.

119 BuddeT, Borggrefe M, Posczek A, Martinez-Rubio A, Breithardt G. Acute and long-term efficacy of oral propafenone in patients with ventricular tachyarrhythmias. *J. Cardiovasc Pharmacol* 1991;**18**:254–60.

120 Connolly SJ, Hoffert DL. Usefulness of propafenone for recurrent paroxysmal atrial fibrillation. *Am. J Cardiol* 1989;**63**:817–19.

121 Dubuc M, Kus T, Campa MA, Lambert C, Rosengarten M, Shenasa M. Electrophysiologic effects of intravenous propafenone inWolff–Parkinson–White syndrome. *Am Heart J* 1989;**117**:370–6.

122 Geibel A, Meinertz T, Zehender M *et al.* Antiarrhythmic efficacy and tolerance of oral propafenone in patients with frequent ventricular arrhythmias: experience of a multi-centre study. *Eur Heart J* (Suppl E) 1989;**10**:81–7.

123 Hernandez M, Reder RF, Marinchak RA, Rials SR, Kowey PR. Propafenone for malignant ventricular arrhythmia: an analysis of the literature. *Am Heart J* 1991;**121**:1178–84.

124 Kus T, Dubuc M, Lambert C, Shenasa M. Efficacy of propafenone in preventing ventricular tachycardia: inverse correlation with rate-related prolongation of conduction time. *J Am Coll Cardiol* 1990;**16**:1229–37.

125 Bigot MC, Debruyne D, Bonnefoy L, Grollier G, Moulin M, Potier JC. Serum digoxin levels related to plasma propafenone levels during concomitant treatment. *J Clin Pharmacol* 1991;**31**:521–6.

126 Lee BL, Dohrmann ML. Theophylline toxicity after propafenone treatment: evidence for drug interaction. *Clin Pharmacol Ther* 1992;**51**:353–5.

127 Harron DWG, Brogden RN, Faulds D, Fitton A. Cibenzoline. A review of its pharmacological properties and therapeutic potential in arrhythmias. *Drugs* 1992;**43**:734–59.

128 Holck M, Osterrieder W. Inhibition of the myocardial Ca^{2+} inward current by the class 1 antiarrhythmic agent, cibenzoline. *Br J Pharmacol* 1986;**87**:705–11.

129 Massé C, Cazes M, Sassine A. Effects of cibenzoline, a novel antiarrhythmic drug, on action potential and transmembrane curents in frog atrial muscle. *Arch Int Pharmacodyn* 1984;**269**:219–35.

130 Sassine A, Massé C, Brugada J, Cazes M, Puech P. Evidence for a class 4 effect of cibenzoline 'in vivo'. *Arch Int Pharmacodyn* 1987;**287**:78–88.

131 Sato T, Wu B, Nakamura S, Kiyosue T, Arita M. Cibenzoline inhibits diazoxide- and 2,4-dinitrophenol-activated ATP-sensitive K+ channels in guinea-pig ventricular cells. *Br J Pharmacol* 1993;**108**:549–56.

132 Sassine A, Massé C, Dufour A, Hirsch JL, Cazes M, Puech P. Cardiac electrophysiologic effects of cibenzoline by acute and chronic administration in the anesthetized dog. *Arch Int Pharmacodyn* 1984;**269**:201–18.

133 Fujiki A, Mizumaki K, Tani M, Yoshida S, Sasayama S. Electrophysiologic effects and efficacy of cibenzoline in patients with supraventricular tachycardia. *J Cardiovasc Pharmacol* 1992;**20**:375–9.

134 Haruno A, Matsuzaki T, Hashimoto K. Antiarrhythmic effects of optical isomers of cibenzoline on canine ventricular arrhythmias. *J Cardiovasc Parmacol* 1990;**16**:376–82.

135 Keefe D, Williams S, Miura D, Rerribile S, Somberg J. A randomized parallel trial of cibenzoline and quinidine for prevention of recurrence of atrial fibrillation or flutter. *J Clin Pharmacol* 1985;**25**:455–74.

136 Kühlkamp V, Meerhof J, Schmidt F *et al*. Electrophysiologic effects and efficacy of cibenzoline on stimulation-induced atrial fibrillation and flutter and implications for treatment of paroxysmal atrial fibrillation. *Am J Cardol* 1990;**65**:628–32.

137 Hoffman E, Mattke S, Haberl R, Steinbeck G. Randomized crossover comparison of the electrophysiologic and antiarrhythmic efficacy of oral cibenzoline and sotalol for sustained ventricular tachycardia. *J Cardiovasc Pharmacol* 1993;**21**:95–100.

138 Gill J, Heel RC, Fitton A. Amiodarone. An overview of its pharmacological properties, and review of its therapeutic use in cardiac arrhythmias. *Drugs* 1992;**43**:69–110.

139 Mason JW. Amiodarone. *N Engl J Med* 1987;**316**:455–66.

140 Balser JR, Bennett PB, Hondeghem LM, Roden DM. Suppression of time-dependent outward current in guinea pig ventricular myocytes. Actions of quinidine and aminodarone. *Circ Res* 1991;**69**:519–29.

141 Moray F, DiCarlo LA Jr, Krol RB, Baerman JM, Debuitler M. Acute and chronic effects of amiodarone on ventricular refractoriness, intraventricular conduction and ventricular tachycardia induction. *J Am Coll Cardiol* 1986;**7**:148–57.

142 Satoh H. Class III antiarrhythmic drugs (amiodarone, bretylium and sotalol) on action potentials and membrane currents in rabbit sino-atrial node preparations. *Naunyn-Schmiedeberg's Arch Pharmacol* 1991;**344**:674–81.

143 Hondeghem LM, Snyders DJ. Class III antiarrhythmic agents have a lot of potential but a long way to go. Reduced effectiveness and dangers of reverse use-dependence. *Circulation* 1990;**81**:686–90.

144 Nattel S, Talajic M, Quantz M, De Roode M. Frequency-dependent effects of amiodarone on atrio-ventricular nodal function and slow-channel action potentials: evidence for calcium channel-blocking activity. *Circulation* 1987;**76**:442–9.

145 Valenzuela C, Bennett PB. Voltage- and use-dependent modulaton of calcium-channel current in guinea pig ventricular cells by amiodarone and des-oxo-amiodarone. *J Cardiovasc Pharmacol* 1991;**17**:894–902.

146 Anderson KP, Walker R, Dustman T *et al*. Rate-related electrophysiologic effects of long-term administration of amiodarone on canine ventricular myocardium *in vivo*. *Circulation* 1989;**79**:948–58.

147 Follmer C, Aomine M, Yez JZ, Singer DH. Amiodarone-induced block of sodium current in isolated cardiac cells. *J Pharmacol Exp Ther* 1987;**243**:187–94.

148 Kodama I, Suzuki R, Kamiya K, Iwata H, Toyama J. Effects of long-term oral administration of amiodarone on the electromechanical performance of rabbit ventricular muscle. *Br J Pharmacol* 1992;107:502–9.

149 Mason JW, Hondeghem LM, Katzung BG. Block of inactivated sodium channels and of depolarization-induced automaticity in guinea pig papillary muscle by amiodarone. *Circ Res* 1984;55:277–285.

150 Honjo H, Kodama I, Kamiya K, Toyama J. Block of cardiac sodium channels by amiodarone studied by using V_{max} of action potential in single ventricular myocytes. *Br J Pharmacol* 1991;102:651–6.

151 Biagetti MO, De Forteza E, Quinteiro RA. Differential effects of amiodarone on V_{max} and conduction velocity in anisotropic myocardium. *J Cardiovasc Pharmacol* 1990;15:918–26.

152 Gagnol JP, Devos C, Clinet M, Nokin P. Amiodarone: biochemical aspects and hemodynamc effects. *Drugs* (Suppl 3) 1985;29:1–10.

153 Nokin P, Clinet M, Schoenfeld P. Cardiac beta adrenoceptor modulation by amiodarone. *Biochem Pharmacol* 1983;32:2473–7.

154 Bjornerheim R, Froysaker T, Hansson V. Effects of chronic amiodarone treatment on human β-adrenoceptor density and adenylate cyclase response. *Cardiovasc Res* 1991;25:503–9.

155 Kadish AH, Chen RF, Schmaltz S, Morady F. Magnitude and time course of beta-adrenergic antagonism during oral amiodarone therapy. *J Am Coll Cardiol* 1990;16:1240–5.

156 Mitchell LB, Wyse G, Gillis AM, Duff HJ. Electropharmacology of amiodarone therapy initiation. Time courses of onset of electrophysiologic and antiarrhythmic effects. *Circulation* 1989;80:34–42.

157 Perret G, Yin YL, Nicolas P *et al.* Amiodarone decreases cardiac β-adrenoceptors through an antagonistic effect on 3,5,3′triodothyronine. *J Cardiovasc Pharmacol* 1992;19:473–8.

158 Yin YL, Perret GY, Nicolas P, Vassy R, Uzzan B, Tod M. *In vivo* effects of amiodarone on cardiac β-adrenoceptor density and heart rate require thyroid hormones. *J Cardiovasc Pharmacol* 1992;19:541–5.

159 Almotrefi AA, Dzimiri N. The influence of potassium concentration on the inhibitory effect of amiodarone on guinea-pig microsomal Na^+-K^+-ATPase activity. *Pharmacol Toxicol* 1991;69:140–3.

160 Munoz A, Karila P, Gallay P *et al.* A randomized hemodynamic comparison of intravenous amiodarone with and without solvent. *Eur Heart J* 1988;9:142–8.

161 Path GJ, Dai XZ, Schwartz JS, Benditt DG, Bache RJ. Effects of amiodarone with and without polysorbate 80 on myocardial oxygen consumption and coronary blood flow during treadmill exercise in the dog. *J Cardiovasc Pharmacol* 1991;18:11–16.

162 Aomine M, Singer DH. Negative inotropic effects of amiodarone on isolated guinea pig papillary muscle. *Cardiovasc Res* 1990;24:182–90.

163 Remme WJ, Kruyssen HACM, Look MP, Van Hoogenhuyze DCA, Krauss XH. Hemodynamic effects and tolerability of intravenous amiodarone in patients with impaired left ventricular function. *Am Heart J* 1991;122:96–103.

164 Singh BN. Amiodarone: electropharmacologic properties. In: Vaughan Williams EM (ed). *Antiarrhythmic drugs.* Berlin: Springer-Verlag :1989:335–64.

165 Liberman BA, Teadsdale SJ. Anaesthesia and amiodarone. *Can Anaesth Soc J* 1985;32:629–38.

166 Mostow ND, Vrobel TR, Noon D, Rakita L. Rapid control of refractory atrial tachyarrhythmias with high-dose oral amiodarone. *Am Heart J* 1990;120:1356–63.

167 Heger JJ, Prystowsky EN, Jackman WM *et al.* Clinical efficacy and electrophysiology of amiodarone during long-term therapy for recurrent ventricular tachycardia or ventricular fibrillation. *N Engl J Med* 1981;305:539–45.

168 Herre JM, Sauve MJ, Malone P *et al.* Long-term results of amiodarone therapy in patients with recurrent sustained ventricular tachycardia or ventricular fibrillation. *J Am Coll Cardiol* 1989;13:442–9.

169 Hohnloser SH, Meinertz T, Dammbacher T *et all.* Electrocardiographic and antiarrhythmic effects of intravenous amiodarone: results of a prospective, placebo-controlled study. *Am Heart J* 1991;121:89–95.

170 McGovern B, Garan H, Malacoff RF et al. Long-term clinical outcome of ventricular tachycardia or fibrillation treated with amiodarone. Am J Cardiol 1984;53:1558–63.

171 Mooss AN, Mohiuddin SM, Hee TT et al. Efficacy and tolerance of high-dose intravenous amiodarone for recurrent, refractory ventricular tachycardia. Am J Cardiol 1990;65:693–714.

172 Myers M, Peter T, Weiss D et al. Benefit and risks of long-term amiodarone therapy for sustained ventricular tachycardia/fibrillation: minimum of three-year follow-up in 145 patients. Am Heart J 1990;119:8–14.

173 Ochi RP, Goldenberg IF, Almquist A et al. Intravenous amiodarone for the rapid treatment of life-threatening ventricular arrhythmias in critically ill patients with coronary artery disease. Am J Cardiol 1989;64:599–603.

174 Vietti-Ramus G, Veglio F, Marchisio U, Burzio P, Latini R. Efficacy and safety of short intravenous amiodarone in supraventricular tachyarrhythmias. Int J Cardiol 1992;35:77–85.

175 Rankin AC, Pringle SD, Cobbe SM. Acute treatment of torsades de pointes with amiodarone: proarrhythmic and antiarrhythmic association of QT prolongation. Am Heart J 1990;119:185–6.

176 Burkart F, Pfisterer M, Kiowski W, Follath F, Burckhardt D. Effects of antiarrhythmic therapy on mortality in survivors of myocardial infarction with asymptomatic complex ventricular arrhythmias: Basel antiarrhythmic study of infarct survival (BASIS). J Am Coll Cardiol 1990;16:1711–18.

177 Strasberg B, Kusniec J, Zlotikamien B, Mager A, Sclarovsky S. Long-term follow-up of postmyocardial infarction patients with ventricular tachycardia or ventricular fibrillation treated with amiodarone. Am J Cardiol 1990;66:673–8.

178 Kerin NZ, Frumin H, Faitel K, Aragon E, Rubenfire M. Survival of patients with nonsustained ventricular tachycardia and impaired left ventricular function treated with low-dose amiodarone. J Clin Pharmacol 1991;31:1112–17.

179 Abdollah H, Brennan FJ, Jimmo S, Brien JF. Relationship between myocardial amiodarone concentration and antiarrhythmic effect in dogs with myocardial infarction and electrically induced ventricular arrhythmias. Can J Physiol Pharmacol 1991;69:812–17.

180 Mayuga RD, Singer DH. Effects of intravenous amiodarone on electrical dispersion in normal and ischaemc tissues and on arrhythmia inducibility: monophasic action potential studies. Cardiovasc Res 1992;26:571–9.

181 Zarembski DG, Nolan PE jr, Slack MK, Caruso AC. Treatment of resistant atrial fibrillation. A meta-analysis comparing amiodarone and flecainide. Arch Intern Med 1995;155:1885–91.

182 Burckhardt D, Robertson A, Hoffmann A, Pfisterer M. Long-term treatment of ventricular tachycardia with amiodarone in presence of severe left ventricular dysfunction. J Clin Pharmacol 1991;31:1105–8.

183 Wilson JS, Podrid PJ. Side effects from amiodarone. Am Heart J 1991;121:158–71.

184 Figge HL, Figge J. The effects of amiodarone on thyroid hormone function: a review of the physiology and clinical manifestations. J Clin Pharmacol 1990;30:588–95.

185 Dusman RE, Stanton MS Miles WM et al. Clinical features of amiodarone-induced pulmonary toxicity. Circulation 1990;82:51–9.

186 Russel DC, Paton L, Douglas AC. Amiodarone associated alveolitis and polyarthropathy. Treatment by plasma exchange. Br Heart J 1983;50:491–4.

187 Weinberg BA, Miles WM, Klein LS et al. Five-year follow-up of 589 patients treated with amiodarone. Am Heart J 1993;125:109–20.

188 Pollak PT, Sharma AD, Carruthers SG. Relation of amiodarone hepatic and pulmonary toxicity to serum drug concentrations and superoxide dismutase activity. Am J Cardiol 1990;65:1185–91.

189 Singh BN, Nademanee K. Use of calcium antagonists for cardiac arrhythmias. Am J Cardiol 1987;59:153B–62B.

190 Atlee JL III. Hallothane: cause or cure for arrythmias? Anesthesiology 1987;67:617–18.

191 Bosjnak ZL, Turner LA. Halothane, catecholamines, and cardiac conduction: Anything new? Anesth Analg 1991;72:1–4.

192 Courtinat C, Blache JL, Borsarelli J, Djiane P, Durand-Gasselin JJ, François G. Effect

comparatif de l'halothane et de l'isoflurane sur les arythmies cardiaques peropératoires. *Ann Fr Anesth Réanim* 1986;5:372–5.

193 Hutchison GL, Davies CA, Main G, Gray G. Incidence of arrhythmias in dental anesthesia, a crossover comparison of halothane and isoflurane. *Br J Anesth* 1989;62:518–21.

194 Katz RL, Bigger JT. Cardiac arrythmias during anesthesia and operation. *Anesthesiology* 1970;33:193–213.

195 Levy W. Clinical evaluation of isoflurane: cardiac arrythmias. *Can Anesth Soc J* 1982;29:528–34.

196 Willats DG, Harrison AR, Groom JF, Crowther A. Cardiac arrhythmias during outpatient dental anaesthesia: comparison of halothane with enflurane. *Br J Anaesth* 1983;55:399–403.

197 Atlee JL III, Bosnjak ZL. Mechanisms for cardiac dysrhythmias during anesthesia. *Anesthesiology* 1990;72:347–74.

198 Atlee JL III, Brownlee SW, Burstrom BS. Conscious state comparisons of the effects of inhalation anesthetics on specialized atrioventricular conduction times in dogs. *Anesthesiology* 1986;64:703–10.

199 Atlee JL III, Rusy BF, Kreul JF, Eby T. Supraventricular excitability in dogs during anesthesia with halothane and enflurane. *Anesthesiology* 1978;48:407–13.

200 Ozaki S, Grokoh Y, Nakaya M, Azuma M, Kanno M. Electrophysiological effects of enflurane and isoflurane on isolated rabbit hearts in the presence and absence of metabolic acidosis. *Anesth Analg* 1985;64:1060–4.

201 Bosjnak ZL, Kampine JP. Effects of halothane, enflurane and isoflurane on the SA node. *Anesthesiology* 1983;58:314–18.

202 Lynch C III, Vogel S, Sperelakis N. Halothane depression of myocardial slow action potentials. *Anesthesiology* 1981;55:360–8.

203 Lynch C III. Effects of halothane and isoflurane on isolated ventricular myocardium. *Anesthesiology* 1988;68:429–32.

204 Bosjnak ZJ, Supan FD, Rusch NJ. The effects of halothane, enflurane, and isoflurane on calcium current in isolated canine ventricular cells. *Anesthesiology* 1991;74:340–5.

205 Drenger B, Quigg M, Blanck TJJ. Volatile anesthetics depress calcium channel blocker binding to bovine cardiac sarcolemma. *Anesthesiology* 1991;74:155–65.

206 Lee DL, Zhang J, Blanck TJJ. The effects of halothane on voltage-dependent calcium channels in isolated Langendorff-perfused rat heart. *Anesthesiology* 1994;81:1212–20.

207 Lynch C III. Are volatile anesthetics really calcium entry blockers? *Anesthesiology* 1984;61:644–6.

208 Nakao S, Hirata H, Yagawa Y. Effects of volatile anesthetics on cardiac calcium channels. *Acta Anaesthesiol Scand* 1989;33:326–30.

209 Puttick RM, Terrar DA. Effects of propofol and enflurane on action potentials, membrane currents and contraction of guinea-pig isolated ventricular myocytes. *Br J Pharmacol* 1992;107:559–65.

210 Carceles MD, Mirailles FS, Laorden ML, Hernandez J. Interactions between diltiazem and inhalation anaesthetics in the isolated heart. *Br J Anaesth* 1989;63:321–5.

211 Kapur PA, Bloor BC, Flacke WE, Olewine SK. Comparison of cardiovascular responses to verapamil during enflurane, isoflurane or halothane anesthesia in the dog. *Anesthesiology* 1984;61:156–60.

212 Katsuaka M, Ohnishi ST. Inhalation anaesthetics decrease calcium content of cardiac sarcoplasmic reticulum. *Br J Anaesth* 1989;62:669–73.

213 Iwatsuki N, Katoh M, Ono K, Amaha K. Antiarrhythmic effect of diltiazem during halothane anesthesia in dogs and in humans. *Anesth Analg* 1985;64:964–70.

214 Turner LA, Bosnjak ZJ, Kampine JP. Actions of halothane on the electical activity of Purkinje fibers observed from normal and infarcted canine hearts. *Anesthesiology* 1987;67:619–29.

215 Ozaki S, Nakaya M, Grokoh Y, Azuma M, Kimmotsa O, Kanno M. Effects of halothane and enflurane on conduction velocity and maximum rate of rise action potential upstroke in guinea pig papillary muscles. *Anesth Analg* 1989;68:219–25.

216 Turner LA, Marijic J, Kampine JP, Bosnjak ZJ. A comparison of the effects of halothane and tetrodotoxin on the regional repolarization characteristics of canine Purkinje fibers.

101

Anesthesiology 1990;73:1158–68.

217 Burt JM, Spray DC. Volatile anesthetics block intercellular communications between neonatal rat myocardial cells. *Circ Res* 1989;65:829–37.

218 Terrar DA, Victory JGG. Influence of halothane on electrical coupling in cell pairs isolated from guinea pig ventricle. *Br J Pharmacol* 1988;94:509–14.

219 Freeman LC, Muir III WW. Effects of halothane on impulse propagation in Purkinje fibers and at Purkinje-muscle junctions: relationship of V_{max} to conduction velocity. *Anesth Analg* 1991;72:5–10.

220 Gallagher JD, Gessman LJ, Nowa P, Kerns D. Electrophysiologic effects of halothane and quinidine on canine cardiac Purkinje fibers: evidence for a synergetic interaction. *Anesthesiology* 1986;65:278–85.

221 Aya GM, Robert E, de La Coussaye JE, Juan JM, Dauzat M, Eledjam JJ. Ventricular electrophysiological and arrhythmogenic effects of enflurane in isolated perfused rabbit hearts. *Br J Anaesth* 1996;76:A135.

222 Gallagher JD. The electrophysiologic effects of amiodarone and halothane on canine Purkinje fibers. *Anesthesiology* 1991;75:106–12.

223 Rooney RT, Stowe DF, Marijic J, Kampine JP, Bosnjak ZJ. Additive depressant effects of amiodarone given with halothane in isolated hearts. *Anesth Analg* 1991;72:474–81.

224 Freeman LC, Li Q. Effects of halothane on delayed afterdepolarization and calcium transients in dog ventricular myocytes exposed to isoproterenol. *Anesthesiology* 1991;74:146–54.

225 Gallagher JD. Effects of isoflurane on ouabain toxicity in canine Purkinje fibers. Comparison with halothane. *Anesthesiology* 1994;81:1500–10.

226 Zuckerman RL, Wheeler DM. Effect of halothane on arrhythmogenic responses induced by sympathomimetic agents in single rat heart cells. *Anesth Analg* 1991;72:596–603.

227 Freeman LC, Muir III WW. Alpha-adrenoceptor stimulation in the presence of halothane: effects on impulse propagation in cardiac Purkinje fibers. *Anesth Analg* 1991;72:11–17.

228 Laszlo A, Polic S, Atlee III JL, Kampine JP, Bosnjak ZJ. Anesthetics and automaticity in latent pacemaker fibers: I. Effects of halothane, enflurane and isoflurane on automaticity and recovery of automaticity from overdrive suppression in Purkinje fibers derived from canine hearts. *Anesthesiology* 1991;75:98–105.

229 Laszlo A, Polic S, Kampine JP, Turner LA, Atlee III JL, Bosnjak ZJ. Halothane, enflurane, and isoflurane on abnormal automaticity and triggered rhythmic activity on Purkinje fibers from 24-hour-old infarcted canine hearts. *Anesthesiology* 1991;75:847–53.

230 Gallagher JD, McClernam CA. The effects of halothane on venticular tachycardia in intact dogs. *Anesthesiology* 1991;75:98–105.

231 Ebert JP, Pearson JD, Gelman S, Harris C, Bradley EL. Circulatory responses to laryngoscopy: the comparative effects of placebo, fentanyl and esmolol. *Can J Anaesth* 1989;36:301–6.

232 Black TE, Kay B, Mealy TEJ. Reducing the haemodynamic responses to laryngoscopy and intubation. A comparison of alfentanil with fentanyl. *Anaesthesia* 1984;39:883–7.

233 Bovill JG, Sebel PS, Stanley T. Opioid analgesics in anesthesia with special reference to their use in cardiovascular anesthesia. *Anesthesiology* 1984;61:731–55.

234 Kirby IZ, Northwood D, Dodson ME. Modification by alfentanil of the haemodynamic response to tracheal intubation in elderly patients. A dose response study. *Br J Anaesth* 1988;60:384–7.

235 Podolakin W, Wells DI. Precipitous bradycardia induced by laryngoscopy in cardiac surgical patients. *Can J Anaesth* 1987;34:618–21.

236 Royster RL, Keeler DK, Haisty WK, Johnston WE, Prough DS. Cardiac electrophysiologic effects of fentanyl and combination of fentanyl and neuromuscular relaxants in pentobarbital anesthetized dogs. *Anesth Analg* 1988;67:15–20.

237 Romero M, Laorden ML, Hernandez J, Serrano JS. Effects of morphine on isolated right atria of the rat. *Gen Pharmacol* 1992;23:1135–8.

238 Blair JR, Pruett JK, Crumnine RS, Balser JS. Prolongation of QT interval in association with the administration of large doses of opiates. *Anesthesiology* 1987;67:442–3.

239 Blair JR, Pruett JK, Introna RPS, Adams RJ, Balser JS. Cardiac electrophysiologic effects of fentanyl and sufentanil in canine cardiac Purkinje fibers. *Anesthesiology*

1989;**71**:565–70.
240 Saini V, Carr DB, Hagestad BL, Lown B, Verrur RL. Antifibrillatory action of the narcotic agonist fentanyl. *Am Heart J* 1988;**115**:598–605.
241 Rabkin SW. Morphine and the endogenous opioid dynorphin in the brain attenuate digoxin-induced arrhythmias in guinea pigs. *Pharmacol Toxicol* 1992;**71**:353–60.
242 Alarcon S, Hernandez J, Laorden M. Effects of morphine: an electrophysiological study on guinea-pig papillary muscle. *J Pharm Pharmacol* 1992;**44**:275–7.
243 Lee AYS. Stereospecific antiarrhythmic effects of naloxone against myocardial ischemia and reperfusion in the dog. *Br J Pharmacol* 1992;**107**:1057–60.
244 Sarne Y, Flitstein A, Oppenheimer E. Antiarrhythmic activities of opioid agonists and antagonists and their stereoisomers. *Br J Pharmacol* 1991;**102**:696–8.
245 Griffin RM, Dimich I, Jurado R, Kaplan JA. Haemodynamic effects of diltiazem during fentanyl-nitrous oxyde anaesthesia. An *in vivo* study in the dog. *Br J Anaesth* 1988;**60**:655–9.
246 Schmeling WT, Kampine JP, Watier DC. Negative chronotropic actions of sufentanil and vecuronium in chronically instrumented dogs pretreated with propranolol and or diltiazem. *Anesth Analg* 1989;**69**:4–14.
247 Deam BK, Soni N. Effects of pipecuronium and pancuronium on the isolated rabbit heart. *Br J Anaesth* 1989;**62**:287–9.
248 Jacobs HK, Salem NR, Rao TLK, Mathru M, Smith BD. Cardiac electrophysiologic effects of pancuronium. *Anesth Analg* 1985;**64**:693–9.
249 Lienhart A, Guggiari M, Tauvent A, Maneglia R, Cousin MT, Viars P. Effets hémodynamiques du bromure de vécuronium chez l'homme. *Ann Fr Anesth Réanim* 1983;**2**:7–13.
250 Marshall RJ, McGrath JC, Miller RD, Docherty JR, Lamar JC. Comparison of the cardiovascular actions of org NC 45 with those produced by other non-depolarizing neuromuscular blocking agents in experimental animals. *Br J Anaesth* 1980;**52**:21S–32S.
251 Narita M, Furukawa Y, Ren LM *et al.* Cardiac effects of vecuronium and its interaction with autonomic nervous system in isolated perfused canine hearts. *J Cardiovasc Pharmacol* 1992;**19**:1000–8.
252 Clayton JC. Asystole associated with vecuronium. *Br J Anaesth* 1986;**58**:937–8.
253 Starr NJ, Sethna DH, Estafanous FG. Bradycardia and asystole following the rapid administration of sufentanil with vecuronium. *Anesthesiology* 1986;**64**:521–3.
254 Urquhart ML, Ramsey FM, Royster RL, Morell RS, Gerr P. Heart rate and rhythm disturbances following an edrophonium/atropine mixture for antagonism of neuromuscular blockade during fentanyl N_2O/O_2 or isoflurane N_2O/O_2 anesthesia. *Anesthesiology* 1987;**67**:561–5.
255 Duarant NN, Nguyen N, Katz RL. Potentiation of neuromuscular blockade by verapamil *Anesthesiology* 1984;**60**:298–303.
256 Ferrick KJ, Power M. Profound exacerbation of neuromuscular weakness by flecainide. *Am Heart J* 1990;**119**:414–15.
257 Boucher M, Dubray C, Li JH, Paire M, Duchene-Marullaz P. Influence of pentobarbital and chloralose anesthesia on quinidine-induced effects on atrial refractoriness and heart rate in the dog. *J Cardiovasc Pharmacol* 1991;**17**:199–206.
258 Komai H, Rusy BF. Calcium and thiopental-induced spontaneous activity in rabbit papillary muscle. *J Mol Cell Cardiol* 1986;**18**:73–9.
259 Alphin RS, Martens JR, Dennis DM. Frequency-dependent effects of propofol on atrioventricular nodal conduction in guinea pig isolated heart. Mechanism and potential antidysrhythmic properties. *Anesthesiology* 1995;**83**:382–94.
260 Pinto JMB, Kirby DA, Johnson DA, Lown B. Diazepam administered prior to coronary artery occlusion increases latency to ventricular fibrillation. *Life Sci* 1991;**49**:587–94.
261 Tanaka H, Habuchi Y, Nishimura M, Sato N, Watanabe Y. Blockade of Na+ current by promethazine in guinea-pig ventricular myocytes. *Br J Pharmacol* 1992;**106**:900–5.
262 Tisdale JE, Kambe JC, Chow MSS, Yeston NS. The effects of haloperidol on ventricular fibrillation threshold in pigs. *Pharmacol Toxicol* 1991;**69**:327–9.
263 Gomez-Arnau J, Marquez-Montes J, Avello F. Fentanyl and droperidol effects on refractoriness of the accessory pathway in the Wolff–Parkinson–White syndrome. *Anesthesiology* 1983;**58**:307–13.

264 Liu WS, Wong KC, Port JD, Andriano KP. Epinephrine-induced arrhythmias during halothane anesthesia with the addition of nitrous oxide, nitrogen, or helium in dogs. *Anesth Analg* 1982;**61**:414–17.

265 Roizen MF, Plummer GO, Lichtor JL. Nitrous oxide and dysrhythmias. *Anesthesiology* 1987;**66**:427–31.

266 Eledjam JJ, Laracine M, de La Coussaye JE *et al*. Effets de la lidocaine aux concentrations plasmatiques obtenues par voie péridurale sur les troubles de la conduction auriculo-ventriculaire. *Ann Fr Anesth Réanim* 1984;**3**:61–2.

267 Coriat P, Harari A, Ducardonnet A, Tarot JP, Viars P. Risk of heart block during extradural anaesthesia in patients with right bundle branch block and left anterior hemiblock. *Br J Anaesth* 1981;**53**:545–8.

268 Eledjam JJ, de La Coussaye JE, Colson P *et al*. Is epidural anaesthesia using bupivacaine safe in patients with atrio-ventricular conduction defects? *Acta Anaesthesiol Scand* 1989;**33**:402–4.

269 Castle NA. Bupivacaine inhibits the transient outward K$^+$ current but not the inward rectifier in rat ventricular myocytes. *J Pharmacol Exp Ther* 1990;**255**:1038–46.

270 Courtney KR, Kendig JJ. Bupivacaine is an effective potassium channel blocker in the heart. *Biochim Biophys Acta* 1988;**939**:163–6.

271 de La Coussaye JE, Massé C, Bassoul BP, Eledjam JJ, Gagnol JP, Sassine A. Bupivacaine-induced slow-inward current inhibition: a voltage clamp study on frog atrial fibres. *Can J Anaesth* 1990;**37**:819–22.

272 de La Coussaye JE, Eledjam JJ, Brugada J *et al*. Les bêta bloquants aggravent-ils la cardiotoxicité de la bupivacaïne? Etude expérimentale. *Ann Fr Anesth Réanim* 1990;**9**:132–6.

273 Howie MB, Mortimer W, Candler EM, McSweeney TD, Frolicher DA. Does nifedipine enhance the cardiovascular depressive effects of bupivacaine? *Reg Anesth* 1989;**14**:19–25.

274 Timour Q, Freycz M, Couzon P *et al*. Possible role of drug interactions in bupivacaine-induced problems related to intraventricular conduction disorders. *Reg Anesth* 1990;**15**:180–5.

275 Edouard AR, Berdeaux A, Ahmad R, Samii K. Cardiovascuar interactions of local anesthetics and calcium entry blockers in conscious dogs. *Reg Anesth* 1991;**16**:95–100.

276 Scheinman MM. Proarrhythmia and primum non nocere. *J Am Coll Cardiol* 1989;**14**:216–17.

277 Anderson JL. Should complex ventricular arrhythmias in patients with congestive heart failure be treated? A protagonist's viewpoint. *Am J Cardiol* 1990;**66**:447–50.

278 Kulick DL, Bhandari AK, Hong R, Petersen R, Leon C, Rahimtoola SH. Effect of acute hemodynamic decompensation on electrical inducibility of ventricular arrhythmias in patients with dilated cardiomopathy and complex nonsustained ventricular arrhythmias. *Am Heart J* 1990;**119**:878–83.

279 Podrid PJ, Wilson S. Should asymptomatic ventricular arrhythmias in patients with congestive heart failure be treated? An antagonists's viewpoint. *Am J Cardiol* 1990;**66**:451–7.

280 Podrid PJ, Tordjman Fuchs T. Left ventricular dysfunction and ventricular arrhythmias: reducing the risk of sudden death. *J Clin Pharmacol* 1991;**31**:1096–104.

281 Pratt CM, Eaton T, Francis M *et al*. The inverse relationship between baseline left ventricular ejection fraction and outcome of antiarrhythmic therapy: a dangerous imbalance in the risk–benefit ratio. *Am Heart J* 1989;**118**:433–40.

282 Libersa C, Caron J, Guedon-Moareau L, Adamantidis M, Nisse C. Adverse cardiovascular effects of antiarrhythmic drugs. Part II: Inotropic effects and specific pharmacokinetic properties. *Therapie* 1992;**47**:199–203.

283 Wilson JR. Use of antiarrhythmic drugs in patients with heart failure: clinical efficacy, hemodynamic resuts, and relation to survival. *Circulation* 1987;**75**(Suppl IV):64–73.

284 Leblanc N, Hume JR. Sodium current-induced release of calcium from cardiac sarcoplasmic reticulum. *Science* 1990;**248**:372–5.

285 de La Coussaye JE, Bassoul BP, Albat B *et al*. Experimental evidence in favor of role of intracellular actions of bupivacaine in myocardial depression. *Anesth Analg* 1992;**74**:698–702.

286 Eledjam JJ, de La Coussaye JE, Brugada J *et al*. *In vitro* study on mechanisms of

bupivacaine-induced depression of myocardial contractility. *Anesth Analg* 1989;**69**:732–5.

287 Garlid KD, Nakashima RA. Studies on the mechanism of uncoupling by amine local anesthetics: evidence for mitochondrial proton transport mediated by lipophilic ion pairs. *J Biol Chem* 1983;**258**:7974–80.

288 Seipel L, Hoffmeister HM. Hemodynamic effects of antiarrhythmic drugs: negative inotropy versus influence of peripheral circulation. *Am J Cardiol* 1989;**64**:37J–40J.

289 Frumin H, Behrens S, Martyn R, Goldberg MJ, Rubenfire M, Kerin N. Hemodynamic effects of antiarrhythmic drugs. *J Clin Pharmacol* 1991;**31**:1070–80.

290 Gottlieb SS, Kukin ML, Medina N, Yushak M, Packer M. Comparative hemodynamic effects of procainamide, tocainide, and encainide in severe chronic heart failure. *Circulation* 1990;**81**:860–4.

291 Hartzell HC, Mery PF, Fischmeister R, Szabo G. Sympathetic reguation of cardiac calcium current is due exclusively to cAMP-dependent phosphorylation. *Nature* 1991;**351**:573–6.

292 Nattel S, Jing W. Rate-dependent changes in intraventricular conduction produced by procainamide in anesthetized dogs. A quantitative analysis based on the relation between phase 0 inward current and conduction velocity. *Circ Res* 1989;**65**:1485–98.

293 Anderson KP, Walker R, Lux RL *et al*. Conduction velocity depression and drug-induced ventricular tachyarrhythmias. Effects of lidocaine in the intact canine heart. *Circulation* 1990;**81**:1024–38.

294 Gay R, Algeo S, Lee R, Olajos M, Morkin E, Goldman S. Treatment of verapamil toxicity in intact dogs. *J Clin Invest* 1986;**77**:1805–11.

295 Wyse DG, Morganroth J, Ledingham R *et al*. New insights into the definition and meaning of proarrhythmia during initiation of antiarrhythmic drug therapy from the Cardiac Arrhythmia Suppression Trial and its pilot study. The CAST and CAPS Investigators. *J Am Coll Cardiol* 1994;**23**:1130–40.

296 Stanton MS, Prystowsky EN, Fineberg NS, Miles WM, Zipes DP, Heger JJ. Arrhythmogenic effects of antiarrhythmic drugs: a study of 506 patients treated for ventricular tachycardia or fibrillation. *J Am Coll Cardiol* 1989;**14**:209–15.

297 Levy MN, Wiseman MN. Electrophysiologic mechanisms for venticular arrhythmias in left ventricular dysfunction: electrolytes, catecholamines and drugs. *J Clin Pharmacol* 1991;**31**:1053–60.

298 Brugada J, Boersma L, Kirchhof C, Allessie MA. Proarrhythmic effects of flecainide: experimental evidence for increased susceptibility to reentrant arrhythmias. *Circulation* 1991;**84**:1808–18.

299 Brugada J, Boersma L, de La Coussaye JE, Allessie M. Mechanisms of the proarrhythmic effects of flecainide and related antiarrhythmic drugs. *N Trends Arrhythmias* 1992;**7**:353–8.

300 Lee JH, Rosen MR. Use-dependent actions and effects on transmembrane action portentials of flecainide, encainide, and ethmozine in canine Purkinje fibers. *J Cardiovasc Pharmacol* 1991;**18**:285–92.

301 Krishnan SC, Antzelevitch C. Flecainide-induced arrhythmia in canine ventricular epicardium. Phase 2 reentry? *Circulation* 1993;**87**:562–72.

302 Robert E, Bruelle P, de La Coussaye JE *et al*. Electrophysiologic and proarrhythmogenic effects of therapeutic and toxic doses of imipramine; a study with high resolution ventricular epicardial mapping in rabbit hearts. *J Pharmacol Exp Ther* 1996;**278**:170–8.

303 Anderson JL, Platia EV, Hallstrom A *et al*. for the Cardiac Arrhythmia Suppression Trial (CAST) Investigators. Interaction of baseline characteristics with the hazard of encainide, flecainide, and moricizine therapy in patients with myocardial infarction. A possible explanation for increased mortality in the Cardiac Arrhythmia Suppression Trial (CAST). *Circulation* 1994;**90**:2843–52.

304 Morganroth J. Early and late proarrhythmia from antiarrhythmic drug therapy. *Cardiovasc Drug Ther* 1992;**6**:11–14.

305 Pfammater JP, Paul T, Lehmann C, Kallfelz HC. Efficacy and proarrhythmia of oral sotalol in pediatric patients. *J Am Coll Cardiol* 1995;**26**:1002–7.

306 Jaillon P, Drici M. Recent antiarrhythmic drugs. *Am J Cardiol* 1989; **64**: 65J–69J.

307 Stratmann HG, Kennedy HL. Torsades de pointes associated with drugs and toxins:

recognition and management. *Am Heart J* 1987;**113**:1470–82.

308 Antzelevitch C, Sicouri S. Clinical relevance of cardiac arrhythmias generated by afterdepolarizations. Role of M cells in the generation of U waves, triggered activity and torsade de pointes. *J Am Coll Cardiol* 1994;**23**:259–77.

309 Charpentier F, Drouin E, Gauthier C, Le Marec H. Early after/depolarizations and triggered activity: mechanisms and autonomic regulation. *Fund Clin Pharmacol* 1993;**7**:39–49.

310 Davidenko JM, Cohen L, Goodrow R, Antzelevitch C. Quinidine-induced action potential prolongation, early afterdepolarizations, and triggered activity in canine Purkinje fibers. Effects of stimulation rate, potassium, and magnesium. *Circulation* 1989;**79**:674–86.

311 El-Sherif N, Bekheit SS, Henkin R. Quinidine-induced long QTU interval and torsades de pointes: role of bradycardia-dependent early afterdepolarizations. *J Am Coll Cardiol* 1989;**14**:252–7.

312 Liu TF. Early afterdepolarization in myocardium and its clinical implications. *Meth Find Exp Clin Pharmacol* 1992;**14**:157–63.

313 Weissenberger J, Davy J-M, Chézalviel F. Experimental models of torsades de pointes. *Fund Clin Pharmacol* 1993;**7**:29–38.

314 Roden DM. Risks and benefits of antiarrhythmic therapy. *N Engl J Med* 1994;**331**:785–91.

315 Wyse KR, Ye V, Campbell TJ. Action potential prolongation exhibits simple dose-dependence for sotalol, buta reverse dose-dependence for quinidine and disopyramide: implications for proarrhythmia due to triggered activity. *J Cardiovasc Pharmacol* 1993;**21**:316–22.

316 Sasyniuk BI, Valois M, Toy W. Recent advances in understanding the mechanisms of drug-induced torsades de pointes arrhythmias. *Am J Cardiol* 1989;**64**:29J–32J.

317 Kadish AH, Weisman HF, Vettri EP, Epstein AE, Slepian MJ, Levine JH. Paradoxical effects of exercise on the QT interval in patients with polymorphic ventricular tachycardia receiving type Ia antiarrhythmic agents. *Circulation* 1990;**81**:14–19.

318 Myerburg RJ, Kessler KM, Cox MM *et al.* Reversal of proarrhythmic effects of flecainide acetate and encainide hydrochloride by propranolol. *Circulation* 1989;**80**:1571–9.

319 Fish FA, Gillette PC, Benson DW. The Pediatric Electrophysiology Group. Proar-rhythmia, cardiac arrest and death in young patients receiving encainide and flecainide. *J Am Coll Cardiol* 1991;**18**:356–65.

320 Coplen SE, Anatman EM, Berlin JA, Hewitt P, Chalmers TC. Efficacy and safety of quinidine therapy for maintenance of sinus rhythm after cardioversion. A meta-analysis of randomized control trials. *Circulation* 1990;**82**:1106–16.

321 Aronow WS, Mercando AD, Epstein S, Kronzon I. Effect of quinidine or procainamide versus no antiarrhythmic drug on sudden cardiac death, total cardiac death, and total death in elderly patients with heart disease and complex ventricular arrhythmias. *Am J Cardiol.* 1990;**66**:423–8.

322 Jackman WM, Wang X, Friday KJ *et al.* Catheter ablation of accessory atrioventricular pathways (Wolff–Parkinson–White syndrome) by radiofrequency current. *N Engl J Med* 1991;**324**:1605–11.

323 Kottkamp H, Hindricks G, Chen X *et al.* Radiofrequency catheter ablation of sustained ventricular tachycardia in idiopathic dilated cardiomyopathy. *Circulation* 1995;**92**:1159–68.

324 Wood MA, Simpson PM, London WB *et al.* Circadian pattern of ventricular tachyarrhythmias in patients with implantable cardioverter–defibrillators. *J Am Coll Cardiol* 1995;**25**:901–7.

325 Nunain SO, Roelke M, Trouton T *et al.* Limitations and late complications of third-generation automatic cardioverter-defibrillators. *Circulation* 1995;**91**:2204–13.

326 Wever EF, Hauer RN, van Capelle FL *et al.* Randomized study of implantable defibrillator as first-choice therapy versus conventional strategy in postinfarct sudden death survivors. *Circulation* 1995;**91**:2195–203.

327 Zhu DW, Maloney JD, Simmons TW *et al.* Radiofrequency catheter ablation for management of symptomatic ventricular ectopic activity. *J Am Coll Cardiol* 1995;**26**:843–9.

328 Woosley RL. Anatiarrhythmic drugs. *Annu Rev Pharmacol Toxicol* 1991;**31**:427–55.
329 O'Kelly B, Browner WS, Massie B, Tubau J, Ngo L, Mangano DT. The Study of Perioperative Ischemia Research Group. Ventricular arrhythmias in patients undergoing noncardiac surgery. *JAMA* 1992;**268**:217–21.
330 Krukemyer JJ, Boudoulas H, Binkley PF, Lima JJ. Comparison of hypersensitivity to adrenergic stimulation after abrupt withdrawal of propranolol and nadolol: influence of half-life differences. *Am Heart J* 1990;**120**:572–9.

5: Alpha$_2$-adrenoceptor agonists

PIERRE-LOUIS DARMON, FRANCIS BONNET

Introduction

For many years, α_2-adrenoceptor agonists have been used principally as hypotensive drugs. They have numerous other properties, stemming from their various interactions with physiological regulation. Indeed, besides their haemodynamic effects, α_2-adrenoceptor agonists can also induce sedation and analgesia. These effects can be considered either as main or side effects depending on the action sought. During the past decade, α_2-adrenergic agonists have been used increasingly in anaesthesia because of their sympatholytic cardiovascular properties. This review will focus on these properties and their clinical implications.

Structural characteristics and pharmacokinetics of α_2-agonists

Alpha$_2$-agonists can be categorised into three main classes: phenyl-ethylamines (for example, methyldopa or guanabenz), imidazolines (for example, clonidine, dexmedetomidine, mivazerol or azepexole) and oxalo-zepines (for example, rilmenidine). Clonidine is considered as the reference drug; it has been identified as a partial agonist, having a 200-fold selectivity for α_2- over α_1- adrenergic receptors. Clonidine is rapidly and almost completely absorbed after oral administration, begins to act after 15–20 minutes and reaches peak plasma concentrations within 60–90 minutes, corresponding to its maximal activity.[1,2] Clonidine bioavailability is close to 70–80%; it is lipid-soluble with a large distribution volume (2 l/kg). It is partly metabolised by the liver into inactive metabolites, and the remainder is excreted unchanged by the kidney. The elimination half-life of clonidine ranges between 12 and 24 hours.[2-4] Guanabenz is a less potent and a shorter-acting substance since it has a shorter (6 hours) half-life.[5] Dexmedetomidine is a highly selective α_2-adrenoceptor agonist having a ten-fold selectivity over clonidine.[6] Dexmedetomidine is the D-enantiomer and active component of medetomidine, a drug used in veterinary anaesthesia. In Europe, dexmedetomidine is in phase III clinical trials for perioperative use. Mivazerol is a highly specific and selective α_2-agonist with an imidazoline structure and possesses myocardial anti-ischaemic activity. Some of the α_2-adrenoceptor agonists have the imidazole ring that enables them to bind to non-adrenergic receptors, with varying haemodynamic effects.[7,8]

Mechanisms of action

Identification of α_2-adrenoceptors

Alpha$_2$-adrenoceptors were identified from the α-adrenoceptor group originally because of their presynaptic site, as opposed to the postsynaptic position of α_1-receptors.[9] They induce a re-uptake of the noradrenaline that is released in the synaptic space during nerve stimulation. There is evidence of post- as well as extra-synaptic locations of α_2-adrenoceptors,[10] so that the classification based on the anatomical location could not be sustained. As more selective α-adrenoceptor antagonists became available, a new pharmacological classification was developed; α_1-adrenoceptors are those antagonised by prazosin, whereas α_2-receptors are antagonised by yohimbine. Alpha$_2$-adrenoceptors were subsequently divided into different categories: α_{2A}-receptors have a higher chemical affinity for rauwolscine than α_{2B}-receptors.[11] A third category, the α_{2C}-receptor, has a high affinity for rauwolscine with an affinity for yohimbine that is intermediate between those of α_{2A}- and α_{2B}-receptors.[12] These categories of α_2-adrenoceptors have their genetic codes located on chromosome II, IV, and X, which are respectively named α_2C_2, α_2C_4, and α_2C_{10}.[13-15]

Cellular effects of α_2-adrenoceptor agonists

Alpha-2 adrenoceptors are transmembrane helicoid proteins presenting an external site which is the agonist binder, and an internal portion associated with a G$_i$ protein by means of reversible links. G proteins are made of three different subunits (α, β, δ) and can be coupled with the α_2-adrenoceptor by the α unit. The α subunit has a single high-affinity binding site for guanine nucleotides and possesses an intrinsic guanosine triphosphatase (GTPase) activity. In the inactive state, the binding site of the α_2-receptor is unoccupied and the α subunit of the G protein is bound by GDP. When the adrenoceptor binds an α_2-agonist, a conformational change occurs in the α subunit of the G protein, and the affinity for GDP decreases; in the presence of Mg^{2+}, GDP is released and replaced by GTP. The GTP-bound α subunit of the G protein dissociates from the adrenoceptor and couples to the effector.

There are five effector mechanisms that are activated by the stimulated

109

α_2-receptor: inhibition of the adenylate cyclase, acceleration of Na^+/H^+ exchange, activation of K^+ channels, inhibition of voltage-sensitive Ca^{2+} channels and modulation of the phosphatidyl inositol turnover. These mechanisms induce a decrease in intracellular cAMP and Ca^{2+}, and generate membrane hyperpolarisation.[16, 17] Alpha₂ adrenoceptors are located in many tissues, including kidney, platelets, bladder, bowel walls, vascular walls, and both central and peripheral nervous systems. High densities of α_2-adrenoceptor binding sites have been found in the central as well as peripheral nervous system. Stimulation of those receptors modifies control mechanisms of vigilance, systemic arterial pressure, heart rate, thermoregulation, muscular tone, and nociceptive perception.

Alpha₂-adrenoceptors and cardiovascular control

Alpha₂-adrenoceptors involved in cardiovascular control are located both in the peripheral and central nervous systems. When stimulated, those sited in the peripheral system, on arteriolar endothelium and on the postjunctional site of vascular smooth muscle, produce vasoconstriction.[18] This peripheral activity explains episodes of transient hypertension following rapid intravenous injection of clonidine, and counteract the vasodilatation induced by the central activity. The overall effect of α_2 adrenergic agonists on the coronary circulation is vasodilatation resulting from opposite peripheral and central activities. The peripheral effects consist of arteriolar vasoconstriction,[19, 20] whereas central activity produces vasodilatation by adenosine and/or NO release,[21, 22] and by metabolic modifications following the α_2-agonist-induced reduction in left ventricular work.

Adrenergic neurones of the central nervous system (CNS) are involved in cardiovascular regulatory mechanisms; stimuli coming from arterial (aortic arch and carotid sinus) baroreceptors are routed via the glossopharyngeal and vagal nerves to the nucleus tractus solitarii (NTS) which is located in the medulla oblongata.[23] Excitatory messages go from the NTS to the dorsal motor nucleus of the vagus nerve from which efferent parasympathetic neurones are activated to decrease heart rate. In addition, the NTS has spinal projections in the C1 area which is located in the rostral ventrolateral medulla, and contains preganglionic sympathetic neurones. The NTS addresses inhibitory impulses to the C1 area that cause inhibition of the sympathetic outflow delivered to the heart, the blood vessels and the adrenal medulla.[24] Stimulation of α_2-adrenoceptors located in the NTS strengthens this inhibitory activity.[25] Alpha₂-agonists, such as clonidine, act within the CNS to increase the gain of the baroreceptor reflex,[26] thus resetting the system so that arterial pressure and heart rate are maintained at a lower level.[27] However, the hypotensive effects of imidazolines, such as clonidine or dexmedetomidine, could be generated by receptors other than the α_2-adrenoceptors.[28]

High densities of α_2-adrenergic receptor binding sites are located on the preganglionic sympathetic neurones of the intermedio-lateral horn of the thoracic spinal cord.[29] At this level, the preganglionic neurones are connected with monoaminergic and catecholinergic neurones originating from the cardiovascular regulatory core which is located in the medulla oblongata.[30, 31] Their sympathetic activity is depressed by local α_2-agonists, which accounts for the hypotensive mechanisms of clonidine.[32-34] Neostigmine counteracts the spinal clonidine-induced hypotension by increasing the number of acetylcholine quanta released from the cholinergic neurones that activate preganglionic sympathetic neurones.[35]

In summary, α_2-adrenergic agonists reduce sympathetic tone but maintain baroreflex responses,[36, 37] predominantly by means of their activity on the CNS. Decreased sympathetic and increased parasympathetic outflows cause lessened adrenergic activity, hypotension, and bradycardia.

Haemodynamic effects of α_2-adrenergic agonists

In young and healthy volunteers, antiadrenergic effects of α_2-agonists are manifested by a significant decrease in plasma concentrations of catecholamines,[38, 39] associated with bradycardia and mild hypotension.[38, 40] Episodes of sinoauricular block following oral dexmedetomidine have been demonstrated in this population, possibly because of its high α_2 selectivity combined with the high level of parasympathetic tone usually encountered in young people. Bradycardia can be treated by atropine, but high doses are sometimes necessary.[41] Adrenergic agents, such as ephedrine, easily counteract the clonidine-induced hypotension and generate an amplified vasoconstrictive response due to the α_2-agonist-induced enhancement of the baroreceptor reflex gain.[42] Nevertheless, transient hypertension, due to stimulation of peripheral vascular receptors, can be observed following rapid intravenous injection of an α_2-agonist.[43]

Alpha$_2$-adrenergic agonists produce decreases in cardiac output, total peripheral resistance, venous return, and myocardial contractility.[44, 45] Reduction in myocardial contractility is related to the reduction in sympathetic tone, and can be deleterious in patients with depressed myocardial function, which relies on a high level of sympathetic tone.[46] However, no direct depressant effect of α_2-adrenergic agonists can be demonstrated in the isolated heart.[47]

The effects of α_2-agonists on the coronary vascular bed are complex and depend upon its anatomical and functional properties. For example, an intracoronary injection of clonidine prevents the sympathetic initiation and aggravation of experimental post-stenotic myocardial ischaemia.[48, 49] However, the overall impact of α_2-agonists on myocardial oxygen balance results from the opposite effects: reduction in myocardial oxygen demand (due to central antiadrenergic activity) and a decrease in coronary perfusion pressure (due to hypotension). Indeed, significant hypotension can reduce coronary blood flow and lead to regional myocardial ischaemia.[50] In a recent animal study, mivazerol reduced myocardial oxygen demand while preserving coronary blood flow, particularly in the inner layers of the ischaemic myocardium.[51]

Sedative effects of α_2-adrenergic agonists

Lowering of CNS catecholamine concentrations induced by α_2-adrenergic agonists produces sedation. The locus coeruleus, which is located in the caudal portion of the fourth ventricle, is the principal cerebral region for the regulation between sleep and arousal.[52] Spontaneous activity of this nucleus is related closely to the state of sleep or wakefulness, with its lowest activity corresponding to paradoxical sleep.[52] Stimulation of α_2-adrenoceptors located in the locus coeruleus induces sedation and sleep.[53–56] Stimulation of α_1-adrenoceptors antagonises the α_2-mediated sedative effect; the sedative effect induced by clonidine is briefer and less potent than that induced by dexmedetomidine.[56] This α_2-sedative effect is mediated by a G protein and consists of hyperpolarisation of the potassium channels.[57] Calcium channels also interfere with the regulatory mechanisms of vigilance because the hypnotic effect induced by clonidine is potentiated by concomitant administration of calcium-channel blockers.[58–60] The activity of α_2-agonists on the locus coeruleus accounts for their anaesthetic-sparing effect and their relevance in opioid withdrawal syndrome.

Analgesic effects of α_2-adrenergic agonists

Alpha$_2$-adrenergic agonists produce analgesia through stimulation of specific receptors located in the dorsal horn of the spinal cord. Depression of the activity of wide dynamic range neurones evoked by stimulation of Aδ and C fibres has been documented after spinal administration. Several animal and human studies have confirmed the analgesic effects of α_2-agonists, during both acute[1] and chronic pain syndromes. Furthermore, α_2-adrenergic receptor stimulation potentiates the analgesic effects of opioids.[22] Oral, transdermal, and intravenous administration of α_2-agonists all induce perioperative analgesia, explaining part of their anaesthetic-sparing effect.

Clinical applications of α_2-adrenergic agonists

It has been known for a long time that abrupt discontinuation of clonidine treatment after prolonged administration may induce a syndrome consisting of severe hypertension, anxiety, headache, nausea and/or vomiting, and possible myocardial ischaemia responsible for myocardial infarction.[61, 62] This 'rebound' syndrome is not expected to occur when α_2-agonists are used only briefly in the perioperative period.

Interactions with anaesthetic agents: sparing effect

Alpha$_2$-adrenergic agonists are used for premedication because of their anxiolytic and sedative properties.[63-67] The classical clonidine doses administered for this goal vary from 2 to 5 µg/kg. A reduction in anaesthetic requirements has been reported consistently by all authors.[63-79] Theoretically, this anaesthetic sparing effect could be attributed to the sedative and/or haemodynamic properties of α_2-agonists because anaesthetic agents are usually administered on the basis of an increased heart rate and/or arterial pressure. However, Ghignone and colleagues have demonstrated that the clonidine-induced sparing effect was still observed when anaesthetic agents were titrated against reduced electroencephalographic activity during induction of anaesthesia.[78] In addition to sedative and haemodynamic properties, a reduction in anaesthetic requirements could also be explained by pharmacokinetic interactions; clonidine prolongs the elimination half-life of opioid drugs and results in, for example, a 60% increase in plasma alfentanil concentration.[68]

In addition to their anaesthetic-sparing effect, α_2-agonists can modify the common cardiovascular consequences of anaesthetic agents, particularly when they are administered simultaneously with sympathetic stimulating drugs such as ketamine[80, 81] or, more recently, desflurane.[82] Intravenous injection of ketamine following administration of clonidine in dogs decreases CNS sympathetic outflow, and results in significant reductions in cardiac output and myocardial contractility that can be attributed to unmasking of the intrinsic negative inotropic effect of ketamine.[80] When patients receive clonidine as part of their premedication, a 30–40% decrease of the tachycardia and hypertension associated with administration of desflurane is observed.[82] Only few interactions have been observed with propofol or etomidate.[80] When administered in association with fentanyl, dexmedetomidine increases the incidence of bradycardia.[83] Despite cardiovascular interactions, α_2-agonists are often well tolerated haemodynamically because they allow a reduction in anaesthetic doses as a result of their sparing effect.

Perioperative haemodynamic stability

Since α_2-adrenergic agonists induce a decrease in CNS sympathetic outflow, their perioperative use could reduce the incidence of episodes of tachycardia and hypertension that may lead to myocardial ischaemia. The first study was conducted in cardiac surgery, with patients receiving a dose of 2–300 µg clonidine as premedication, and repeated 5 hours later.[73] Clonidine administration reduced plasma concentrations of noradrenaline before induction of anaesthesia as well as during the course of surgery. In patients receiving clonidine, arterial pressure and heart rate were significantly lower on arrival in the operating room, after skin incision, and after sternotomy. Sternotomy was responsible for an increase in systemic vascular resistance that was not observed in the patients who received clonidine. In addition, cardiac output was higher in the clonidine group, presumably because of the clonidine-induced reduction in afterload. These results have been confirmed in high-risk patients scheduled for cardiac[84] and non-cardiac surgery.[75, 76] Similar results have been observed using pre- and/or peroperative administration of dexmedetomidine that was responsible for a 20% decrease in arterial pressure.[66, 85, 86] Studies focused on tracheal intubation have demonstrated that laryngoscopy-induced tachycardia and hypertension were prevented by premedication using clonidine or dexmedetomidine,[63, 87, 88] although the effect of clonidine was incomplete in cases of sustained stimulation during tracheal intubation.[89]

All these data suggest that α_2-adrenergic agonists should be useful to obviate haemodynamic instability and myocardial ischaemia in high-risk surgical patients.[90] However, although the mean values of arterial pressure and heart rate were lower in patients receiving clonidine premedication, the relative variations of these values throughout the perioperative period were not demonstrated to be significantly different.[77, 91] Thus, if clonidine can prevent tachycardia and hypertension, episodes of hypotension are frequently observed and may be responsible for myocardial ischaemia by themselves. In addition, the elimination half-life of clonidine is long which might be a disadvantage if prolonged hypotension results, even if episodes of bradycardia or hypotension are easily treated. In a recent study,[92] the incidence of bradycardia requiring atropine administration was 44% in patients receiving perioperative dexmedetomidine, confirming previous reports.[93] Finally, since all published studies rely on small sample sizes, α_2-agonists have not yet been demonstrated conclusively to reduce perioperative myocardial ischaemia or cardiovascular morbidity in high-risk surgical patients.

Kent and colleagues found a shorter duration of ischaemic events in a small series of patients scheduled for coronary artery bypass grafting who received premedication of clonidine 200 µg.[94] In a similar series of cardiac surgery patients, Quintin and colleagues, and Dorman and colleagues reported a clonidine-induced reduction in the total number of episodes of ST-depression indicative of ischaemia.[95, 96] Fulgencio and colleagues obtained comparable results in vascular surgery patients who received epidural clonidine.[97] Conversely, in a series of 61 patients scheduled for major, non-cardiac surgery who received transdermal clonidine or placebo, Ellis and colleagues could not find any difference in the total number of patients exhibiting ECG modifications indicative of myocardial ischaemia.[98] Lipszyc and colleagues did not find a difference in the total number of episodes of ST-depression in carotid surgery patients receiving premedication of clonidine 4 μg/kg.[99] However, in that study, ischaemic events were noticed particularly during tachycardic or hypertensive episodes in the control group, whereas myocardial ischaemia occurred usually during hypotension in the clonidine-treated group. In a preliminary study of vascular surgery patients,[92] perioperative dexmedetomidine did not reduce the occurrence of ischaemic events. However, the sample size of that study was small ($n=24$) and it is not possible to reach a negative conclusion regarding failure of dexmedetomidine to prevent myocardial ischaemia in the perioperative period.

The recovery time is characterised by an increase in sympathetic activity associated with a high incidence of myocardial ischaemia. During that period, frequent shivering episodes are noticed which generate increases in left ventricular work and myocardial oxygen consumption. Since α_2-agonists reduce the adrenergic, metabolic, and haemodynamic responses to shivering,[100–102] they could decrease the incidence of myocardial ischaemia related to that specific mechanism.[44, 103, 104] This would imply that administration of α_2-agonists should be repeated, without limiting their use to the preoperative period.

Other cardiovascular properties of α_2-adrenergic agonists

Alpha₂-adrenergic agonists have antiarrhythmic properties. Dexmedetomidine prevents the adrenaline-induced arrhythmias observed with halothane;[105] clonidine reduces the systemic toxicity of intravenous bupivacaine and augments its toxicity threshold in respect of ventricular arhythmias.[106–108]

Clonidine and dexmedetomidine reduce acute cocaine toxicity; in laboratory animals, clonidine premedication decreases mortality, episodes of seizure and haemodynamic collapse after cocaine administration.[109, 110] Cocaine is known to increase heart rate, arterial pressure, end-systolic and end-diastolic left ventricular pressures, and myocardial oxygen consumption. All these haemodynamic alterations are partly attenuated by dexmedetomidine except for that on systemic vascular resistance, which is augmented.[111] In addition, dexmedetomidine antagonises cocaine-related coronary artery vasoconstriction.[111]

Alpha₂-adrenergic agonists also diminish cerebral blood flow, presumably by reducing cerebral oxygen consumption.[112, 113] A beneficial effect of α_2-agonists on cerebral ischaemia has been suspected and demonstrated experimentally. Several pathophysiological mechanisms could be involved: prevention of the hypertensive episodes following cerebral ischaemia, or cellular effects associated with inactivation of NMDA receptors and the resulting inhibition of NO synthesis.[114–116] These properties could offer new therapeutic indications for α_2-adrenergic agonists, particularly in patients at risk for cerebral ischaemia (for example during carotid artery surgery).

115

Summary and conclusions

Alpha$_2$-adrenergic agonists possess a number of proved applications and have several potential clinical uses in the anaesthesiology field, but suffer from side effects that restrict their utilisation. They could be considered as the reference sympathoadrenolytic agents in every pathological condition where excessive sympathoexcitation is involved.[40] However, precise guidelines regarding their use remain to be defined. Development of new selective agents that can dissociate between sedative, analgesic, and haemodynamic effects should facilitate their perioperative use and allow a more precise definition of indications.

1 Bonnet F, Boico O, Rostaing S, Loriferne JF, Saada M. Clonidine-induced analgesia in post-operative patients: epidural versus intramuscular administration. *Anesthesiology* 1990;**72**:423–27.
2 Arndts D, Stähle H, Förster HJ. Development of a RIA for clonidine and its comparison with the reference methods. *J Pharmacol Methods* 1981;**6**:295–307.
3 Arndts D. New aspects of the clinical pharmacology of clonidine. *Chest* 1983;**83**:397–400.
4 Arndts D, Doevendans KR, Heintz B. New aspects of the pharmacokinetics and pharmacodynamics of clonidine in man. *Eur J Clin Pharmacol* 1983;**24**:21–30.
5 Scheinin H, Virtanen R, MacDonald E, Lammintausta R, Scheinin M. Medetomidine – a novel α_2-adrenoceptor agonist: a review of its pharmacodynamic effects. *Progr Neuropsychopharmacol Biol Psychiatr* 1989;**13**:635–51.
6 Virtanen R, Savola JM, Saano V, Nyman L. Characterization of the selectivity, specificity and potency of metedomidine, an α_2-adrenoceptor agonist. *Eur J Pharmacol* 1988;**150**:9–14.
7 Ernsberger P, Meeley MP, Mann JJ, Reis DJ. Clonidine binds to imidazoline binding sites as well as α_2-adrenoceptors in the ventrolateral medulla. *Eur J Pharmacol* 1987;**134**:1–13.
8 Tibirica E, Feldman J, Mermet C, Gonen F, Bousquet P. An imidazoline-specific mechanism for the hypotensive effect of clonidine. A study with yohimbine and idazoxan. *J Pharmacol Exp Ther* 1991;**256**:606–13.
9 Van Zwieten PA, Timmermans PB. Central and peripheral α-adrenoceptors. Pharmacological aspects and clinical potential. *Adv Drug Res* 1979;**13**:221–53.
10 Drew GM. Effect of α-adrenoceptors agonists and antagonists on pre- and post-synaptically located α-adrenoceptors. *Eur J Pharmacol* 1976;**36**:313–20.
11 Michel AD, Loury DN, Whiting RL. Assessment of imiloxan as a selective α_{2B}-adrenoceptor antagonist. *Br J Pharmacol* 1990;**99**:560–4.
12 Murphy TJ, Bylund DB. Characterization of α_2-adrenergic receptors in the OK cell, and opossum kidney cell line. *J Pharmacol Exp Ther* 1988;**244**:571–8.
13 Kobilka BK, Matsui H, Kobilka TS *et al.* Cloning, sequencing and expression of the gene coding for the human platelet α_2-adrenergic receptor. *Science* 1987;**238**:650–6.
14 Lomasney JW, Lorenz W, Allen LF *et al.* Expansion of the α_2-adrenergic receptor family: cloning and characteriztion of a human α_2-adrenergic receptor subtype, the gene for which is located on chromosome 2. *Proc Natl Acad Sci USA* 1990:**87**:5094–8.
15 Regan JW, Kobilka TS, Yang-Freng TL *et al.* Cloning and expression of the human kidney cDNA for an α_2-adrenergic receptor subtype. *Proc Natl Acad Sci USA* 1988;**85**:6301–5
16 Limbird LE. Receptors linked to inhibition of adenylcyclase: additional signaling mechanisms. *FASEB J* 1988;**2**:2686–95.
17 Codina J, Yatani A, Grenet D. The a subunit of the GTP binding protein Gk opens atrial potassium channels. *Science* 1987;**236**:442–5.
18 Sakakibara Y, Fujiwara M, Maramatsu I. Pharmacological characterization of the α-adrenoceptors of the dog basilar artery. *Naunyn Schmiedbergs Arch Pharmacol*

1982;**319**:1–7.

19 Woodam DL, Vatner SF. Coronary vasoconstriction mediated by α_1- and α_2-adrenoceptors in conscious dogs. *Am J Physiol* 1987;**253**:H388–H393.

20 Heusch G, Deussen A, Schippfke T, Thämer V. Alpha$_1$- and α_2-adrenoceptor mediated vasoconstriction of large and small coronary arteries *in vivo*. *J Cardiovasc Pharmacol* 1984;**6**:961–8.

21 Coughlan MG, Lee JG, Bosnjak ZJ, Schmeling WT, Kampine JP, Warltier DC. Direct coronary and cerebral vascular responses to dexmedetomidine: significance of endogenous nitric oxide synthesis. *Anesthesiology* 1992;**77**:998–1006.

22 Solomon RE, Gebhart GF. Intrathecal morphine and clonidine: antinociceptive tolerance and cross-tolerance and effects on blood pressure. *J Pharmacol Exp Ther* 1988;**245**:444–54.

23 Reis DJ, Granata AR, Joh TH. Brain stem catecholamine mechanisms in tonic and reflex control of blood pressure. *Hypertension* 1984;**II**(Suppl):87–93.

24 Reis DJ, Morrison SM, Ruggiero D. The C1 area of the brainstem in tonic and reflex control of blood pressure. *Hypertension* 1988;**11**:8–13.

25 Kubo T, Misu Y. Pharmacological characterisation of the α-adrenoreceptor responsible for a decrease of blood pressure in the nucleus tractus solitarii of the rat. *Naunyn Schmiedebergs Arch Pharmacol* 1981;**317**:120–5.

26 Kitagawa H, Walland A. Augmentation of vagal reflex bradycardia by central α_2-adrenoceptors in the cat. *Naunyn Schmiedebergs Arch Pharmacol* 1982;**321**:44–7.

27 Harron DWG, Riddell JG, Shanks RG. Effects of azepexole and clonidine on baroreceptor mediated reflex bradycardia and physiological tremor in man. *Br J Clin Pharmacol* 1985;**20**:431–6.

28 Ernsberger PR, Meeley MP, Mann JJ, Reis DJ. Clonidine binds to imidazole binding sites as well as α_2-adrenoceptors in the ventrolateral medulla. *Eur J Pharmacol* 1988;**134**:1–14.

29 Seybold VS, Elde RP. Receptor autoradiography in thoracic spinal cord: correlation of neurotransmitters binding sites with sympathoadrenal neurons. *J Neurosci* 1984;**4**:2533–42.

30 Fuxe K, Tinner B, Bjelke B. Monoaminergic and peptidergic innervation of the intermedio-lateral horn of the spinal cord: I Distribution patterns of nerve terminal networks. *Eur J Neurosci* 1990;**2**:430–50

31 Fuxe K, Tinner B, Bjelke B. Monoaminergic and peptidergic innervation of the intermedio-lateral horn of the spinal cord: II. Relationship to preganglionic sympathetic neurons. *Eur J Neurosci* 1990;**2**:451–60.

32 Eisenach JC, Tong C. Site of hemodynamic effects of intrathecal α_2-adrenergic agonists. *Anesthesiology* 1991;**74**:766–71.

33 Guyenet PG, Cabot JB. Inhibition of sympathetic preganglionic neurons by catecholamines and clonidine: mediation by an α_2-adrenergic receptor. *J Neurosci* 1981;**1**:908–17.

34 Calvillo O, Ghignone M. Presynaptic effect of clonidine on unmyelinated afferent fibers in the spinal cord of the cat. *Neurosci Letter* 1986;**64**:335–9

35 Williams JS, Tong C, Eisenach JC. Neostigmine counteracts spinal clonidine-induced hypotension in sheep. *Anesthesiology* 1993;**78**:301–7.

36 Muzi M, Goff DR, Kampine JP, Roerig DL, Ebert TJ. Clonidine reduces sympathetic activation but maintains baroreflex responses in normotensive humans. *Anesthesiology* 1992;**77**:864–71.

37 Walland A, Kobinger W, Csongrady A. Action of clonidine on baroreceptor reflexes in conscious dogs. *Eur J Pharmacol* 1974;**26**:184–90.

38 Kallio A, Scheinin M, Koulu M *et al.* Effects of dexmedetomidine, a selective α_2-adrenoceptor agonist, on hemodynamic control mechanisms. *Clin Pharmacol Ther* 1989;**46**:33–42.

39 Scheinin H, Karhuvaara S, Olkkola KT *et al.* Pharmacodynamics and pharmacokinetics of intramuscular dexmedetomidine. *Clin Pharmacol Ther* 1992;**52**:537–46.

40 Flacke JW, Flacke WE. Clonidine prevention of myocardial ischemia: will this change outcome? *J Cardiothorac Anesth* 1993;**7**:383–5.

41 Nishikawa T, Dohi S. Oral clonidine blunts the heart rate response to intravenous

117

atropine in humans. *Anesthesiology* 1991; **75**:217–22.

42 Nishikawa T, Kimura T, Taguchi N, Dohi S. Oral clonidine preanesthetic medication augments the pressor responses to intravenous ephedrine in awake or anesthetized patients. *Anesthesiology* 1991;**74**:705–10.

43 Savola JM, Ruskohaho H, Puurunen J, Salonen JS, Karki NT. Evidence for metedomidine as a selective and potent agonist at α_2-adrenoceptor. *J Auton Pharmacol* 1986;**5**:275–84.

44 Proctor LT, Schmeling WT, Roerig D, Kampine JP, Warltier DC. Oral dexmedetomidine attenuates hemodynamic responses during emergence from general anesthesia in chronically instrumented dogs. *Anesthesiology* 1991;**74**:108–14.

45 Brest AN. Haemodynamic and cardiac effect of clonidine. *J Cardiovasc Pharmacol* 1980;**2**:S39–S46.

46 Abi-Jaoude F, Brusset A, Ceddaha A, Schlumberger S, Dubois C, Fischler M. Clonidine premedication for coronary artery bypass grafting under high dose alfentanil anesthesia: intraoperative hemodynamic study. *J Cardiothorac Vasc Anesth* 1993;**7**:35–40.

47 Flacke WE, Flake JW, Blow K, McIntee DF, Bloor BC. Effect of dexmedetomidine, an α_2-adrenergic agonist, in the isolated heart. *J Cardiothorac Vasc Anesth* 1992;**6**:418–23.

48 Seitelberger R, Guth BD, Heusch G. Intracoronary α_2-adrenergic blockade attenuates ischemia in conscious dogs during exercise. *Circ Res* 1988;**62**:436–42.

49 Heusch G, Schipke J, Thämer V. Clonidine prevents the sympathetic initiation and aggravation of poststenotic myocardial ischemia. *J Cardiovasc Pharmacol* 1985;**7**:1176–82.

50 Kono M, Morita S, Hayashi T, Saitoh M, Fuke N, Rubsamen R. The effects of intravenous clonidine on regional myocardial function in a canine model of regional myocardial ischemia. *Anesth Analg* 1994;**78**:1047–52.

51 Roekaerts PMHJ, Prinzen FW, Willigers HMM, De Lange S. The effects of α_2-adrenergic stimulation with mivazerol on myocardial blood flow and function during coronary artery stenosis in anesthetized dogs. *Anesth Analg* 1996;**82**:702–11.

52 Aston-Jones G, Chiang C, Alexinsky T. Discharge of noradrenergic locus coeruleus neurons in behaving rats and monkeys suggests a role in vigilance. In: Barnes CD, Pompeiano O. *Neurobiology of the locus coeruleus. Progress in Brain Research*. Amsterdam: Elsevier, 1991;**88**:187–95.

53 Angel A, Majeed ABA. Alterations of 'sleeping time' in the rat induced by drugs which modulate central monoaminergic systems. *Br J Anaesth* 1990;**64**:594–600.

54 Correa-Sales C, Rabin BC, Maze M. A hypnotic response to dexmedetomidine, an α_2-agonist, is mediated in the locus coeruleus in rats. *Anesthesiology* 1992;**76**:948–52.

55 Doze VA, Chen BX, Maze M. Dexmedetomidine produces a hypnotic-anesthetic action in rats via activation of central α_2-adrenoceptors. *Anesthesiology* 1989;**71**:75–9.

56 De Sarro GB, Asciotic F, Libri V, Nistico G. Evidence that locus coeruleus is the site where clonidine and drugs acting at α_1- and α_2-adrenoceptors affect sleep and arousal. *Br J Pharmacol* 1987;**90**:675–85.

57 Doze VA, Chen B X, Tinklenberg JA, Maze M. Pertussis toxin and 4-amidopyridine differential affect the hypnotic-anesthetic action of dexmedetomidine and pentobarbital. *Anesthesiology* 1990;**73**:304–7.

58 Horvath G, Benedek G, Szikszay M. Enhancement of fentanyl analgesia by clonidine plus verapamil in rats. *Anesth Analg* 1990;**70**:284–8.

59 Horvath G, Szikszay M, Benedek G. Calcium channels are involved in the hypnotic-anesthetic action of dexmedetomidine in rats. *Anesth Analg* 1992;**74**:884–8.

60 Horvath G, Szikszay M, Benedek G. Potentiated hypnotic action with a combination of fentanyl, a calcium channel blocker and an α_2-agonist in rats. *Acta Anaesthesiol Scand* 1992;**36**:170–4.

61 Berge KH, Lanier WL. Myocardial infarction accompanying acute clonidine withdrawal in a patient without a history of ischemic coronary artery disease. *Anesth Analg* 1991;**72**:259–61.

62 Bruce DL, Croley TF, Lee JS. Preoperative clonidine withdrawal syndrome. *Anesthesiology* 1979;**51**:90–2.

63 Aanta RE, Kanto JH, Scheinin M *et al.* Dexmedetomidine premedication for minor gynecologic surgery. *Anesth Analg* 1990;**70**:407–13.

64 Aanta R, Aakola ML, Kallio A, Kanto J, Scheinin M, Vuorinen JA. A comparison of dexmedetomidine, an α_2-adrenoceptor agonist and midazolam as IM premedication for minor gynaecological surgery. *Br J Anaesth* 1991;**647**:402–9.

65 Aanta R, Kanto J, Scheinin M. Intramuscular dexmedetomidine, a novel α_2-adreno-ceptor agonist, as premedication for minor gynaecological surgery. *Acta Anaesthesiol Scand* 1991;**35**:283–8.

66 Aanta RE, Kanto JH, Scheinin M, Kallio AM, Scheinin H. Dexmedetomidine, an α_2-adrenoceptor agonist, reduces anesthetic requirements for patients undergoing minor gynecologic surgery. *Anesthesiology* 1990;**73**:230–5.

67 Kallio A, Salonen M, Forssell H, Scheinin H, Scheinin M, Tuominen J. Medetomidine premedication in dental surgery – a double-blind cross-over study with a new α_2-adrenoceptor. *Acta Anaesthesiol Scand* 1990;**34**:171–5.

68 Richards MJ, Skues MA, Prys-Roberts APJ. Total IV anaesthesia with propofol and alfentanil: dose requirements for propofol and the effect of premedication with clonidine. *Br J Anaesth* 1990;**65**:157–63.

69 Jaakola ML, Kanto J, Scheinin H, Kallio A. Intramuscular dexmedetomidine premedica-tion – an alternative to midazolam fentanyl combination in elective hysterectomy? *Acta Anaesthesiol Scand* 1994;**38**:238–43.

70 Filos, KS, Patroni O, Goudas CC, Bosas O, Kassaras A, Guartanis S. A dose–response study of orally administered clonidine as premedication in the elderly: evaluating hemodynamic safety. *Anesth Analg* 1993;**77**:1185–92.

71 Scheinin H, Jaakola ML, Sjövall S, Ali-Melkkliä T, Kaukinen S, Turunen J, Kanto J. Intramuscular dexmedetomidine as premedication for general anesthesia. *Anesthesiology* 1993;**78**:1065–75.

72 Mikawa K, Mackawa N, Nishina K, Takao Y, Yaku H, Obara H. Efficacy of oral cloni-dine premedication in children. *Anesthesiology* 1993;**79**:926–31.

73 Flacke JW, Bloor BC, Flacke WE *et al.* Reduced narcotic requirements by clonidine with improved hemodynamic and adrenergic stability in patients undergoing coronary bypass surgery. *Anesthesiology* 1987;**67**:11–19.

74 Segal IS, Jarvis DJ, Duncan SR, White PF, Maze M. Clinical efficacy of oral-transdermal clonidine combination during the perioperative period. *Anesthesiology* 1991;**74**:220–5.

75 Ghignone M, Calvillo O, Quintin L. Anesthesia and hypertension: the effect of clonidine on perioperative hemodynamics and isoflurane requirements. *Anesthesiology* 1987;**67**:3–10.

76 Quintin L, Bonnet F, Macquin I, Szekely B, Becquemin JP, Ghignone M. Aortic surgery: effect of clonidine on intraoperative catecholaminergic and circulatory stability. *Acta Anaesthesiol Scand* 1990;**34**:132–7.

77 Engelman E, Lipszyc M, Gilbart E, *et al.* Effects of clonidine on anesthetic drug requirements and hemodynamic response during aortic surgery. *Anesthesiology* 1989;**71**:178–87.

78 Ghignone M, Noe C, Calvillo O, Quintin L. Anesthesia for ophthalmic surgery in the elderly: the effects of clonidine on intraocular pressure, perioperative hemodynamics, and anesthetic requirements. *Anesthesiology* 1988;**68**:707–16.

79 Bellaiche S, Bonnet F, Sperandio M, Lerouge P, Cannet G, Roujas F. Clonidine does not delay recovery from anaesthesia. *Br J Anaesth* 1991;**66**:353–7.

80 Proctor LY, Schmeling WT, Warltier DC. Premedication with oral clonidine alters hemodynamic action of intravenous anesthetic agents in chronically instrumented dogs. *Anesthesiology* 1992;**77**:554–62.

81 Doak GJ, Duke PC. Oral clonidine premedication attenuates the haemodynamic effects associated with ketamine anaesthetic induction in humans. *Can J Anaesth* 1994;**40**:612–8.

82 Devcic A, Muzi M, Ebert TJ. The effects of clonidine on desflurane-mediated sympathoexcitation in humans. *Anesth Analg* 1995;**80**:773–9.

83 Salmenpera MT, Szlam F, Hug CC. Anesthetic and hemodynamic interactions of dexmedetomidine and fentanyl in dogs. *Anesthesiology* 1994;**80**:837–46.

84 Kulka PJ, Tryba M, Zenz M. Dose-response effects of intravenous clonidine on stress response during induction of anesthesia in coronary artery bypass graft patients. *Anesth Analg* 1995;**80**:263–8.

85 Aho M, Lehtinen AM, Erkola O, Kallio A, Korttila K. The effect of intravenously administered dexmedetomidine on perioperative hemodynamics and isoflurane requirements in patients undergoing abdominal hysterectomy. *Anesthesiology* 1991;74:997–1002.

86 Bloor BC, Ward DS, Belleville JP, Maze M. Effects of intravenous dexmedetomidine in humans: II Hemodynamic changes. *Anesthesiology* 1992;77:1134–42.

87 Carabine UA, Wright PMC, Moore J. Preanaesthetic medication with clonidine: a dose-response study. *Br J Anaesth* 1991;67:79–83.

88 Scheinin B, Lindgren L, Randell T, Schneinin H, Scheinin M. Dexmedetomidine attenuates sympathoadrenal responses to tracheal intubation and reduces the need for thiopentone and peroperative fentanyl. *Br J Anaesth* 1992;68:126–31.

89 Laurito CE, Baughman VL, Becker GL. Oral clonidine blunts the hemodynamic responses to brief but not prolonged laryngoscopy. *J Clin Anesth* 1993;5:54–7.

90 Longnecker DE. Alpine anesthesia: can pretreatment with clonidine decreases the peaks and valleys? *Anesthesiology* 1987;67:1–2.

91 Pluskwa F, Bonnet F, Saada M *et al.* Effect of clonidine on changes in blood pressure during carotid artery surgery. *J Cardiothorac Anesth* 1991;5:431–6

92 Talke P, Ii J, Jain U, Leung J, Drasner K, Hollenberg M, Mangano DT. Effects of perioperative dexmedetomidine infusion in patients undergoing vascular surgery. The study of perioperative ischemia research group. *Anesthesiology* 1995;82:620–33.

93 Scheinin H, Jaakkola MJ, Sjövall S *et al.* Intramuscular dexmedetomidine as premedication for general anesthesia. *Anesthesiology* 1993;78:1065–75.

94 Kent M, Thomsen B, Cicala R. Clonidine decreases ischemic events during coronary artery surgery. *Anesthesiology* 1990;73:A129.

95 Quintin L, Cicala R, Kent M, Thomsen B. Effect of clonidine on myocardial ischemia: a double-blind pilot trial. *Can J Anaesth* 1993;40:85–6.

96 Dorman BH, Zucker JR, Verrier ED, Gartman DM, Slachman FN. Clonidine improves perioperative myocardial ischemia, reduces anesthetic requirements, and alters hemodynamic parameters in patients undergoing coronary artery bypass surgery. *J Cardiothorac Vasc Anesth* 1993;7:386–95.

97 Fulgencio JP, Rimaniol JP, Catoire P, Bonnet F. Clonidine and postoperative myocardial ischaemia. *Can J Anaesth* 1994;41:550–1.

98 Ellis JE, Drijvers G, Pedlow S *et al.* Premedication with oral and transdermal clonidine provides safe and efficacious postoperative sympatholysis. *Anesth Analg* 1994;79:1133–40.

99 Lipszyc M, Engelman E. Clonidine does not prevent myocardial ischemia during noncardiac surgery. *Anesthesiology* 1991;75:A93.

100 Delaunay L, Bonnet F, Duvaldestin Ph. Clonidine decreases postoperative oxygen consumption in patients recovering from general anaesthesia. *Br J Anaesth* 1991;67:397–401.

101 Delaunay L, Bonnet F, Liu N, Beydon L, Catoire P, Sessler DI. Clonidine comparably decreases the thermoregulatory thresholds for vasoconstriction and shivering in humans. *Anesthesiology* 1993;79:470–4.

102 Joris J, Banache M, Bonnet F, Sessier D, Lamy M. Chlonidine and ketanserin both are effective treatment for postanesthetic shivering. *Anesthesiology* 1993;79:532–9.

103 Quintin L, Roudot-Thoraval F, Roux C *et al.* Effect of clonidine on the circulation and vasoactive hormones after aortic surgery. *Br J Anaesth* 1991;66:108–15.

104 Quintin L, Viale JP, Annat G *et al.* Oxygen uptake after major abdominal surgery: effect of clonidine. *Anesthesiology* 1991;74:236–41.

105 Hayashi Y, Sumikawa K, Maze M *et al.* Dexmedetomidine prevents epinephrine-induced arrhythmias through stimulation of central alpha-2 adrenoceptors in halothane anesthetized dogs. *Anesthesiology* 1991;75:113–17.

106 De Koch M, Le Polain B, Henin D, Vandewalle F, Scholtes JL. Clonidine pretreatment reduces the systemic toxicity of intravenous bupivacaine in rats. *Anesthesiology* 1993;79:282–9.

107 de la Coussaye J, Bassoul B, Brugada J *et al.* Reversal of electrophysiologic and hemodynamics effects induced by high doses of bupivacaine by the combination of clonidine and dobutamine in anesthetized dogs. *Anesth Analg* 1992;74:703–11.

108 De La Coussaye J, Eledjam JJ, Bassoul B *et al.* Receptor mechanisms for clonidine reversal of bupivacaine-induced impairment of ventricular conduction in pentobarbital-anesthetized dogs. *Anesth Analg* 1994;78:624–37.

109 Tella SR, Korupolu GR, Schindler CW, Goldberg SR. Pathophysiological and pharmacological mechanisms of acute cocaine toxicity in conscious rat. *J Pharmacol Exp Ther* 1992;262:936–46.

110 Derlet RW, Albertson TE. Acute cocaine toxicity: antagonism by agents interacting with adrenoceptors. *Pharmacol Biochem Behav* 1990;36:225–31.

111 Kersten J, Pagel PS, Hettrick A, Warltier DC. Dexmedetomidine partially attenuates the sympathetically mediated systemic and coronary hemodynamic effects of cocaine. *Anesth Anal* 1995;80:114–21.

112 Karlsson BR, Forsman M, Roald OK, Heir MS, Steen PA. Effect of dexmedetomidine, a selective and potent α_2-agonist, on cerebral blood flow and oxygen consumption during halothane anesthesia in dogs. *Anesth Anal* 1990;71:125–9.

113 Zornow MH, Fleischer JE, Scheller MS, Nakakimura K, Drummond JC. Dexmedetomidine, an α_2-adrenergic agonist decreases cerebral blood flow in the isoflurane-anesthetized dog. *Anesth Analg* 1990;70:624–30.

114 Hoffman WE, Cheng MA, Thomas C, Baughman VL, Albrecht RF. Clonidine decreases plasma catecholamines and improves outcome from incomplete ischemia in the rat. *Anesth Analg* 1991;73:460–4.

115 Hoffman WE, Kochs E, Werner C, Thomas C, Albrecht RF. Dexmedetomidine improves neurologic outcome from incomplete ischemia in the rat. *Anesthesiology* 1991;75:328–32.

116 Hoffman WE, Lingamneni P, Minshall R, Miletich DJ, Albrecht F. Brain α_2-adrenergic receptor binding during incomplete cerebral ischemia in the rat. *Anesth Analg* 1993;76:274–8.

Part Two

Use of cardiovascular agents in anaesthesia and intensive care

6: Treatment of intraoperative hypotension

AXEL W. GOERTZ

Intraoperative arterial hypotension is considered to be the most frequently occurring anaesthesia-related complication. In a series of 18 350 consecutive anaesthetic procedures, Schwilk and co-workers observed episodes of arterial hypotension that required therapy in 1485 cases, representing about one-quarter of all complications and an overall incidence of 8%.[1] An even higher incidence has been reported in a series of patients receiving spinal anaesthesia.[2] Carpenter et al. observed a decrease in systolic arterial pressure to 90 mmHg or below in 33% of 1000 patients.

In a minority of patients, intraoperative hypotension may be due to a severe chronic or subacute impairment of cardiovascular function such as decompensated cardiac failure or septic shock; these are usually patients who have been treated in an intensive care unit and who present, for example, for emergency laparotomy or for tracheostomy. Invasive monitoring techniques are usually used to guide continuous cardiovascular therapy in these patients. Isotropes and vasopressors or even vasodilators are employed not only to restore organ perfusion pressure but also to optimise oxygen delivery and consumption. The intraoperative care for these patients typically means a continuation of intensive care therapy, using the same monitoring devices and treatment regimens (Figure 6.1).

There are numerous other chronic diseases that may be associated with arterial hypotension and orthostatic syncope. These relatively rare conditions include diseases of the autonomic nervous system (for example, Shy–Drager syndrome, Riley–Day syndrome, peripheral neuropathies) as well as endocrine disorders (for example, Addison's disease). The perioperative care of these patients may require invasive monitoring in order to optimise intravascular volume status. In some cases, continuous administration of sympathomimetics may be necessary.

The great majority of patients suffering from episodes of intraoperative hypotension, however, show well-compensated cardiovascular function preoperatively. In these patients, causes of intraoperative hypotensive episodes can be attributed to:

- anaesthesia;
- the surgical procedure;
- an acute impairment of the patient's condition.

Factors that are related to anaesthesia may be direct or indirect influences of anaesthetic drugs on cardiac contractility, peripheral vascular tone and integrity of cardiovascular reflex mechanisms. Examples of factors related to the surgical procedure are head-up positioning of the patient, intra-operative bleeding, pneumoperitoneum or intraoperative release of vasoactive substances, such as in 'mesenteric traction syndrome'. The most frequently occurring factor attributable to the patient's condition other than chronic disease is intravascular volume depletion. Typically, a combination of several factors is responsible for the hypotensive episode. Obviously, a patient who receives extensive spinal blockade for a procedure that requires head-up positioning is likely to develop some degree of hypotension. Often, such hypotensive episodes are transient in nature. In some cases, however, the hypotension may be of a magnitude that requires rapid intervention. An intravenous bolus injection of a vasopressor or inotrope is generally used for treatment. Without data from invasive monitoring techniques, changes of arterial pressure are most often used to

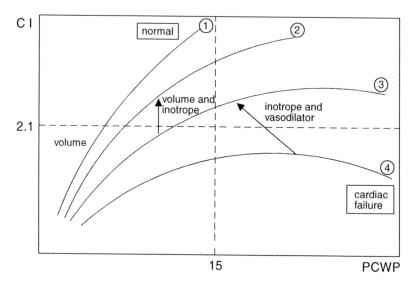

Fig 6.1 Data from invasive monitoring guide therapy in patients with severe impairment of left ventricular function. Cardiac function curves – relationship between cardiac index (CI) and pulmonary capillary wedge pressure (PCWP) – are shown in patients with normal (1), moderately (2), and severely altered (3) left ventricular function. In patients with severe cardiac failure (4), a combination of drugs is often needed to produce satisfactory correction of states of hypotension, hypoperfusion, and venous congestion

guide therapy. Here we will discuss the adrenergic substances that are frequently administered as an intravenous bolus and give a rationale for their use in the following typical clinical situations:

- Hypotension during epidural or spinal anaesthesia.
- Hypotension induced by a volatile anaesthetic.
- Intraoperaive postural hypotension.
- Mesenteric traction syndrome as an example for the intraoperative release of vasoactive substances.

Frequently used substances

Phenylephrine

Phenylephrine is probably one of the substances most frequently used to restore arterial pressure intraoperatively. It is administered usually as an intravenous bolus of $1-2$ μg/kg. Its mechanism of action is predominantly a vasopressor effect mediated via α_1-adrenergic receptors. The use of phenylephrine has been proposed in a wide range of clinical situations, including various forms of general anaesthesia,[3] epidural anaesthesia,[4] and combinations of both.[5] The use of phenylephrine has even been reported during epidural anaesthesia for a caesarean section.[6] During cardiac surgery, phenylephrine has been employed to restore coronary perfusion pressure, particularly in patients with coronary artery disease[7] and those with aortic stenosis.[8] There has been a recent debate about the use of phenylephrine in the presence of severe coronary artery disease. The continuous infusion of phenylephrine or intravenous bolus injection may lead to severe increases of left ventricular wall stress associated with a decrease in cardiac output (Figure 6.2).[3, 9, 10] Smith and associates observed the development of left ventricular wall motion abnormalities in response to phenylephrine infusion, that were believed to indicate myocardial ischaemia.[9]

Ephedrine

Like phenylephrine, ephedrine has gained widespread use. Most often it is employed in the treatment of hypotension during epidural or spinal anaesthesia. Ephedrine has direct and indirect stimulating properties on adrenergic α- and β-receptors.[11, 12] The mechanism of its indirect effect is believed to be central nervous stimulation, peripheral postsynaptic noradrenaline release and, possibly, an inhibition of neuronal noradrenaline reuptake.[12, 13] The effect of ephedrine on arterial pressure is based on an increase of cardiac output, which is the result of positive inotropism[11, 12] and an increase of left ventricular preload due to constriction of venous capacitance vessels.[14] There appears to be some controversy about the effect of ephedrine on systemic vascular resistance. Systemic vascular resistance

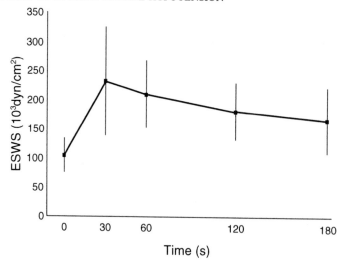

Fig 6.2   Time course of left ventricular end-systolic wall stress (ESWS) following intravenous bolus administration of phenylephrine (1 μg/kg) given to patients with severe coronary artery disease and normal left ventricular function to restore arterial pressure. The diagram shows a transient but severe increase in left ventricular end-systolic wall stress which outlasted the effect on arterial pressure. Note the large variability of values, indicating that some individuals are particularly susceptible to a sudden rise in left ventricular afterload. (Modified from Goertz *et al.*, 1993[10])

has been reported to be increased,[12, 14–16] unchanged[6] or even reduced[11, 12, 18] in response to ephedrine. There is some indication that there is a biphasic action, with an initial decrease in systemic vascular resistance due to predominant β-adrenergic stimulation, followed by an increase in systemic vascular resistance back to normal caused by α-receptor stimulation.[16, 17]

Similarly, the influence of ephedrine on heart rate is the subject of some debate.[13] In our experience, moderate cardioacceleration can be expected under most circumstances. It might be of particular interest that ephedrine appears to normalise regional perfusion of the splanchnic area, which is impaired during epidural anaesthesia.[15]

Etilefrine

Like ephedrine, etilefrine is a combined α- and β-receptor stimulant which increases cardiac output. Its influence on systemic vascular resistance is a moderate increase and, as with ephedrine, the time course of systemic vascular resistance may be biphasic.[16] Both substances appear to be equally suited to counteract the haemodynamic consequences of epidural[16] or spinal anaesthesia.[18] In contrast to ephedrine, however, the effect of etilefrine on venous capacitance vessels appears to be relatively small.[19–21]

Norfenefrine

The haemodynamic effects of norfenefrine are similar to those of phenylephrine, with the main mechanism of action being an α-receptor-mediated increase in systemic vascular resistance.[16, 19] In response to the increase in arterial pressure, there are baroreceptor reflex-mediated decreases in heart rate and cardiac output. The effect of norfenefrine following intravenous bolus injection seems to be less sustained compared to ephedrine or etilefrine.[16]

Angiotensin

Although a commercial preparation of angiotensin II has been available for clinical use since the early 1960s it has never gained widespread use. Angiotensin II increases systemic vascular resistance and arterial pressure by a direct effect on arteriolar tone. Compared to noradrenaline it has a more pronounced ability to produce splanchnic vascular constriction while reducing muscle blood flow to a lesser degree.[22] The administration of angiotensin has been advocated in situations of profound hypotension due to low systemic vascular resistance which proves refractory to conventional vasopressor therapy. These situations include hypotension caused by angiotensin-converting enzyme (ACE) inhibitor therapy[23] and hypotension secondary to therapy with the antiarrhythmic agent amiodarone.[24] In partricular, ACE inhibitor or amiodarone therapy in patients undergoing prolonged cardiopulmonary bypass (CPB) may cause profound hypotension during and after CPB which has been shown to be reversed effectively using an infusion of angiotensin at a rate of 6–7 µg/min.[23, 24]

Clinical applications

Hypotension during central neural blockade

It has long been recognised that spinal and epidural anaesthesia may have major influences on cardiovascular function. The degree of haemodynamic depression is known to be dependent on the extent of sympathetic block. The blockade of sympathetic outflow to capacitance and resistance vessels is compensated for by vasoconstriction in unblocked segments.[25] As a result, systemic vascular resistance usually remains within normal limits unless the upper level of a lumbar block exceeds the mid-thoracic segments.[26] It is worth noting that, even if the epidural block is confined to a few thoracic segments, a reduction in sympathetic tone in distal segments occurs.[27, 28] Usually, venous pooling occurs even with low-level lumbar epidural or spinal blocks. Unless intravascular volume is augmented, this leads to decreases of systemic venous return and cardiac preload, and consequently to reduced cardiac output. If the block includes cardiac segments, decreases in heart rate and left ventricular contractility, and a

127

further decrease in cardiac output, can be expected,[29] together with impairment of baroreceptor-reflex control of heart rate.[30]

There is relatively little information about the interaction between epidural or spinal anaesthesia and cardiopulmonary reflexes originating from receptors of the central low-pressure system. A decrease of systemic venous return induced by epidural anaesthesia or reversed Trendelenburg positioning of the patient is believed to increase the sensitivity of arterial baroreceptor reflex in such a way that the response to an increase as well as a decrease in blood pressure is augmented.[31, 32] In general, it appears that the low-pressure cardiopulmonary reflexes and arterial baroreceptor reflex interact such that the sensitivity of one is increased when the influence of the other is diminished.[33]

Finally, the systemic actions of local anaesthetic drugs must be considered. The absorption of local anaesthetic solution from the epidural space into the systemic circulation is known to be similar to that after intramuscular administration.[34] With lower plasma concentrations there may be excitatory influences on the cardiovascular system caused by central nervous stimulation. With higher plasma concentrations, depressant effects on the cardiovascular system can be expected to dominate.[35]

There have been reports of syncope and asystole during spinal anaesthesia. Some of these episodes appeared to be simply emotionally induced and 'vasovagal' in nature[36] but others required cardiopulmonary resuscitation and were associated with high mortality.[37] It has been speculated that the Bezold–Jarish reflex may be involved; left ventricular mechanoreceptors are activated when the left ventricle collapses, leading to vagal stimulation and thereby to sudden bradycardia/asystole combined with a sudden decrease in peripheral vascular tone.[38]

Numerous substances have been used to counteract the cardiovascular effects of spinal or epidural anaesthesia, including dopamine,[39] dobutamine,[40] adrenaline,[41] noradrenaline,[42] ephedrine,[5, 15, 43, 44] phenylephrine,[5, 6] methoxamine,[5, 17] isoprenaline,[41] etilefrine,[16, 20] norfenefrine,[16] theodrenaline/cafedrine,[16] amezinium,[16] and dihydroergotamine.[20] Substances with almost pure β-mimetic effects (for example isoprenaline) are obviously disadvantageous since in most cases they cannot be expected to increase arterial pressure. Substances with a predominantly vasopressor effect (like phenylephrine, methoxamine, and norfenefrine) also appear to be unsuitable in many cases; they may increase the compensatory vasoconstriction that occurs in unblocked segments and could possibly contribute to splanchnic organ hypoperfusion. In patients with high thoracic block, the use of a pure vasopressor might even be associated with an increase in left ventricular wall stress together with a transient impairment of left ventricular systolic function (Figure 6.3).[45] As a result, a further decrease in cardiac output could occur with further deterioration of organ perfusion. Substances with combined cardiostimulating and vasopressor effects (such

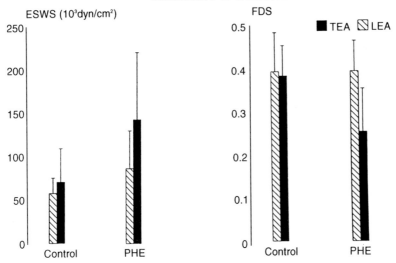

Fig 6.3 Effect of bolus administration of phenylephrine (PHE) on left ventricular end-systolic wall stress (ESWS) and fractional diameter shortening (FDS) in a group of patients with lumbar epidural anaesthesia (LEA) and a group with high thoracic epidural anaesthesia (TEA), both combined with general anaesthesia. Phenylephrine was given to restore arterial presure from hypotensive to normo-tensive values. There is an increase in left ventricular end-systolic wall stress following intravenous phenylephrine associated with a decrease in fractional diameter shortening in the patients with TEA but not in those with LEA. This was interpreted as transient impairment of left ventricular systolic function. Obviously, the use of vasopressor agents is poorly tolerated by patients with high thoracic epidural anaesthesia. Although no differences in left ventricular performance were identified before phenylephrine was given, it was speculated that cardiac con-tractility must have been reduced as a result of cardiac sympathetic block. (Modified from Lundberg et al., 1991[42])

as ephedrine) appear to be best suited. They restore arterial pressure and cardiac output at the same time, the latter mainly by augmenting venous return and by a positive inotropic action (Figure 6.4).

The arterial hypotension that occurs during epidural or spinal anaes-thesia for obstetric procedures is of particular importance. Even short episodes of hypotension may result in severe impairment of utero-placental perfusion, an effect that persists after normal blood pressure has been restored.[17] As a consequence, simple fluid administration does not appear to be sufficient once hypotension is present. Intravenous bolus injection of a substance that rapidly increases arterial pressure without increasing the vascular resistance in the utero-placental circulation is appropriate. Ephedrine, which has been used widely for this purpose, appears to be a reasonable choice.[46] There are reports of the use of phenylephrine[6] or methoxamine[17] in this setting. Although no negative influences on the

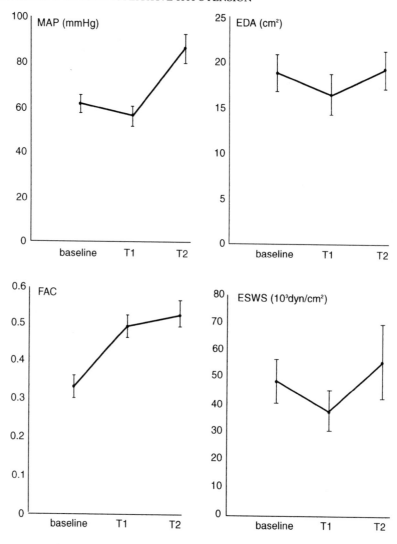

Fig 6.4 Influence of ephedrine administration on left ventricular function in hypotensive patients during high thoracic epidural anaesthesia. A biphasic action of ephedrine is shown. There are transient further decreases in mean arterial pressure (MAP), left ventricular filling measured as end-diastolic area (EDA), and left ventricular afterload measured as end-systolic wall stress (ESWS), with minimum values reached 30 s after injection (T1). This brief initial phase was followed by a sustained improvement of mean arterial pressure that was caused mainly by an increase in left ventricular global systolic function measured as fractional area change (FAC). Left ventricular pre- and afterloads (EDA and ESWS, respectively) were restored to baseline values (T2). Excessive increases of ESWS as seen following phenylephrine injection were not observed. (Modified from Goertz et al., 1993[47])

neonate's outcome have been found in these clinical studies, substances without predominant vasoconstrictor properties are preferred.

Resuscitation from astyole occurring during spinal anaesthesia may be particularly difficult. Assuming that the Bezold–Jarish reflex is the major mechanism, immediate restoration of cardiac filling appears to be crucial. Although, for obvious reasons, there are no data from controlled studies, administration of a potent vasopressor (such as noradrenaline) appears to be indicated if a high dose of atropine does not immediately restore heart rate to an acceptable level.

Hypotension induced by inhalational anaesthetics

Arterial hypotension occurring during inhaltional anaesthesia in a patient who is normovolaemic and without pre-existing cardiac disease is based principally on two mechanisms: peripheral vasodilatation and a reduction in cardiac output. Peripheral vasodilatation is a predominant feature during isoflurane or desflurane anaesthesia whereas the influence on cardiac output is minimal.[48] In contrast, halothane severely reduces cardiac output with only minor changes in peripheral vascular tone.[48] The effects of enflurane on both parameters are intermediate. It appears tempting to consider vasopressor therapy during isoflurane or desflurane anaesthesia. However, it must be noted that even these two anaesthetic agents possess considerable negative inotropic properties, although these are masked by the reduction in left ventricular afterload that occurs at the same time.[49, 50] Intravenous bolus injection of phenylephrine in patients under isoflurane-induced hypotension causes a transient reduction in left ventricular ejection faction and a decrease in cardiac output.[51] As a consequence, substances with combined α- and β-adrenergic properties (such as ephedrine, etilefrine or theodrenaline/cafedrine) should be preferred, irrespective of the volatile anaesthetic used.

Intraoperative postural hypotension

Some operative procedures require head-up positioning of the anaes-thetised patient. This is often associated with a decrease in arterial pressure which sometimes, in spite of prophylactic fluid loading, requires pharmaco-logical intervention.[52] The major mechanism of hypotension is a decrease in systemic venous return and thus decreased cardiac filling. Often the critical period is short: for example, the time between positioning of the patient and skin incision. To restore cardiac filling and blood pressure, a bolus injection of a vasopressor agent (such as phenylephrine or norfenefrine) may be appropriate (Figure 6.5).[53] If cardiac slowing is present at the same time (possibly mediated by cardiopulmonary reflexes originating from cardio-pulmonary receptors of the low-pressure system) a substance like ephedrine is preferable.

131

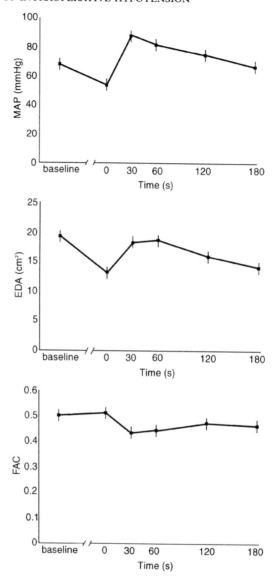

Fig 6.5 Effect of intravenous phenylephrine bolus administration on left ventricular function in patients with postural hypotension. Repositioning of an anaesthetised patient from a horizontal (baseline) to a 30-degree reverse Trendelenburg position (time 0) causes a decrease in cardiac filling measured as mean arterial pressure (MAP) and end-diatolic area (EDA). Intravenous phenylephrine restores left ventricular filling and arterial pressure without altering left ventricular systolic function measured as fractional area change (FAC). The effect is transient in nature. Pre-phenylephrine values were reached again 3 minutes following injection. (Modified from Pagel et al., 1991[50])

Mesenteric traction syndrome

Intraoperative abdominal mesenteric traction may result in considerable decreases in arterial pressure and systemic vascular resistance combined with (possibly baroreceptor-reflex-induced) increases in heart rate and cardiac output.[54] Another typical feature of mesenteric traction syndrome is a decrease in arterial oxygen partial pressure, which is believed to be secondary to increased intrapulmonary shunting.[54] These reactions are caused by a release of prostacyclin into the systemic circultion. A 30-fold increase in the plasma concentration of 6-keto-PGF$_{1\alpha}$ (a stable metabolite of prostacyclin) has been found after mesenteric traction.[55] After pretreatment with the cyclooxygenase inhibitor ibuprofen, 6-keto-PGF$_{1\alpha}$ plasma concentrations stay within normal limits and haemodynamic variables remain stable.[55] The tretment of mesenteric traction syndrome-induced hypotension can be difficult. In our experience, application of an ephedrine-type substance often results in a further increase in heart rate without sufficiently stabilising arterial pressure. Substances with predominant vasopressor properties (such as phenylephrine) may be appropriate in these cases. In patients with severe coronary artery disease, mitral or aortic valvular stenosis, or carotid artery stenosis, pretreatment with a cyclooxygenase inhibitor may be indicated.

Conclusions

Among other factors, vasodilatation is present in most instances of intraoperative hypotension leading to relative hypovolaemia. In addition, moderate to severe dehydration is a frequently observed feature in patients presenting for surgery. Therefore, intravascular volume augmentation is effective as prophylaxis and remains the first-line measure for treatment: '*if in doubt, give volume*'.

In most cases of intraoperative arterial hypotension, a negative inotropic influence on the heart, with a resulting decrease in cardiac output, cannot be excluded. Consequently, substances with mixed β- and α-receptor agonist properties should be used, if pharmacological intervention appears to be indicated.

In some instances, in which systemic vascular resistance can be assumed to be grossly diminished, ephedrine-type substances may be ineffective. Under these circumstances, agents with a predominantly vasopressor effect (for example, phenylephrine) should be preferred.

1 Schwilk B, Muche R, Bothner U, Goertz A, Friesdorf W, Georgieff M. Prozessqualität in der Anästhesiologie. Ergebnisse einer prospektiven Erhebung nach den Empfehlungen der DGAI. *Anaesthesist* 1995;44:242–9.
2 Carpenter RL, Caplan RA, Brown DL, Stephenson C, Wu R. Incidence and risk factors for side effects of spinal anaesthesia. *Anesthesiology* 1992;76:906–16.
3 Schwinn DA, Reves JG. Time course and hemodynamic effects of alpha-1-adrenergic

bolus administration in anesthetized patients with myocardial disease. *Anesth Analg* 1989;**68**:571–8.

4 Chestnut DH, Vincent RD, Sipes SL, DeBruin CS, Bleuer SA, Chatterjee P. Which vasopressor should one give to treat hypotension during magnesium sulfate infusion and epidural anesthesia (Abstract)? *Anesthesiology* 1991;**75**:A824.

5 Wright PMC, Fee JPH. Cardiovascular support during combined extradural and general anaesthesia. *Br J Anaesth* 1992;**68**:585–9.

6 Ramanathan S, Grant GJ. Vasopressor therapy for hypotension due to epidural anaesthesia for cesarean section. *Acta Anaesthesiol Scand* 1988;**32**:559–65.

7 O'Connor JP, Wynands JE. Anesthesia for myocardial revascularization. In: Kaplan JA (ed). *Cardiac anesthesia*, 2nd edn, vol 2. New York: Grune & Stratton, 1987:551–88.

8 Jackson JM, Thomas SJ. Valvular heart disease. In: Kaplan JA (ed). *Cardiac anesthesia*, 2nd edn, vol 2. New York: Grune & Stratton, 1987:589–633.

9 Smith JS, Roizen MF, Cahalan MK, Benefiel DJ, Beaupre PN, Sohn YJ *et al*. Does anesthetic technique make a difference? Augmentation of systolic blood pressure during carotid endarterectomy: effects of phenylephrine versus light anesthesia and of isoflurane versus halothane on the incidence of myocardial ischemia. *Anesthesiology* 1988;**69**:846–53.

10 Goertz AW, Lindner KH, Seefelder C, Schirmer U, Beyer M, Georgieff M. Effect of phenylephrine bolus administration on global left ventricular function in patients with coronary artery disease and patients with valvular aortic stenosis. *Anesthesiology* 1993;**78**:834–41.

11 Andersen TW, Gravenstein JS. Mephenteramine and ephedrine in man. A comparative study on cardiovascular effects. *Clin Pharmacol Ther* 1964;**5**:281–5.

12 Cohn JN. Comparative cardiovascular effects of tyramine, ephedrine, and norepinephrine in man. *Circ Res* 1965;**61**:174–82.

13 Smith NT, Corbascio AN. The use and misuse of pressor agents. *Anesthesiology* 1970;**33**:58–101.

14 Butterworth JF, Piccone W, Berrizbeitia LD, Dance G, Shemin RJ, Cohn LH. Augmentation of venous return by adrenergic agonists during spinal anesthesia. *Anesth Analg* 1986;**65**:612–16.

15 Greitz T, Andreen M, Irestedt L. Effects of ephedrine on haemodynamics and oxygen consumption in the dog during high epidural block with special reference to the splanchnic region. *Acta Anaesthesiol Scand* 1984;**28**:557–62.

16 Müller H, Brähler A, Börner U, Boldt J, Stoyanov M, Hempelmann G. Hämodynamische Veränderungen nach der Bolusgabe verschiedener Vasopressiva zur Blutdruckstabilisierung bei Periduralanästhesie. *Regional-Anästhesie* 1985;**8**:43–9.

17 Wright PMC, Iftikhar M, Fitzpatrick KT, Moore J, Thompson W. Vasopressor therapy for hypotension during epidural anesthesia for cesarean section: effects on maternal and fetal flow velocity ratios. *Anesth Analg* 1992;**75**:56–61.

18 Taivainen T. Comparison of ephedrine and etilefrine for the treatment of arterial hypotension during spinal anesthesia in elderly patients. *Acta Anaesthesiol Scand* 1991;**35**:164–70.

19 Boldt J, Müller H, Börner U, Kling D, Moosdorf R, Hempelmann G. Untersuchungen zur isolierten Beeinflussung des Gefässsystems durch verschiedene blutdrucksteigernde Medikamente (Akrinor®, Etilefrin, Ephedrin, Norfenefrin, Amezinium) während der extrakorporalen Zirkulation beim Menschen. *Anaesthesist* 1986;**35**:93–8.

20 Stanton-Hicks M, Höck A, Stühmeier K-D, Arndt JO. Vasoconstrictor agents mobilize blood from different sources and increase intrathoracic filling during epidural anesthesia in supine humans. *Anesthesiology* 1987;**66**:317–25.

21 Yamazaki R, Tzuchida K, Otomo S. Effects of dihydroergotamine and etilefrine on experimentally induced postural hypotension in dogs. *J Pharmacobio Dyn* 1990;**13**:519–26.

22 Del Greco F, Johnson DC. Clinical experience with angiotensin II in the treatment of shock. *JAMA* 1961;**178**:994–9.

23 Thaker U, Geary V, Chalmers P, Sheikk F. Low systemic vascular resistance during cardiac surgery: case reports, brief review, and management with angiotensin II. *J Cardiothorac Anesth* 1990;**4**:360–3.

134

24 Geary VM, Thaker UN, Chalmers PC, Sheikh F. The use of angiotensin II to treat hypotension in a patient taking amiodarone. *J. Cardiothorac Anesth* 1990;4:364–7.

25 Arndt JO, Höck A, Stanton-Hicks M, Stühmeier KD. Peridural anesthesia and the distribution of blood in supine humans. *Anesthesiology* 1985;63:616–23.

26 Bonica JJ, Berges PU, Marikawa K. Circulatory effects of peridural block: effects of level of analgesia and dose of lidocaine. *Anesthesiology* 1979;33:619–26.

27 Hopf HB, Weissbach B, Peters J. High thoracic segmental epidural anesthesia diminishes sympathetic outflow to the legs despite restriction of sensory blockade to the upper thorax. *Anesthesiology* 1990;73:882–9.

28 Peters J, Kousoulis L, Arndt JO. Effects of segmental thoracic extradural analgesia on sympathetic block in conscious dogs. *Br J Anaesth* 1989;63:470–6.

29 Goertz A, Seeling W, Heinrich H, Lindner KH, Schirmer U. Influence of high thoracic epidural anaesthesia on left ventricular contractility assessed using the end-systolic pressure-length relationship. *Acta Anaesthesiol Scand* 1993;37:38–44.

30 Goertz A, Heinrich H, Seeling W. Baroreflex control of heart rate during high thoracic epidural anesthesia. *Anaesthesia* 1992;47:984–7.

31 Baron J-F, Decaux-Jacolot A, Edouard A, Berdeaux A, Samili K. Influence of venous return on baroreflex control of heart rate during lumbar epidural anesthesia in humans. *Anesthesiology* 1986;64:188–93.

32 Billman GE, Dickey DT, Teoh KK, Stone HL. Effects of central venous blood volume shifts on arterial baroreflex control of heart rate. *Am J Physiol* 1981;241:H571–H575.

33 Abbould FM. Interaction of cardiovascular reflexes in circulatory control. In: Shepherd JT, Abboud FM. *Handbook of physiology*, section 2: *The cardiovascular system*, vol. 3. Bethesda, MD: American Physiological Society, 1983:675–753.

34 Wattwil M, Sundberg A, Arvill A, Lennquist C. Circulatory changes during high thoracic epidural anaesthesia – influence of sympathetic block and of systemic effect of local anaesthetic. *Acta Anaesthesiol Scand* 1985;29:849–55.

35 Sundberg A, Wattwil M, Wiklund L. Haemodynamic effects of intravenous bupivacaine during high thoracic epidural anaesthesia. *Acta Anaesthesiol Scand* 1987;31:143–7.

36 McConachie I. Vasovagale asystole during spinal anaesthesia. *Anaesthesia* 1991;46:281–2.

37 Caplan RA, Ward RJ, Posner K, Cheney FW. Unexpected cardiac arrest during spinal anesthesia: a closed claims analysis of predisposing factors. *Anesthesiology* 1988;68:5–11.

38 Mackey DC, Carpenter RL, Thomson GE, Brown DL, Bodily MN. Bradycardia and asystole during spinal anesthesia: a report of three cases without morbidity. *Anesthesiology* 1989;70:866–8.

39 Lundberg J, Nogren L, Thomson D, Werner O. Hemodynamic effects of dopamine during thoracic epidural anesthesia in man. *Anesthesiology* 1987;66:641–52.

40 Takasaki M, Hatano M, Nakamura Y, Kosaka Y. Evaluation of ephedrine, dopamine and dobutamine for circulatory depression with thoracic epidural analgesia in geriatric patients. *Masui* 1986;35:1212–20.

41 Ottensen S, Renck H, Jynge P. Cardiovascular effects of epidural analgesia and their modification by plasma expansion, adrenaline, isoproterenol and hypoxia: an experimental study in open-chest sheep. *Acta Anaesthesiol Scand* 1978;69:1–16.

42 Lundberg J, Biber B, Martner J, Raner C, Vinsö O. Dopamine or norepinephrine infusion during thoracic epidural anesthesia? Differences in hemodynamic effects and plasma norepinephrine levels (Abstract). *Anesthesiology* 1991;75:A740.

43 Engberg G, Wiklund L. The circulatory effects of intravenously administered ephedrine during epidural blockade. *Acta Anaesthesiol Scand* 1978;66(Suppl):27–36.

44 Engberg G, Wiklund L. The use of ephedrine for the prevention of arterial hypotension during epidural blockade. *Acta Anaesthesiol Scand* 1978;66(Suppl):1–26.

45 Goertz AW, Seeling W, Heinrich H, Lindner KH, Rockemann MG, Georgieff M. Effect of phenylephrine bolus administration on left ventricular function during high thoracic and lumbar epidural anesthesia combined with general anesthesia. *Anesth Analg* 1993;76:541–5.

46 Ralston DH, Shnider SM, DeLorimer AA. Effects of equipotent ephedrine, mephenter-amine and methoxamine on uterine blood flow in the pregnant ewe. *Anesthesiology* 1974;40:354–69.

47 Goertz AW, Hübner C, Seefelder C, Seeling W, Lindner KH, Rockemann MG *et al*. The

effect of ephedrine bolus administration on left ventricular loading and systolic performance during high thoracic epidural anesthesia combined with general anesthesia. *Anesth Analg* 1993;**78**:101–5.

48 Rouby J-J, Léger P, Andreev A, Arthaud M, Landau C, Vicaut E *et al*. Peripheral vascular effects of halothane and isoflurane in humans with an artificial heart. *Anesthesiology* 1990;**72**:462–9.

49 Coetzee A, Fourie P. Effect of halothane, enflurane, and isoflurane on the end-systolic pressure-length relationship. *Can J Anesth* 1987;**34**:351–7.

50 Pagel PS, Kampine JP, Smeling WT, Warltier DC. Influence of volatile anesthetics on myocardial contractility *in vivo*: desflurane versus halothane. *Anesthesiology* 1991;**74**:900–7.

51 Goertz AW, Schmidt M, Seefelder C, Lindner KH, Georgieff M. The effect of phenylephrine bolus administration on left ventricular function during isoflurane-induced hypotension. *Anesth Analg* 1993;**77**:227–31.

52 Marshall WK, Bedford RF, Miller ED. Cardiovascular responses in the seated position – impact of four anesthetic techniques. *Anesth Analg* 1983;**62**:648–56.

53 Goertz AW, Schmidt M, Lindner M, Seefelder C, Georgieff M. Effect of phenylephrine bolus administration on left ventricular function during postural hypotension in anesthetized patients. *J Clin Anesth* 1993;**5**:408–13.

54 Seeling W, Heinrich H, Öttinger W. Das Eventerationssyndrom: Prostacyclinfreisetzung und PaO$_2$-Abfall durch Dünndarmeventeration. *Anaesthesist* 1986;**35**:738–43.

55 Brinkmann A, Seeling W, Wolf CF, Kneitingen E, Junger S, Rockemann M *et al*. Der Einfluss der thorakalen Epiduralanästhesie auf die Pathophysiologie des Eventerationssyndroms. *Anaesthesist* 1994;**43**:235–44.

7: Treatment of acute postoperative hypertension

CHRIS DECLERCK, PIERRE CORIAT

Several factors promote the occurrence of acute postoperative hypertensive episodes. Their incidence varies with the type of operation, and the patient's age and history. The deleterious effects of these acute hypertensive episodes are implicated in the pathogenesis of postoperative cardiorespiratory complications. Verification of systemic blood pressure is therefore all the more crucial when the patient presents with cardiovascular disease (hypertension, ischaemic heart disease, heart failure) as a baseline problem. Treatment must be based on the well-established pathophysiological data regarding postoperative hypertension *and* on the underlying heart disease which may be present in the individual patient.

Pathophysiological mechanisms of postoperative hyptertension

To understand the mechanisms responsible for acute postoperative hypertensive episodes more precisely, it is necessary to consider, first, the haemodynamic characteristics of hypertension, and secondly, those factors which specifically promote it in the postoperative period.

Haemodynamic characteristics of essential hypertension

The vast majority of cases of hypertension are characterised haemodynamically by a pathological rise in the tone of arterial and arteriolar smooth muscle, which increases resistance in the resistant vascular system, and by a decrease in venous capacitance.[1, 2] An absolute or relative rise in systemic vascular resistance, typical of hypertensive disease, reflects a homogenous increase in vascular resistance in all the organs. In parallel with these abnormalities of the peripheral vessels, increased tone in the capacitory venous system redistributes the blood towards the cardiopulmonary beds and reinforces the transmural pressure of left ventricular distension. The effect of this rise in left ventricular preload is an increase in the systolic stroke volume, which is frequently observed in the first stages of hypertension. Calculated absolute values for systemic vascular resistance are normal; in fact, these values are inappropriate since they lead to a pathological rise in blood pressure. Secondarily, hypovolaemia occurs and cardiac output returns to normal, while venous tone remains raised.[3] Thus, in the majority of cases of essential hypertension, especially when of long standing, cardiac output is not increased and total peripheral resistance is high.

Cardiac and vascular structural modifications develop in response to a prolonged rise in systemic vascular resistance. They are characterised by an increase in the cardiac muscle mass (an adaptive mechanism to mechanical overload of the ventricle) and, especially, by hypertrophy of arteriolar smooth muscle. Concurrently, increased tone in the resistant and capacitory systems decreases volaemia. Water and sodium retention occurs only at a later stage, once cardiac output reserves have become limited, and particularly if hypertension has impaired renal function.

Hypertension episodes in the perioperative period result from abrupt accentuation of arteriolar vasoconstriction, under the effect of noradrenergic hyperactivity[4] caused by the nociceptive stimuli of tracheal intubation, surgery itself, and the recovery period.[5] A significantly marked increase in the plasma concentration of noradrenaline during these stimuli has been quantified in a number of studies.[6-8] The degree of arteriolar vasoconstriction depends on the extent of the nociceptive stimulus and the vascular reactivity of the patient being operated on. Increased sensitivity of the resistant vascular system of the hypertensive subject to catecholamines[9] accounts for the high incidence of peri- and especially postoperative hypertensive episodes in these patients. Increased reactivity of the arterial muscle cell in hypertensive subjects has been demonstrated in several studies which suggest that an increased sodium concentration within the smooth muscle cells increases their sensitivity to vasoconstrictors.[2, 9]

Moreover, in hypertensive subjects in whom blood pressure has not been controlled by appropriate treatment, reactive hypertrophy of the arteriolar smooth muscles occurs; this reinforces vasoconstriction induced by plasma catecholamines.[9]

Myocardial hypertrophy secondary to hypertension-induced mechanical overload is a contributory factor in the pathogenesis of acute hypertensive episodes. Increased myocardial mass effectively exaggerates the increase in the left ventricular stroke volume which results from catecholamine release.[2]

If present water and sodium retention increases blood pressure. Although a fall in venous return is generally observed during the operative period due to the effect of anaesthetic agents and mechanical ventilation, it should be recalled that excessive vascular filling in hypertensive patients, in whom venous compliance is generally diminished, may be involved to a significant degree in the aetiology of acute hypertensive episodes.

138

Abnormalities of the baroreflex arc, very commonly found in hypertensive patients, contribute to the pathogenesis of peri- and postoperative blood pressure surges. Activity of the barosensor reflex arc is depressed by negative feedback control. Stimulation of the baroreceptors by raised blood pressure has an inhibitory effect on bulbar vasomotor centres, manifested essentially by reduced sympathetic nervous system activity leading to a fall in blood pressure. In hypertensive subjects, the depressant effect of a blood pressure rise on the sympathetic nervous system is attenuated. A rise in the blood pressure threshold at which these reflex mechanisms come into play also occurs. This phenomenon, which is invariably found in hypertension, reflects baroreflex readjustment to a higher blood pressure level, termed resetting of the baroreflex.[10, 11]

Factors promoting postoperative hypertension

Acute postoperative hypertensive episodes are due essentially to abrupt accentuation of the phenomenon of arteriolar vasoconstriction under the combined effect of several factors characteristic of the operative period and/or the incapacity of the resistant vascular system to vasodilate in response to the raised cardiac output which is constant during the recovery period.[12] The various factors promoting acute perioperative hypertensive episodes – which we will now consider, and which are highly specific to the recovery period – influence either directly or indirectly the conditions defining left ventricular load, myocardial contractility, and baroreflex response. These factors may be summarised thus:

1 Increased tone of the resistant vascular system promoted by the major release of catecholamines which is characteristic of the recovery period.
2 Secondary increase in venous return:
   – on removal of the paralytic effect of the anaesthetic agent on vascular smooth muscle;
   – on increased release of adrenaline and noradrenaline;
   – on fluid redistribution during rewarming and after ceasing mechanical ventilation.
3 Volaemic abnormalities, both hypervolaemia and hypovolaemia.
4 Increased myocardial contractility linked to sympathetic stimulation.
5 In chronic hypertensive subjects, other mechanisms intervene after surgery:
   – reduction in the plasma level of antihypertensive medications prescribed prior to the operation;
   – 'resetting of the baroreflex', which does not intervene when there is a rise in blood pressure to higher levels;
   – accentuation of arteriolar vasoconstriction when challenged by catecholamine release;

   – a major increase in myocardial contractility in hypertrophic heart disease due to catecholamine release.

Acute hypertensive episodes are thus more frequent in patients with chronic hypertension who undergo surgery.

An understanding of pathophysiological data forms the basis for identifying the effects which might be expected of an antihypertensive agent appropriate for the postoperative period.

Impact on organ systems

Impact on the myocardium

The fact that acute hypertensive episodes alter ventricular systolic ejection at the end of systole depends on cardiac inotropism and the sum of factors which counter myocardial fibre shortening. The postsystolic residue is increased when baseline inotropism is impaired, for the same rise in blood pressure.[13] It is for this reason that when starting treatment of acute hypertensive episodes, medications should be administered which directly or indirectly diminish arteriolar resistance and improve left ventricular systolic emptying.[14]

The increased end-systolic volume reduces each stroke volume and the left ventricular ejection fraction. It compromises the energy balance of the myocardium by increasing the systolic transmural pressure, the key determinant of myocardial oxygen consumption. In addition, left ventricular hypertrophy, if present, may limit perfusion of subendocardial layers. Should the hypertensive episode induce myocardial ischaemia, reduction in the ejection fraction secondary to an acute hypertensive episode is even more marked since the ischaemic territory loses its contractile function.

Even in the absence of underlying heart disease, hypertensive episodes promote the onset of atrial or ventricular dysrhythmias, namely atrial extrasystoles, complete arrhythmia due to paroxysmal atrial fibrillation, and ventricular extrasystoles. These rhythm disorders are due to an increase in the atrial or ventricular transmural pressures.[15]

Impact on the brain

The cerebral arteries are subjected directly to blood pressure surges since they are poor in precapillary sphincters. This is particularly the case in the cerebrum, which is the only organ system exposed in this way.[16] Excessive blood pressure in the cerebral vascular beds causes altered vascular permeability leading to the development of interstitial cerebral oedema. Cerebrovascular accidents secondary to mural rupture of small arteries subjected to high pressure are rare, except in association with surgery for carotid stenosis;[17] in this situation, cerebral haemorrhage is a real possibility if there is a precipitate rise in blood pressure during endarterectomy.

Impact on the kidneys

The accentuation of vasoconstrictive phenomena which are responsible for acute hypertensive episodes also affects the vasculature of the kidney. Renal ischaemia may result from such episodes, with a reduction in renin–angiotensin system activity and further worsening of the blood pressure rise. There may be a real risk of acute postoperative renal failure.

Treatment of acute hypertensive episodes

It is of prime importance to provide rapid treatment, and better still to prevent such hypertensive episodes from occurring. There may be a rationale for prevention in a number of specific preoperative situations, such as patients who have had heart surgery, patients with restricted cardiac output, and patients who have undergone carotid endarterectomy.

In patients with limited coronary artery or cardiac reserves, the occurrence of significant fluctuations in blood pressure increases the incidence of myocardial ischaemic episodes, rhythm disorders, congestive left heart failure, and acute postoperative myocardial necrosis. The greater the impairment in baseline left ventricular systolic function, the more likely it is that increased blood pressure will affect left ventricular function. The frequency with which blood pressure increases – and their potentially harmful effects – occur in the immediate postoperative period after carotid endarterectomy has been well established.[5] Apart from their myocardial effects, acute hypertensive episodes after carotid endarterectomy carry the risk of causing haematoma at the vascular suture site, haemorrhagic cerebrovascular accidents, and revascularisation-type cerebral oedema.

Principles of treatment

Acute postoperative hypertensive episodes are characterised pathophysiologically by maladaptation of systemic arterial resistance to a given haemodynamic state.[5] Hypertension may occur when cardiac output increases to meet the oxygen requirements of the body during the operative period, while systemic arterial resistance remains normal. In fact, this normal response of systemic arterial resistance is inappropriate since it leads to hypertension.[18] In most cases, postoperative hypertension results from arteriolar vasoconstriction with pathological elevation of systemic arterial resistance. Treatment is therefore based on vasodilators, which reduce factors counteracting left ventricular ejection. Intravenous administration of a β-blocker such as low-dose propranolol should therefore be considered only if vasodilator treatment promotes the development of a hyperkinetic syndrome with marked acceleration of heart rate.[19]

A specification for the ideal antihypertensive medication for controlling acute postoperative hypertensive episodes is given below.

141

Profile of the ideal drug for the treatment of acute perioperative hypertensive episodes

1   Can be administered intravenously to produce a dose-dependent effect.
2   Rapid-acting.
3   Vasodilator predominantly on the resistant vascular system.
4   No effect on venous tone.
5   No reflex hypertonic sympathetic effect.
6   No reflex tachycardia.
7   No negative inotropic effect.
8   No harmful effect on the myocardial oxygenation of compromised areas.
9   No rebound effect.
10 With a pharmacokinetic profile which matches the operative period from the haemodynamic viewpoint (duration of action no longer than 1 hour after intravenous injection).

Antihypertensive agents

We will consider below the utility and limitations of drugs that have been suggested for treatment of postoperative hypertension.

Dihydralazine

Two factors restrict the use of this medication during acute postoperative hypertensive episodes: its pharmacokinetics and its effect on the energy balance of the myocardium.[20]

The latency time and the occasionally prolonged duration of its effects may be troublesome if a dangerous blood pressure rise occurs postoperatively, and if surgery exposes the subject to significant volaemic changes. Its action on the energy balance of the myocardium has been described previously.

Glyceryl trinitrate and sodium nitroprusside

Both of these extremely potent intravenous vasodilators may be used for the treatment of some types of acute postoperative hypertensive episodes. Their administration following heart surgery has been proposed by a number of authors.[19, 21, 22]

Sodium nitroprusside (SNP) is a potent vasodilator, which acts both on the arterial and venous vascular smooth muscle.[22] Its action on blood pressure is particularly rapid since it is apparent less than 40 seconds after a continuous infusion is started. The vasodilator effect disappears less than 2 minutes after stopping the infusion. SNP is broken down by non-enzymatic processes, principally within the red blood cells. This gives rise to increased production of methaemoglobin, and especially to the release of cyanide ions, the plasma concentration of which will be proportional to the dose of SNP injected.[23] There is a more than theoretical risk of poisoning with cyanide ions if more than 200 mg of SNP is administered, especially where renal or hepatic function is impaired.[24] When administered as a long-term infusion, the plasma concentration of cyanide ions should be monitored.[25]

The blood pressure decrease induced by SNP is dose-dependent, and affects both systolic and diastolic blood pressures.[22] The reflex rise in heart rate, secondary to hypotension, is usually moderate. The potential harmful effects of SNP on the energy balance of the myocardium, and the risk of shunting blood flow from areas distal to coronary stenoses to dilated healthy coronary arteries (coronary steal), are factors which limit its use in patients with coronary artery disease.[22]

The main action of glyceryl trinitrate (GTN) is to relax all the smooth muscle fibres in the body, irrespective of their innervation and their responses to stimulation.[26] Its main therapeutic effects result from its action on smooth muscle in the coronary artery network, resistant peripheral arterial system and capacitory venous system. At a dose of less than 1·5 mg/h, vasodilatation affects mainly the capacitory venous system. Veins which are more than 5 mm in diameter have been noted to possess highly extensive smooth muscle fibres. At a dose of greater than 2 mg/h, vasodilatation extends to involve the resistant vascular system.[26]

Reduction in blood pressure is slower with GTN than with SNP. The effect disappears gradually 4–7 minutes after stopping the infusion.

The fall in the mean blood pressure is dose-dependent. Systolic blood pressure falls much more markedly than diastolic blood pressure. Coronary artery perfusion thus often remains intact. The anti-ischaemic effects of GTN administered intravenously have been widely established. They stem not only from reduced oxygen consumption of the myocardium,[27] but also from increased coronary flow into the compromised myocardial area. This medication is therefore particularly useful in patients with limited coronary reserves.[28]

Studies that have provided an understanding of the haemodynamic effects of GTN and/or SNP administered in the control of perioperative hypertension have been conducted mostly during aortic-coronary artery bypass surgery under anaesthesia induced using high doses of fentanyl.[28–31]

Modifications of cardiac output induced by these vasodilators essentially depend on the dosage at which they are administered, and on left ventricular function and volaemic status in surgical patients.[30, 32, 33] If left ventricular kinetic patterns and contractility are normal, a perioperative rise in blood pressure has little effect on ventricular systolic emptying. Administration of GTN or SNP returns the blood pressure to normal, but lowers left ventricular end-systolic volume very little, since systolic emptying is already satisfactory. The decreases in venous return and ventricular transmural distension pressure reduce the end-diastolic volume considerably. The general result of these modifications is a slight fall in stroke volume, often with a reactive tachycardia secondary to increased sympathetic system tone.

Several studies have shown that haemodynamic modifications secondary to administration of GTN and SNP when used to control acute postoperative hypertensive episodes can be superimposed. We will therefore examine these changes in tandem.

Arteriolar vasodilatation induced by GTN or SNP provides an appropriate counterbalance to rises in postoperative blood pressure. Reduced tone in the capacitory system decreases left ventricular end-diastolic volume and pulmonary capillary pressure. If the patient develops absolute or relative volaemic overload following surgery, the vasodilatory effect of GTN or SNP is entirely beneficial, and returns the pulmonary capillary pressure to normal. If the patient is hypovolaemic, however, and not in heart failure, a reduced venous return may lead to a hyperkinetic state with a significant diminution of stroke volume.

In general surgery, rapid treatment of acute postoperative hypertensive episodes may be achieved by administering a bolus of GTN (0·5 mg), repeated every 30 seconds until blood pressure returns to normal. The development of a significant fall in blood pressure during the first bolus is rare, but may be observed in hypovolaemic patients; fluid replacement should be given. The beneficial effect of the GTN bolus lasts for only 5–10 minutes. To prolong the antihypertensive effect, GTN must be administered intravenously at a constant flow rate. The dosage of GTN required in this setting is extremely variable; the infusion flow rate should be titrated in relation to the blood pressure changes obtained.

SNP can be administered only as a continuous infusion and close monitoring of blood pressure is required, preferably by means of an indwelling radial catheter.

It should not be forgotten that during an infusion with GTN or SNP cardiac output is extremely dependent on the volaemic state, and that the insidious development of hypovolaemia may reduce blood pressure and stroke volume to dangerously low levels, thus compromising peripheral oxygenation. It is often difficult following a procedure in general surgery to know the relative volaemic state other than by appropriate haemodynamic monitoring. This explains why it is sometimes difficult to determine the optimum dosage of GTN or SNP to be administered by infusion. Monitoring of left ventricular filling pressure and cardiac output may produce very useful data in these cases. The dosage of these vasodilators should then be titrated in relation to venous return, which may fluctuate widely following surgery. Initially, venous return increases due to catecholamine release. Thereafter, occasionally large-scale fluid shifts from the vascular compartment to the extravascular space lead to hypovolaemia, which may develop insidiously. This can then induce an accelerated heart rate and reduced stroke volume.

144

Continuous monitoring of pulmonary capillary pressure and cardiac output is of particular benefit when intending to treat acute postoperative hypertensive episodes with GTN or SNP since these vasodilators are commonly used in hypertensive patients. It is difficult to control blood pressure postoperatively in these patients because they often have impaired cardiac output reserves.

It should finally be noted that it is necessary to step up the infusion rate of GTN with time to maintain the reduction in systolic blood pressure. This effect of GTN on blood pressure may be described as a habituation phenomenon.[26] Although tachyphylaxis has been described when SNP is used to obtain profound perioperative hypotension, this phenomenon has not been observed when this vasodilator is used to control postoperative hypertension.[22] Cyanide toxicity can occur in long-term therapy and the metabolism of cyanide is dependent on the availability of thiosulphate. Thiosulphate donates sulphur to cyanide to convert it to thiocyanate, which has a renal clearance. Thiosulphate storage is limited in the liver, which may result in a reduced clearance of cyanide. This is particularly the case in patients with hepatic failure, following recent surgery, in chronic diuretic use, and in malnutrition.[34] However, the most important factor for cyanide toxicity is the dose of SNP. A maximum dose of 10 μg/kg per min over two or three hours is recommended. First signs of cyanide toxicity are tachyphylaxis, lactic acidosis, and a narrowed arteriovenous oxygen difference. To avoid cyanide toxicity, 1 g of sodium thiosulphate per 100 mg of SNP can be given.[35] When cyanide toxicity is suspected, the poisoning can be treated with the Lilly Cyanide Antidote Kit.

Several *in vitro* studies have shown platelet inhibition with the use of SNP. This has been confirmed *in vivo*, and must be taken into consideration if a patient has undergone surgery which might expose them to the risk of postoperative haemorrhagic complications.

Clonidine

During the recovery period, it has been shown that administration of clonidine can limit the increased plasma concentration of noradrenaline generally observed in the immediate postoperative period.[36] This neuro-endocrinological modification partly accounts for the beneficial effect of this medication on postoperative hypertension.

However, few studies have analysed the haemodynamic effects of clonidine when administered as a continuous intravenous infusion in the treatment of acute postoperative hypertensive episodes.

The sedative effect of clonidine may limit its use within the immediate postoperative period.

Calcium antagonists

Calcium-channel blockers or antagonists, in particular those of the dihydropiridine group such as nifedipine and nicardipine and, to a lesser

145

degree, intravenous diltiazem, assume an increasingly larger role in the treatment of acute postoperative hypertensive episodes. The mechanisms of action and haemodynamic effects of these drugs are particularly suited to the treatment of hypertensive episodes that threaten the hypertensive patient after surgery. The risk of causing a precipitate fall in blood pressure when initiating treatment of acute postoperative hypertension with calcium antagonists is very small.[37] In fact, the degree of vasodilator effect is dependent on the tone of the resistant vascular system.

In addition, drug interactions between calcium antagonists and agents that may be used for postoperative sedation do not carry the risk of producing postoperative haemodynamic complications.[38]

Nifedipine and nicardipine have even been suggested for treatment of congestive left ventricular failure if blood pressure is raised.[39, 40] In this indication, improved systolic emptying due to the reduced left ventricular afterload peredominates very markedly over any possible negative inotropic effect.

The many pharmacokinetic and pharmacodynamic advantages of the calcium inhibitors of the dihydropiridine group have resulted in nifedipine now being administered intranasally or sublingually as a first-line treatment of acute postoperative hypertensive episodes in general surgery, and most especially, in vascular surgery.

The recent marketing of nicardipine, which can be administered intravenously,[41, 42] has been followed by its increasingly wider use in the treatment of acute postoperative hypertensive episodes, since this calcium antagonist is currently the only agent in the dihydropiridine group which can be administered by this route. Moreover, administered at dosages of 0·5–20 mg by repeated bolus of 0·5 mg or 1 mg, nicardipine has a dose-dependent hypotensive effect.[41, 42] This finding has been confirmed by a recent study demonstrating that there is a linear reduction in systolic, diastolic, and mean blood pressures, both resting and on exercise, when successive boluses of 1·25, 2·5, and 5 mg are administered.[43]

After aortobifemoral bypass, nifedipine has been used successfully in the treatment of acute hypertensive episodes.[44] In parallel with a return of systemic blood pressure to normal, pulmonary artery pressure falls by 20%. In several studies, nifedipine has proved to be highly effective in the treatment of raised blood pressure, both during and after carotid endarterectomy. Monitoring of mixed venous blood oxygen saturation measured in the pulmonary artery ($S_{\bar{v}}O_2$) using a pulmonary artery catheter during the operative period in patients undergoing carotid endarterectomy showed that a significant fall in $S_{\bar{v}}O_2$ was frequently associated with the onset of a systolic blood pressure surge to more than 170 mmHg.[45] Administration of nifedipine 10 mg intranasally enabled the rise in blood pressure to be controlled within a few minutes. A rise of more than 30% in the cardiac output and an improvement in the $S_{\bar{v}}O_2$ was noted concurrently

146

with the return to baseline blood pressure values; this reflects an improvement in the pre-existing balance between cardiac output and the metbolic requirements of the body.

Intravenously administered nicardipine currently appears to be supplanting intranasally administered nifedipine in the treatment of acute postoperative hypertensive episodes. This method of administering nicardipine permits the desired blood pressure level to be obtained with precision,[41, 42, 46] and protects the patient from the risk of a fall in blood pressure at the beginning of treatment. Like nifedipine, nicardipine lowers blood pressure by reducing systemic vascular resistance,[47] which leads to reflex activation of the sympathetic system, and acceleration of the heart rate.[41]

Although the negative inotropic effect of nifedipine is moderate *in vivo*, that of nicardipine appears to be even more limited, as confirmed by a study in which calcium antagonists were administered into the coronary arteries. Whereas nifedipine decreases ventricular function, in this setting nicardipine had no myocardial depressant effect.[48]

It is therefore not surprising that in clinical practice administration of nicardipine is particularly beneficial in hypertensive subjects with impaired cardiac function.[39, 40, 49] In patients with an ejection fraction of between 20 and 40%, administration of nicardipine improved the cardiac output. These patients experienced a very clear-cut benefit from the reduced left ventricular afterload.[39, 49] In parallel with these antihypertensive effects, nicardipine has other beneficial effects. It improves the energy balance of the myocardium by decreasing its oxygen consumption, and by exerting a direct effect on the coronary circulation.[41, 50] Intravenous administration of nicardipine to patients with acute angina reduces the myocardial lactate production, indicating better oxygenation of the ischaemic myocardial beds.[50, 51]

These beneficial effects on the energy balance of the myocardium have been confirmed during coronary angioplasty.[52] The onset of myocardial ischaemia in coronary artery occlusion could be prevented or markedly delayed in 7 out of 10 patients included in the study by Rousseau, who administered nicardipine preventively (2 mg bolus over 1 minute followed by an infusion of 25–50 µg/min) during coronary angioplasty. In addition, coronary blood flow was improved.

Arterial vasodilatation also affects the cerebral vasculature,[53] and nicardipine increases renal blood flow and glomerular filtration.[54]

In the perioperative period, nicardipine is used mostly for curative treatment of postoperative hypertension.[42, 55] Nicardipine is generally administered as a slow bolus over 2–10 minutes, followed by a continuous infusion of doses ranging from 4 to 8 mg/h; in some cases, maintenance doses of 15 mg/h have been reported.[41, 42]

We compared the effects of intravenously administered nicardipine and

GTN on haemodynamics and left ventricular function assessed by transoesophageal echocardiography.[56] Both these vasodilators were used for treating episodes of hypertension occurring in the period immediately after aortic surgery while patients were still receiving mechanical ventilation of the lungs and morphine sedation. Haemodynamic and echocardiogram parameters were compared in both groups after blood pressure had been restored to its normal value following intravenous GTN or nicardipine. Analysis of end-diastolic and end-systolic surface area modifications obtained by transoesophageal echocardiography provided a more exact understanding of the impact of decreased left ventricular loading conditions, as induced by GTN, on myocardial function and output (Figure 7.1).

With GTN, although left ventricular systolic emptying is improved, reduction of preload leads to a moderate but significant fall in the systolic index. Reduced venous return with GTN is also reflected by decreased pulmonary capillary pressure. However, in patients receiving nicardipine for treatment of acute postoperative hypertensive episodes, a rise in stroke volume secondary to improved left ventricular systolic emptying was noted, although the left ventricular preload remained the same, as shown by the absence of any changes in end-diastolic surface area and pulmonary capillary pressure. In both groups, treatment of the hypertensive episode led to sharply improved ventricular function, as demonstrated by the clear-cut improvement in the ejection fraction (Figure 7.2).

Calcium inhibitors of the dihydropiridine group therefore provide rapid and effective treatment of raised postoperative blood pressure, without compromising the adjustment of cardiac output to the metabolic requirement of the body, and while improving left ventricular function.

Diltiazem, administered as successive boluses of 0·4 mg/kg, is indicated mainly for acute hypertensive episodes complicated by atrial fibrillation. It enables the hypertensive episode to be corrected by slowing the heart rate, although it is nevertheless unable to promote a return to sinus rhythm.[57]

Beta-blockers

Pathophysiologically, acute postoperative hypertensive episodes are characterised by an inappropriate absolute or relative rise in systemic vascular resistance. As explained above, the antihypertensive effect of β-blockers results essentially from a reduced cardiac output due chiefly to slowing of the heart rate, and to a lesser degree, to a negative inotropic effect. Beta-blockers therefore have no place in the first-line treatment of acute postoperative hypertensive episodes. To diminish cardiac output without removing, or indeed while worsening peripheral arteriolar constriction, by hampering myocrdial contractility – the function of which is to overcome the state of mechanical overload represented by hypertension – exposes the patient to a risk of left ventricular failure, and does not in any

148

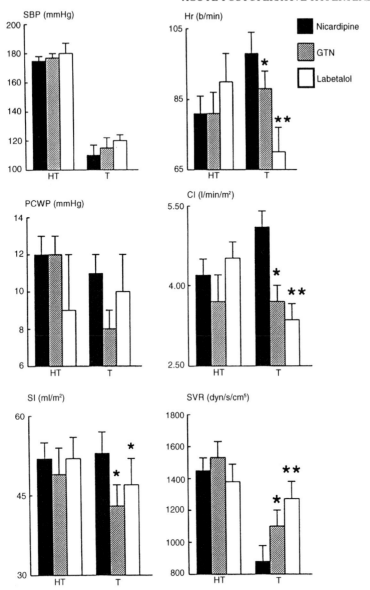

Fig 7.1 Treatment of postoperative hypertension: comparative efficacy of three antihypertensive agents. An intravenous bolus of Nicardipine, or glyceryl trinitrate (GTN), or labetabol was given to control blood pressure. Haemodynamic parameters are presented at the time of hypertension (HT) and after treatment (T). SBP, systolic blood pressure; HR, heart rate; PCWP, pulmonary capillary wedge pressure; CI, cardiac index; SI, stroke index; SVR, systemic vascular resistance. * versus hypertension; ** versus the two other agents. (Adapted from Ben Ammar et al, 1987[56] and Lebret et al, 1992[65].)

way correspond to the requirements of an aetiological treatment.[58] However, once peripheral vasoconstriction has been offset by a vasodilator drug, a β-blocker may be administered intravenously to limit any likelihood of a hyperkinetic syndrome. Beta-blockers should not be administered for this indication except at low, divided doses (no more than 0·5 mg propranolol every 30 seconds).

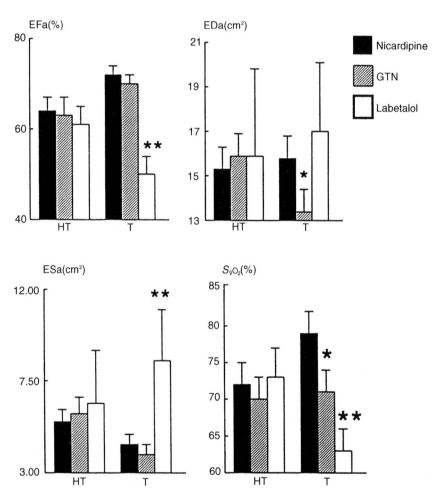

Fig 7.2 Left ventricular function response to treatment (T) of postoperative hypertension (HT). Left ventricular function indices were determined using transoesophageal echocardiography and mixed venous oxygen saturation continuously measured using a pulmonary artery catheter. EFa, ejection fraction area; EDa, end-diastolic area; ESa, end-systolic area, $S_{\bar{v}}O_2$, mixed venous oxygen saturation. * versus hypertension; ** versus the two other agents. (Adapted from Ben Ammar et al, 1987[56] and Lebret et al, 1992[65].)

150

In the postoperative period with a gret deal of haemodynamic activity, it is useful to have a short-acting agent available.

Esmolol has been proposed for the treatment of acute hypertensive episodes associated with tachycardia.[59] It is a cardioselective β_1-blocker devoid of any sympathomimetic activity or 'membrane stabilising' properties. Its elimination half-life is 9 minutes, due to the fact that it is rapidly hydrolysed by red cell esterases. As a continuous infusion, steady-state levels are reached within 5 minutes after a loading dose of 300 µg/kg per minute administered over 2–3 minutes according to heart rate response; maintenance is provided by a continuous infusion at a dose of 100 µg/kg/min. The drug effect ceases 20 minutes after stopping the infusion. It is also possible to use a single 100 mg injection (i.e. one ampoule) over 3–4 minutes.[60]

Esmolol may be used on a preventive basis when it is absolutely essential to control blood pressure and heart rate when the trachea is extubated, for example, following a neurosurgical operation.

If β-blockers are used postoperatively, it should be recalled that these drugs have a negative inotropic effect that is all the more marked when myocardial contractility is impaired, and that they restrict adaptation of cardiac output to increased metabolic requirements of the body. These requirements can then be met only at the expense of greater peripheral extraction of oxygen.

Labetalol has been recommended for the treatment of rises in blood pressure occurring after various surgical procedure.[61-63] Its α-antagonist effects reduce the tone of the resistant system, while its β-effects decrease cardiac output and left ventricular function, while improving the energy balance of the myocardium.[61, 63, 64] According to some authors, its half-life of 4 hours enables labetalol to limit its effects to the first few hours of the operative period, those in which patients are subject to the haemodynamic constraints responsible for postoperative pressure rises.[62] The role played by increased plasma catecholamine concentrations in the pathogenesis of acute postoperative hypertensive episodes has led some authors to suggest the use of labetalol for treating this problem. In fact, even when administered to treat acute postoperative hypertensive episodes, the β-antagonist effects of labetalol largely outweigh its α-antagonist effect.[65] This finding is in agreement with pharmacological studies which report that the β-antagonist effect of labetalol is four- to sixteen-fold more potent than the α-effect.[64, 66, 67]

Findings of a recent study which examined the effects of labetalol on haemodynamics and ventricular function when used to treat hypertensive episodes after aortic surgery also support the hypothesis of a clearly predominant β-antagonist effect[65] (see Figure 7.1). Transoesophageal echocardiographic monitoring of ventricular kinetic patterns demonstrated a significant decrease in the left ventricular ejection fraction despite return of blood pressure to normal[65] (*see Figure 7.2*). Administration of labetalol for the treatment of acute hypertensive episodes should therefore be undertaken with caution in surgical patients with limited cardiac reserves in whom reserves of cardiac output (preload reserve, accelerated heart rate) or peripheral oxygen extraction reserves will already have been called upon to meet postoperative metabolic constraints during the acute hypertensive episode. Labetalol would, however, appear appropriate for coronary surgery patients in whom cardiac output reserves have not been impaired by coronary artery disease.

Curative treatment of acute postoperative hypertensive episodes with labetalol requires bolus administration which may be followed if need be by the injection of additional boluses or a continuous infusion.[68] Although several studies in the literature have cited initial boluses of 0·5–1 mg/kg,[61, 68] it is categorically not recommended that treatment be commenced with a bolus of more than 20 mg, to avoid the occurrence of haemodynamic complications. It is preferable to administer an initial bolus of 20 mg over 2 minutes and to administer bluses of 40 mg every 5 minutes to a maximum of 1·5 mg/kg if systolic blood pressure remains above the desired value. This dosage protects the subject from hypotensive episodes at the beginning of treatment. Subsequently, boluses of 20–40 mg may be administered on demand, depending on the blood pressure, to reinforce or sustain if need be the antihypertensive effect of labetalol. Some authors have suggested the use of a continuous infusion at a dosage of between 0·15 and 0·2 mg/kg per hour,[68] which would require that the patient remain in the intensive care unit after operation.

Urapidil

This is a new intravenous antihypertensive agent (a derivative of phenylpiperazine and amino-4-uracil). Its mechanism of action is based on inhibition of central[69] and peripheral[70] postsynaptic α_1-receptors. It differs from prazosin in terms of its agonist action on serotoninergic receptors ($5HT_1$), with a resultant reduction in sympathetic tone and increase in parasympathetic tone. This property accounts for the lack of reflex tachycardia when blood pressure is reduced using urapidil.[71]

After injection of a bolus of 25–100 mg, blood pressure control is achieved within 2–5 minutes in approximately 75% of patients;[72] the effect can be maintained with a continuous infusion at a dose of between 60 and 180 mg/h.

On stopping the infusion there is no tachyphylaxis phenomenon or rebound effect. The absence of any rise in intracranial pressure makes this a drug of choice when extubating the trachea after neurosurgery.

Absence of reflex tachycardia suggested to us that urapidil might be of value in coronary surgery patients. We therefore evaluated the effect of urapidil on haemodynamics and left ventricular 'pump' function (analysed by echocardiography) in this type of patient.[73]

Reductions in vascular tone, in pulmonary artery occlusion pressure, and in end-diastolic surface area, which is the accepted preload index, reflect inhibition of α_1-adrenoceptors. This decreased preload requires careful monitoring should hypovolaemia occur; this is particularly frequent in the recovery period and requires appropriate fluid replacement. Improved emptying, manifested by a decreased end-systolic surface area, accounts for the increased cardiac index. The pump function expressed as the left ventricular ejection fraction suggests that the effect on the afterload is greater than that on the preload.

Urapidil has also been proposed as a vasodilator for use in congestive heart failure.

Ketanserin

Ketanserin is a selective S_2-serotonin receptor antagonist with α_1-adrenergic blocking effects. Ketanserin lowers the blood pressure in hypertensive patients by reducing the elevated systemic vascular resistance. It is able to reduce pulmonary hypertension by decreasing pulmonary vascular resistance. There is no change in pulmonary shunt fraction in contrast to treatment with sodium nitroprusside (SNP).[74, 75] Neither reflex tachycardia[76] nor tachyphylaxis occurs with ketanserin administration.

Ketanserin may decrease myocardial oxygen consumption by reducing preload and afterload but few recent clinical studies are available. Perioperative treatment with ketanserin reduces postoperative hypertension without influencing the cerebral blood flow or metabolism.[77] Intermittent doses of 5 mg can be given iv to a maximum of 30 mg; the dose by continuous infusion is 2–6 mg/h. Our experience with ketanserin is that the antihypertensive effect is not always reached despite administering the maximum dose.

The prevalence of ventricular arrhythmias, induced by a prolonged QT-interval, is a dose-dependent effect of ketanserin. Therefore ketanserin should not be administered with class I_a, I_c or III anti-arrhythmics. Care must be taken in patients with hypokalaemia.

Angiotensin-converting enzyme (ACE) inhibitors

ACE inhibitors prevent the conversion of angiotensin I to angiotensin II, a potent vasoconstrictor which stimulates aldosterone secretion. The pharmacological action of ACE inhibitors results in vasodilatation, a reduction in blood pressure, and a reduction in aldosterone secretion.

Enalaprilat is the only available ACE inhibitor which can be given intravenously. Enalaprilat is effective in reducing blood pressure in patients with coronary artery disease, without causing reflex tachycardia. Myocardial oxygen consumption is reduced through a reduction in left ventricular afterload and the absence of tachycardia.[78]

The concentrations of isoflurane required for induced hypotension in cerebral aneurysm surgery are much lower after ACE inhibition by enalaprilat.[79]

Usually ACE inhibitors are titrated to an antihypertensive effect and a recommended initial dose of enalaprilat in hypertensive crisis is 0·625 mg iv. No significant differences were found with doses above 0·625 mg in hypertensive patients.[80]

Care should be taken with the first-dose effect, especially in volume-depleted patients and in patients receiving diuretics. Hypokalaemia and hypotension are dose-related side effects in patients with renal failure. Therefore monitoring of potassium levels is recommended in patients treated with an ACE inhibitor.

Conclusions

The development of antihypertensive agents which can be administered intravenously has greatly simplified the treatment of acute postoperative hypertensive episodes. This treatment returns subjects to a satisfactory haemodynamic status both safely and effectively if due consideration is given to the pathophysiological origin of acute postoperative hypertensive episodes and to the pharmacodynamic properties of antihypertensives administered intravenously in the postoperative period (Table 7.1). Since acute postoperative hypertensive episodes are characterised haemodynam-ically by an absolute or relative rise in systemic vascular resistance, their first-line treatment is based on vasodilators. In this situation, calcium antagonists (resistant vasodilators) have pride of place. Urapidil, a mixed-type vasodilator, when used to re-establish blood pressure control is characterised by the fact that it does not accelerate the heart rate, a useful property in patients with coronary artery disease. Once arterial vasocon-striction has been treated, the use of a β-blocker such as labetalol would

Table 7.1 Comparative effects of some agents used for curative treatment of acute postoperative hypertensive episodes

	NFP	NCP	DTZ	LBT	GTN
Arterial vasodilator effect	+++	++++	++	+	+++
Reduced capacitory tone	0	0	0	0	++++
Rapid action	++	++++	+++	+++	++++
Short duration of action	+	+++	++	+	++++
Improved energy balance of the myocardium	++	++	++++	+++	+++
Heart rate	+++	+++	−	− − −	++++
Dosage of initial bolus to repeat until desired effect achieved	10 mg Intra-nasal	1 mg iv	20 mg iv	20 mg iv	0·5 mg iv

NFP, nifedipine; NCP, nicardipine; DTZ, diltiazem; LBT, labetalol; GTN, glyceryl trini-trate.

154

appear appropriate in order to reduce any likelihood of a hyperkinetic syndrome.

1 Frohlich ED. Cardiovascular disease, pathophysiology of essential hypertension. In: Zella R (ed). *The peripheral circulations*, vol. 1. New York: Grune and Stratton, 1985:261–82.

2 Frohlich ED. Haemodynamics of hypertension. In: Genest P, Kolw N, Kuchel P (eds). *Hypertension: physiopathology and treatment*. New York: McGraw Hill, 1977:15–49.

3 Tarazi RC, Dustan HP, Frohlich ED *et al.* Plasma volume and chronic hypertension. Relationship to arterial pressure levels in different hypertensive diseases. *Arch Intern Med* 1970;**125**:835–9.

4 Peterson FD, Brown AM. Pressor reflexes produced by stimulation of afferent fibers in the cardiac sympathetic nerves of the cat. *Circ Res* 1971;**28**:605–10.

5 Prys-Roberts C. Anesthesia and hypertension. *Br J Anaesth* 1984;**56**:711–21.

6 Low JM, Harvey JT, Prys-Roberts C, Dagnino J. Studies of anaesthesia in relation to hypertension. VII: Adrenergic response to laryngoscopy. *Br J Anaesth* 1986;**58**:471–7.

7 Roizen MF, Hamilton WK, Sohn YJ. Treatment of stress-induced increases in pulmonary capillary wedge pressure using volatile anesthetics. *Anesthesiology* 1981;**55**:446–50.

8 Turner DAB, Shribman AJ, Smith G *et al.* Effect of halothane on cardiovascular and plasma catecholamine responses to tracheal intubation. *Br J Anaesth* 1986;**58**:1365–70.

9 Abboud FM. The sympathetic system in hypertension. State of the art review. *Hypertension* 1982;**4**:208–25.

10 Bristow JD, Honour AJ, Pickering GW *et al.* Diminished baroreflex sensitivity in high blood pressure. *Circulation* 1969;**39**:48–54.

11 Gribbin B, Pickering TG, Sleight P, Peto R. Effect of age and high blood pressure on baroreflex sensitivity in man. *Circ Respir* 1971;**29**:424–31.

12 Desmonts JM, Bohm G, Couderc E. Hemodynamic responses to low doses of naloxone after narcotic-nitrous oxide anesthesia. *Anesthesiology* 1978;**49**:12–16.

13 Sagawa K. Editorial: The end-systolic pressure-volume relation of the ventricle: definition, modifications and clinical use. *Circulation* 1981;**63**:1223–7.

14 Cohn JN. Blood pressure and cardiac performance. *Am J Med* 1973;**55**:351–61.

15 Frohlich ED, Tarazi RC, Dustan HP. Clinical physiological correlations in the development of hypertensive heart disease. *Circulation* 1971;**44**:446–51.

16 Strandgaard S, Olesen J, Skinho J *et al.* Autoregulation of brain circulation in severe arterial hypertension. *Br Med J* 1973;**1**:507–10.

17 Caplan LR, Skillman J, Ojemann R *et al.* Intracerebral hemorrhage following carotid endarterectomy: a hypertensive complication? *Stroke* 1978;**9**:457–60.

18 Frohlich ED, Tarazi RC, Dustan HP. Re-examination of the hemodynamics of hypertension. *Am J Med Sci* 1968;**257**:9–17.

19 Fyman PN, Cottrel JE, Kushins L, Casthely PA. Vasodilator therapy in the perioperative period. *Can Anesth Soc J* 1986;**33**:629–43.

20 Sladen RN, Rosenthal MD. Specific afterload reduction with parenteral hydralazine following cardiac surgery. *J Thorac Cardiovasc Surg* 1979;**78**:125–202.

21 Herling M. Intravenous nitroglycerin clinical pharmacology and therapeutic considerations. *Am Heart J* 1984;**108**:141–9.

22 Tinker JH, Michenfelder JD. Sodium nitroprusside: pharmacology, toxicology and therapeutics. *Anesthesiology* 1976;**45**:340–54.

23 Vesey CJ, Cole PV, Simpson PJ. Cyanide and thicyanate concentrations following SNP infusion in man. *Br J Anaesth* 1976;**48**:651–60.

24 Davies DW, Greiss L, Kadar D *et al.* Sodium nitroprusside in children: observations on metabolism during normal and abnormal responses. *Can Anaesth Soc J* 1975;**22**:553–60.

25 Michenfelder JD, Tinker JH. Cyanide toxicity and thiosulfate protection during chronic administration of SNP in the dog: correlation with a human case. *Anesthesiology* 1977;**47**:441–8.

26 Sorkin EM, Brogden RN, Romankiewicz JA. Intravenous glyceryl trinitrate (nitroglycerin). A review of its pharmacological properties and therapeutic efficacy. *Drugs* 1984;**27**:45–80.

27 Sethna DH, Moffitt EA, Bussel JA *et al.* Intravenous nitroglycerin and myocardial

155

metabolism during anesthesia in patients undergoing myocardial revascularisation. *Anesth Analg* 1982;**61**:828–33.

28 Kaplan JA, Dunbar RW, Jones EL. Nitroglycerin infusion during coronary artery surgery. *Anesthesiology* 1976;**45**:14–21.

29 Chiariello M, Gold HK, Leinbach RC *et al.* Comparison between the effects of nitroprusside and nitroglycerin on ischemic injury during acute myocardial infarction. *Circulation* 1976;**54**:766–73.

30 Fyman PN, Cottrell JE, Kushins L, Casthely PA. Vasodilator therapy in the perioperative period. *Can Anaesth Soc J*, 1986;**33**:629–43.

31 Kaplan JA, Jones EL. Vasodilator therapy during coronary artery surgery. *J Thorac Cardiovasc Surg* 1979;**77**:301–9.

32 Ludbrook PA, Tiefenbrunn AJ, Reed FR *et al.* Acute hemodynamic responses to sublingual nifedipine: dependence on left ventricular function. *Circulation*, 1982;**65**:489–98.

33 Miller RR, Vismara L, Williams DO *et al.* Pharmacological mechanisms for left ventricular unloading in clinical congestive heart failure. Different effects of nitroprusside, phentolamine, and nitroglycerin on cardiac function and peripheral circulation. *Circ Res* 1976;**39**:127–33.

34 Curry SC, Arnold-Capell P, Nitroprusside, nitroglycerin and ace inhibitors. *Crit Care Clin* 1991;**7**:555–8.

35 Rindone J, Sloane E. Cyanide toxicity from sodium nitroprusside: risks and management. *Ann Pharmacother* 1992;**26**:515–19.

36 Flacke JW, Bloor BC, Wong DC *et al.* Effects of clonidine upon hyperadrenergic responses and narcotic requirements in patients undergoing CABG surgery. *Anesthesiology* 1986;**65**:3A.

37 Lederballe-Pedersen O, Christensen NJ, Ramsch KD. Comparison of acute effects of nifedipine in normotensive and hypertensive man. *J Cardiovasc Pharmacol* 1980;**2**:357–66.

38 Reves JG, Kissin I, Lell WA, Tosone S. Calcium entry blockers: uses and implications for anesthesiologists. *Anesthesiology* 1982;**57**:504–18.

39 Burlew B, Jafri SM, Goldberg AD *et al.* Haemodynamic effects of nicardipine hydrochloride in patients with chronic congestive heart failure. *Clin Res* 1986;**34**:285A.

40 Greenbaum RA, Wan S, Evans TR. The acute haemodynamic effects of nicardipine in patients with chronic left ventricular failure. *Eur J Clin Pharmacol* 1986;**30**:383–6.

41 Sorkin EM, Clissold SP. Nicardipine: a review of its pharmacodynamic and pharmacokinetic properties, and therapeutic efficacy, in the treatment of angina pectoris, hypertension and related cardiovascular disorders. *Drugs* 1987;**33**:296–345.

42 Turlapaty P, Vary R, Kaplan JA. Nicardipine, a new intravenous calcium antagonist: a review of its pharmacology, pharmacokinetics, and perioperative applications. *J Cardiothorac Anesth* 1989;**3**:344–55.

43 Silke B, Verma SP, Hafizullah M *et al.* Hemodynamic effects of nicardipne in acute myocardial infarction. *Postgrad Med J* 60 (Suppl 4):29–34.

44 Sodeyama O, Ikeda K, Matsuda I, Fukunaga AF, Bishay EG. Nifedipine for control of postoperative hypertension. *Anesthesiology* 1983;**59**:A18.

45 Ghignone M, Quintin L, Duke PC, Kehler CH, Calvillo O. Effects of clonidine on narcotic requirements and haemodynamic response during induction of fentanyl anesthesia and endotracheal intubation. *Anesthesiology* 1986;**64**:36–42.

46 Liopoulou A, Turner P, Warrington SJ. Acute hemodynamic effects of a new calcium antagonist, nicardipine, in man. A comparison with nifedipine. *Br J Clin Pharmacol* 1983;**15**:59–66.

47 Frishman WH, Weinberg P, Peled HB *et al.* Calcium entry blockers for the treatment of severe hypertension and hypertensive crisis. *Am J Med* 1984;**77**:35–45.

48 Rousseau H, Pouleur H. Calcium antagonism free of negtive inotropic effects? A comparison of intracoronary nifedipine and nicardipine. *Circulation* 1984;**70**(Suppl. II): II-304.

49 Lahiri A, Robinson CW, Caruana MP *et al.* Acute and chronic effects of nicardipine on systolic and diastolic left ventricular performance in patients with heart failure: a pilot study. *Clin Cardiol* 1986;**9**:257–61.

50 Pepine CJ, Lambert CR. Effects of nicardipine on coronary blood flow. *Am Heart J*

1988;**116**:248–54.

51 Hanet C, Rousseau MF, Vincent MF *et al.* Effects of nicardipine on myocardial metabolism and coronary haemodynamics: a review. *Br J Clin Pharmacol* 1986;**22**:215S–229S.

52 Rousseau MF, Renkin J, Pardonge EF *et al.* Myocardial protection by intracoronary injection of nicardipine during transluminal coronary angioplasty. *Circulation* 1985;**72**(Suppl):400.

53 Takenaka T, Handa J. Cerebrovascular effects of YC-93, a new vasodilator, in dogs, monkeys and human patients. *Int J Clin Pharmacol Biopharmacy* 1979;**17**:1–11.

54 Abe Y, Komori T, Mirura K *et al.* Effects of the calcium antagonist nicardipine on renal function and renin release in dogs. *J Cardiovasc Pharmacol* 1983;**5**:254–9.

55 Reves JG, Kissin I, Lell WA *et al.* Calcium entry blockers: uses and implications for anesthesiologist. *Anesthesiology* 1982;**57**:504–18.

56 Ben Ammar M, Coriat P, Houissa M *et al.* Nicardipine vs trinitrine for treatment of postoperative hypertension: effects on haemodynamics and left ventricular function. *Anesthesiology* 1987;**67**:A139.

57 Britt A. Diltiazem (review) *Can Anaesth Soc J* 1985;**32**:30–44.

58 Bazaral MG, Wagner R, Abi Nader E, Estafanous FG. Comparison of effects of 15 and 60 μg/kg used for induction of anesthesia in patients with coronary artery diseases. *Anesth Analg* 1985;**64**:312–18.

59 Gold ML, Sacks DJ, Grosnoff DB *et al.* Use of esmolol during anesthesia to treat tachycardia and hypertension. *Anesth Analg* 1989;**68**:101–4.

60 Kaplan JA. Role of ultrashort acting beta-blockers in the perioperative period. *J Cardiothorac Anesth* 1988;**2**:683–91.

61 Leslie JB, Kalayjian RW, Sirgo MA *et al.* Intravenous labetalol for treatment of postoperative hypertension. *Anesthesiology* 1987;**67**:415–16.

62 Golberg ME, Seltzer J, Azad SS, Smullens SN, Marr AT, Larijani GE. Intravenous labetalol for treatment of hypertension after carotod endarterectomy. *J Cardiothorac Anesth* 1939;**3**:411–17.

63 Brogden RN, Heel RC, Speight TM *et al.* Labetalol: a review of its pharmacology and therapeutic use in hypertension. *Drugs* 1978;**15**:251–70.

64 Richards DA, Tuckman J, Prichard BNC. Assessment of alpha and beta adrenoceptor blocking actions of labetalol. *Br J Clin Pharmacol* 1976;**3**:849–55.

65 Lebret F, Coriat P, Gosgnach M, Baron JF, Reiz S, Viars P. Transesophageal echocardiography assessment of LV function response to labetalol when given to control postoperative hypertension. *J Cardiothorac Anesth* 1992;**6**:443–7.

66 Carter BL. Labetalol. *Drug Intell Clin Pharmacol* 1983;**17**:704–12. Mehta J, Cohn JN. Haemodynamic effects of labetalol, an alpha and beta adrenergic blocking agent in hypertensive subjects. *Circulation* 1977;**55**:370–5.

68 Chauvin M, Deriaz H, Viars P. Continuous intravenous infusion of labetalol for postoperative hypertension. *Br J Anesth* 1987;**59**:1250–6.

69 Gillis RA, Dretchen KL, Namath I *et al.* Hypotensive effect of urapidil: CNS site and relative contribution. *J Cardiovasc Pharmacol* 1987;**9**:103–9.

70 Eltze M. Investigations on the mode of action of a new antihypertensive drug urapidil in the isolated rat vas deferens. *Eur J Pharmacol* 1979;**59**:1–9.

71 Belz GG, Matthews J, Graf D *et al.* Dynamic responses to intravenous urapidil and dihydralazine in normal subjects. *Clin Pharmacol Ther* 1985;**37**:48–54.

72 Hess W, Schulte-Sasse V, Tarnow J, Veit S. Comparison of phentolamine and urapidil in controlling acute intra-operative hypertension in patients subject to coronary artery bypass surgery. *Eur J Anaesthesiol* 1985;**2**:21–2.

73 Le Bret F, Vrints Y, Daas G *et al.* Traitement des accès hypertensifs postopératoires par l'urapidil chez le patient coronarien: effets sur la fonction cardiaque évaluée par l'échocardiographie transoesophagienne. *Ann Fr Anesth Réanim* 1990;**9**:R103.

74 Van Der Starre JA, Feld R, Reneman R. Ketanserin in the treatment of pulmonary hypertension after valvular surgery: a comparison with sodium nitroprusside. *Crit. Care Med* 1989;**17**:613–18.

75 Möllhoft T, Van Aken H, Mulier JP *et al.* Effects of urapidil, ketanserin and sodium nitroprusside on venous admixture and arterial oxygenation following coronary artery

bypass grafting. *Br J Anesth* 1990;**64**:493–7.

76 Vandenbroucke G, Foubert L, Coddens J *et al.* Use of ketanserin in the treatment of hypertension following coronary artery surgery. *J Cardiothorac Anesth* 1994;**8**:324–9.

77 Felding M, Cold GE, Jacobsen C *et al.* The effect of ketanserin upon postoperative blood pressure, cerebral blood flow and oxygen metabolism in patients subjected to craniotomy for cerebral tumours. *Acta Anaesthesiol. Scand.* 1995;**39**:582–5.

78 Boldt J, Schindler E, Wollbrück M. Cardiorespiratory response of intravenous angiotensin-converting enzyme inhibitor enalaprilat in hypertensive cardiac surgery patients. *J Cardiothorac Anesth* 1995;**9**:44–9.

79 Van-Aken J, Leusen I, Lacroix E. Influsion of converting enzyme inhibition on isoflurane-induced hypotension for cerebral aneurysm surgery. *Anaesthesia* 1992;**47**:261–4.

80 Hirschl MM, Binder M, Bur A *et al.* Clinical evaluation of different doses of intravenous enalaprilat in patients with hypertensive crises. *Arch Intern Med* 1995;**155**(20):2217–23.

8: Perioperative management of myocardial ischaemia and coronary artery bypass graft spasm

PHILIPPE OLIVIER, NICOLA D'ATTELLIS, JEAN-FRANÇOIS BARON

Anaesthesia and management of myocardial revascularisation by coronary artery bypass graft (CABG) surgery have been the subject of innumerable research and review articles, with extensive commentary on epidemiology, outcome, effects of anaesthetic agents, and monitoring of the patient.[1, 2]

In addition to the goals of providing anaesthesia and muscle relaxation, a major concern of the anaesthesiologist is the prevention and treatment of myocardial ischaemia. In the past decade, numerous laboratory and clinical studies have examined the incidence of myocardial ischaemia in the pre-bypass period, as it relates to the administration of anaesthetics or muscle relaxants. While the incidence of pre-bypass ischaemia in patients appears to be between 10 and 50% it is not at all clear that the anaesthetic drug combination *per se* is a determinant of this incidence.[3-6] The majority of ischaemic episodes are unrelated to changes in blood pressure or heart rate.[3] This argument has been used at least partly to explain the recent finding of a similar incidence of ischaemia occurring in patients managed with several different anaesthetic techniques in large outcome studies.[7, 8]

During recent years, the extensive use of arterial conduits, internal mammary, gastroepiploic, and radial arteries, has become common practice since this is accompanied by excellent long-term results.[9] However, since the first reported coronary artery spasm immediately after CABG,[10] there have been numerous descriptions of this problem. Many hypotheses have been put forward to explain the origin of coronary artery spasm. Accordingly, prevention and treatment of arterial graft spasm is a major objective of post-cardiopulmonary bypass and postoperative care.

Perioperative myocardial ischaemia

While it would seem logical that the focus should be on the pre-bypass period, as after cardiopulmnary by-pass the heart has been 'revascularised', recent studies have shown that there is a higher incidence of ischaemia after rather than before cardiopulmonary bypass.[3, 5] When compared to the preoperative and postoperative periods, the intraoperative period appears to be the least likely time for ischaemic events. Mangano *et al.* have reported that continuing anaesthesia into the postoperative period with an infusion of sufentanil reduced the incidence of postoperative ischaemic events.[11]

An association exists between tachycardia and the development of myocardial ischaemia. This has been demonstrated by Slogoff and Keats in studies assessing the effect of preoperative antianginal medication.[6] In this study, the incidence of ischaemia was related to peak heart rate. Several investigations have demonstrated that infusion of esmolol, a short-acting cardioselective β-receptor antagonist, attenuates the heart rate response to stressful stimuli during CABG.[12, 13]

The association of tachycardia with hypotension, or hypertension in response to surgical stress, can be associated with pulmonary hypertension and elevated pulmonary capillary wedge pressure. While ECG changes occur later, these early haemodynamic abnormalities almost certainly are the result of ischaemic left ventricular dysfunction. Close attention to haemodynamic control and rapid treatment of abnormalities is a fundamental principle of intraoperative management of the patient with coronary artery disease. The mean arterial pressure–heart rate quotient has been suggested as an indicator of an impaired myocardial oxygen balance,[14] decreased rate quotient indicating decreased supply relative to demand; however, the clinical utility and sensitivity of this index has been as disappointing as the rate–pressure product.

However, if reversible physiological variables could be identified that are indicators of myocardial ischaemia, treatment might be instituted early to prevent cardiac morbidity. In patients undergoing elective coronary artery bypass graft surgery, Urban *et al.* studied the relationship between several premorbid patient characteristics, selected haemodynamic variables, intraoperative myocardial ischaema, and perioperative myocardial infarction.[15] One hundred consecutive patients for elective coronary artery bypass graft surgery were studied prospectively before the initiation of cardiopulmonary bypass. Neither the selected haemodynamic variables nor the premorbid patient characteristics were significantly associated with a perioperative myocardial infarction. No sensitive clinically available haemodynamic indicator of intraoperative myocardial ischaemia was identified. The clinical implication for the anaesthesiologist is that careful ECG monitoring with

ST segment analysis must continue after byass and into the surgical intensive care unit.

Coronary artery spasm

The extensive use of arterial grafts is now common practice and is accompanied by excellent long-term results without increased operative mortality and morbidity.[9] Since 1981, when Buxton *et al.*[10] first reported coronary artery spasm immediately after CABG, there have been numerous descriptions of this problem. Spasm has usually been associated with profound ST segment elevation on the ECG, hypotension, severe venticular dysfunction, and myocardial irritability. Many hypotheses have been put forward to explain the origin of coronary artery spasm; some of the mechanisms that may play a role are shown in Figure 8.1.

Internal mammary artery spasm

Several authors have suggested that native coronary artery spasm remote from the site of anastomosis is responsible for episodes of perioperative haemodynamic collapse in patients undergoing CABG.[16] Occasionally, the phenomenon has been documented angiographically as it occurs.[17]

Sarabu *et al.*[18] described two typical case reports of patients suffering profound haemodynamic instability as a result of intractable spasm of a left internal mammary artery bypass graft in the immediate postoperative period. The location of the spasm at the site of the distal anastomosis of the internal mammary artery graft suggests the extemely important role of local trauma to the vessel. Reports of native coronary artery spasm in the immediate postoperative period have been remarkable for the relatively

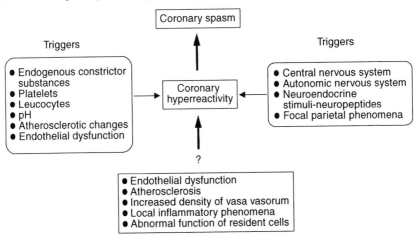

Fig 8.1   Pathogenesis of coronary artery spasm in variant angina pectoris

intractable nature of this phenomenon. Many patients require direct intracoronary infusions of glyceryl trinitrate (GTN) or papaverine, or direct application of papaverine, and the majority require sublingual administration of nifedipine for adequate resolution of graft spasm. Both patients described by Sarabu et al. sustained catastrophic physiological insults as a result of protracted spasm of the internal mammary artery graft at a time when homeostasis generally is maintained in a somewhat precarious fashion. Rebound vasoconstriction has been described in native coronary arteries when calcium-channel blockade is abruptly withdrawn.

The dynamic responses of a native coronary artery and an internal mammary artery graft to pharmacological intervention were examined by arteriography in five patients with variant angina who had undergone CABG with an *in situ* internal mammary artery to the left anterior descending coronary artery.[19] All patients had severe fixed lesions in addition to marked spasm of the left anterior descending coronary artery after stimulation by the administration of ergonovine. Postoperatively, after ergonovine stimulation, complete occlusion or marked subtotal narrowing was again observed at the primary fixed lesion in the proximal portion of the left anterior descending coronary artery, but the internal mammary artery graft and the coronary artery distal to the anastomotic site maintained satisfactory patency with no further occurrence of anginal pain or ST segment elevation. The diameter of the internal mammary artery showed only small changes during infusion of GTN in contrast to the marked vascular reactivity of the coronary artery. These findings indicate that the internal mammary artery graft is unresponsive to ergonovine at least in amounts required to produce coronary artery spasm in patients with variant angina and fixed lesions. The internal mammary artery graft appears from a clinical and pharmacological viewpoint to function well in patients with variant angina.

Several studies have been designed to assess and establish the most appropriate vasodilator agent. The most striking results are those of He et al.[20] The authors studied the reactivity of ring segments of human internal mammary artery in organ baths to various constrictor and dilator agents. Thromboxane-A_2 was the most potent internal mammary artery constrictor agent followed by noradrenaline, serotonin, phenylephrine, and potassium chloride. Reports in the literature suggest that the thromboxane-A_2 level, measured as the stable, inactive metabolite, thromboxane-B_2, is elevated during cardiopulmonary bypass. Increased plasma concentrations of other vasoconstrictors have also been reported during cardiopulmonary bypass. The important results of this work may be summarised as follows: human internal mammary artery contracts strongly to stimulation by thromboxane and α-adrenoreceptor agonists; GNT rapidly and fully relaxes a precontracted internal mammary artery, but this dilator agent is a very weak inhibitor if applied before the constrictor stimulus; calcium-channel blocking drugs have a slow onset time but fully relax a precontracted internal mammary artery; and pretreatment with calcium-channel blockers is very effective in inhibiting contraction induced by membrane depolarisation but is less effective against thromboxane-induced contraction.

These findings in isolated ring segments have, for the first time, characterised the reactivity of human internal mammary artery to a range of constrictor agents, some of which may play an important role in the perioperative period. In particular, platelet-derived thromboxane and serotonin are two potential constrictor mediators. Another important constrictor agent is noradrenaline. The function of β-adrenoreceptors on the human internal mammary artery was studied in vitro to predict the manner in which internal mammary artery grafts would respond to β-adrenergic agonists and antagonists administered in the perioperative period.[21] Ring segments of the distal internal mammary artery obtained from patients not receiving β-blocker therapy were mounted in organ baths and isometric wall force was measured. For comparison, similar experiments were conducted on segments of canine coronary artery, a vessel known to have powerful β-adrenoceptor function. In the human internal mammary artery, the maximum relaxation induced by isoprenaline was weak compared with relaxation measured in the corresponding experiments on canine coronary arteries. These studies suggest that human internal mammary artery has only a small number of β-adrenoceptors that contribute little to the reactivity of human internal mammary artery grafts to sympathomimetic drugs. Clinical implications are that the isolated human internal mammary artery responds poorly to β-adrenoceptor stimulation. This implies that perioperatively administered β-adrenergic catecholamines (for example dobutamine) are most unlikely to dilate the internal mammary artery. As a corollary, β-adrenoceptor antagonists will not uncover constrictor activity on the internal mammary artery and are therefore unlikely to induce spasm, as has been reported for coronary arteries. The study by He et al.[21] suggests that circulating noradrenaline or adrenaline (both α- and β-adrenoceptor agonists) would predominantly contract these vessels. This work indicates that noradrenaline may stimulate α_1- and α_2-adrenoceptors mediating contraction because the α_2-selective agonist, phenylephrine, causes a significantly lower maximal response.

Relativity of the gastroepiploic artery

The right gastroepiploic artery is an alternative coronary artery bypass graft. However, several studies have suggested that the gastroepiploic artery has a higher reactivity and sensitivity to catecholamines.[22-24] In Yang's study,[23] the right gastroepiploic artery exhibited better contractility than the internal mammary artery but comparable endothelium-dependent and endothelium-independent relaxation. The good endothelial function of the gastroepiploic artery might be important for graft function and patency, whereas the enhanced contractility may facillitate vasospasm, especially in the presence of high circulating levels of catecholamines. Dignan et al.,[22] using a similar model, demonstrated that gastroepiploic artery segments have stronger contractions to potassium chloride, adrenergic stimulation (noradrenaline), and product of platelet aggregation (serotonin). However, the gastroepiploic and internal mammary arteries showed equal sensitivity, measured by the concentration causing half-maximal contraction to noradrenaline and serotonin. There was no difference in relaxation to sodium nitroprusside. These data suggest that prevention of platelet-, adrenergic-, or potassium-induced contraction may be more important when the gastroepiploic artery is used as an alternate conduit for coronary artery bypass grafting.

Flow characteristics of the gastroepiploic artery originating from the descending aorta could be another important factor involved in graft patency.[25] Indeed, the inferior capacity of flow through grafts which originate in the descending aorta compared with those that originate in the ascending aorta, is mainly attributed to reduced diastolic pressure in the arterial grafts and is caused by anatomical characteristics. There may be instances, for example intraoartic balloon counterpulsation, in which arterial grafts originating from a systolic-dominant circulation far away from the heart have some limitations in the ability to supply blood to the diastolic-dominant coronary circulation.

Radial artery reactivity

Coronary artery bypass grafting with the radial artery was first proposed and performed by Carpentier in 1973.[26] Later, he recommended that this technique be abandoned because of a 35% incidence of narrowing or occlusion of the conduit at control arteriography. He suggested that graft failure was due to spasm of the denervated artery. Several patients belonging to the early series and having shown some degree of obstruction or occlusion were reinvestigated at a later date and showed a patent radial artery conduit. These observations, together with new antispastic drugs available today, stimulated the reinvestigation of the technique in carefully selected patients.

One hundred and four patients who underwent myocardial revascularisation using 122 radial artery grafts were studied by Acar et al.[27] All patients received intravenous diltiazem intraoperatively and oral diltiazem after discharge. In addition, aspirin (100 mg/day) was prescribed on discharge. Early angiographic controls, within two weeks, were obtained in the first 50 consecutive patients and revealed 100% patent radial artery grafts, left and right internal mammary artery grafts, while 14 out of 18 free internal mammary artery grafts, and 8 out of 9 saphenous vein grafts were patent. Six patients had localised narrowing of the radial artery conduit unrelated to the anastomotic site (spasm). Acar *et al.* believed that failure of the initial experience with the radial artery graft was due to the combination of two mechanisms, vasospasm of the radial artery conduit and intimal hyperplasia. These angiographic studies clearly demonstrated the propensity of the radial artery to undergo spasm. This radiological aspect was noted in 6 patients on the early postoperative angiograms. These spasms were due to a strong contraction of the arterial wall that could not be consistently relieved by vasodilators. However, these spasms were reversible in at least 2 patients, in whom they disappeared 6–12 months later.

After this initial series of patients in whom the radial artery was used as a conduit for CABG, an *in vitro* study was designed to analyse the vasoreactive properties of the radial artery and to compare them with those of the internal mammary and the gastroepiploic arteries.[28] Human radial, internal mammary, and gastroepiploic artery ring segments were studied. The radial artery had stronger contractions to potassium chloride than the other vessels. The radial and gastroepiploic arteries with intact endothelium presented a higher contraction force than the internal mammary artery in response to noradrenaline and serotonin. The three vessels had equal sensitivities to noradrenaline and serotonin. The gastroepiploic artery had a lower sensitivity to a thromboxane-A_2 mimetic than the other two vessels.

The radial artery is very sensitive to mechanical stimuli and reacts instantaneously by producing spasm. Both the harvesting technique and graft preparation have been markedly improved. No intraluminal instruments are used. A recent study by He *et al.* suggests that the combination of verapamil and GTN may provide a rapid onset, complete relaxation, and a long-lasting relaxant effect when used to prepare the radial artery for grafting.[29] The same combination has been suggested to be effective also in saphaneous vein harvesting.[30] The increased reactivity of the radial artery explains its propensity to spasm and emphasises the need for antispastic drugs and platelet inhibitors when the radial artery is used for coronary artery bypass grafting.

Saphenous vein reactivity

Little is known regarding specific biological and pharmacological differences between the human internal mammary artery and saphenous vein. Weinstein *et al.*[31] designed a study to define the role of α-adrenoceptor-mediated vasoconstriction in human internal mammary arteries and saphenous veins. Fresh specimens of both vessels were obtained from 32 patients undergoing CAGB. For consistency, however, the endothelium was purposely removed by gentle abrasion with a rubber-coated applicator. Dose–response curves were generated for the relatively selective α_1-receptor agonist phenylephrine, an α_2-receptor agonist, and the α_1- and α_2-receptor agonist noradrenaline. Phenylephrine elicited similar contractile response in both internal mammary artery and saphenous vein. Selective stimulation of α_2- receptors with an α_2-agonist elicited a marked contractile response in saphenous veins only. Dose–response curves for phenylephrine and the α_2-agonist were shifted to the right for both vessels in the presence of the α_1-receptor antagonist prazosin and the α_2-receptor antagonist yohimbine, respectively. Noradrenaline elicited contraction at a lower concentration in saphenous veins than in the internal mammary arteries. The results suggest that α-adrenoceptor-mediated vasoconstriction is caused primarily by α_1-receptors in human internal mammary arteries and by α_1- and α_2-receptors in human saphenous veins.

Clinical evaluation of coronary artery graft flow

What little data are available concerning regulation of the coronary circulation in humans suggest that under normal conditions the control of the coronary circulation in large mammals is reasonably similar to that observed in man. The opposite is true in the presence of disease. Pathological states simulated in animals (hypertrophy, coronary obstruction, myocardial ischaemia, and coronary collaterals) produce alterations in the coronary circulation that are markedly different from those observed in patients with similar disease processes.[32]

After the initial clinical application of videodensitometry by Rutishauser,[33] a new approach using similar assumptions involving measurements of bypass graft flow reserve with ultrafast computed tomography[34] has been described. Measurements of volume flow or blood flow velocity with Doppler technology have several advantages over electromagnetic flow probes for studies in patients.[35, 36] Finally, a small 3 FG Doppler catheter has been developed recently.[37] This instrument is a significant improvement over the previously described Doppler technique because it measures flow selectively in major coronary vessels rather than in only the left main coronary artery or proximal right coronary artery.

Payen et al.[36] contributed greatly to developing Doppler techniques for the perioperative measurement of graft blood flow. An initial study has been designed in patients with angiographically proven stenosis of the proximal left anterior descending coronary artery of over 90% and a preoperative left ventricular ejection fraction over 45%. After patients were weaned off cardiopulmonary bypass and were haemodynamically stable, implantation of the microprobes was performed. The essential features of the 8 MHz transducer and the zero-cross pulsed Doppler flowmeter have been described and validated. With such a system it is possible to measure the vessel diameter, cross-sectional blood flow velocity and blood flow. Diameter values measured on the first postoperative day are in accordance with the few data published in the literature.[38] Coronary graft velocities recorded are also in agreement with those in previous reports.[25, 39]

Treatment and prevention of myocardial ischaemia and coronary artery bypass graft spasm

When a haemodynamic abnormality is temporally related to the onset of ischaemia, this abnormality should be treated immediately. For example, hypotension should be treated by administration of volume, vasoconstrictors, and/or inotropes; the hypertensive response to surgical stress should be treated by deepening anaesthesia or vasodilator therapy. Inhaled anaesthetic agents may be useful in this respect; there are reports of their use in treatment of acute myocardial dysfunction, most likely secondary to ischaemia and in reducing the ischaemia associated with rapid atrial pacing. However, they could also worsen ischaemia.

Vasodilator therapy, which has beneficial effects on the coronary circulation, is the treatment of choice if the depth of anaesthesia is appropriate. Haemodynamic treatment ensuring an adequate coronary artery perfusion pressure (mean aortic diastolic pressure minus left ventricular end-diastolic pressure) should be a priority, as should control of heart rate, the single most important treatable determinant of myocardial oxygen consumption. Tachycardia not only increases oxygen demand but also reduces the supply, especially to the subendocardium, by reducing diastolic perfusion time. Table 8.1 summarises the treatment of acute perioperative haemodynamically related myocardial ischaemia.

Glyceryl trinitrate (GTN) has been the drug of choice for relieving myocardial ischaemia for more than a century. Intravenous GTN acts immediately, reducing left ventricular preload and wall tension primarily by decreasing venous tone at lower doses, while at larger doses it may also

Table 8.1   Treatment of suspected intraoperative myocardial ischaemia

Associated haemodynamic finding	Therapy
Hypertension, tachycardia	Deepen anaesthesia Beta-blockade iv
Normotension, tachycardia	Assure adequate anaesthesia/change anaesthetic regimen Beta-blockade iv
Hypertension, normal heart rate	Deepen anaesthesia Nicardipine Glyceryl trinitrate iv
Hypotension, tachycardia	Lighten anaesthetic regimen Phenylephrine iv Noradrenaline iv
Hypotension, bradycardia	Lighten anaesthesia Ephedrine iv Adrenaline iv
Hypotension, normal heart rate	Lighten anaesthesia Noradrenaline iv Adrenalaine iv
No abnormality	Glyceryl trinitrate iv Nicardipine iv

decrease arterial resistance.[40] GTN has been shown consistently to decrease left ventricular filling pressure, systemic blood pressure, and myocardial oxygen consumption, and to improve left ventricular performance in patients with severe dysfunction.[41, 42] It is most effective in the treatment of acute myocardial ischaemia associated with induced ventricular dysfunction accompanied by sudden elevations in left ventricular end-diastolic volume and pressure. These elevations in left ventricular preload and wall tension further exacerbate perfusion deficits to the ischaemic subendocardium and usually respond immediately to iv GTN.

In hypovolaemic states, however, higher doses of GTN may markedly reduce systemic blood pressure to dangerous levels. A reflex increase in heart rate may occur at arterial vasodilating doses.

GTN has several important effects on the coronary circulation. It is a potent epicardial coronary artery vasodilator in both normal and diseased vessels.[43] Stenotic lesions dilate with GTN, reducing the resistance to coronary blood flow and improving myocardial ischaemia. Smaller coronary arteries may dilate relatively more than larger coronary vessels; however, the degree of dilatation may depend on the baseline tone of the vessel. This drug is also effective in reversing or preventing coronary artery vasospasm in patients with normal or stenotic coronary vessels. Total coronary blood flow may increase initially, but eventually decreases with GTN despite coronary vasodilatation. Coronary arteriographic studies in humans demonstrate that coronary collateral vessels increase in size after administration of GTN.[44] The improvement in blood flow to the subendocardium, the most vulnerable area to develop ischaemia, is secondary both to improvement in collateral flow and reduction in wall stress, which reduces subendocardial resistance to blood flow.

Preoperatively, GTN is used to treat patients with unstable angina or ischaemic mitral regurgitation, or to limit the size of an evolving myocardial infarction, reduce associated complications, and reverse segmental wall motion abnormalities. During coronary artery bypass grafting, iv GTN is used in the pre-bypass and post-bypass periods. Prior to cardiopulmonary bypass, iv GTN is used to treat signs of ischaemia such as ST segment depression, hypertension uncontrolled by the anaesthetic technique, ventricular dysfunction, or coronary artery spasm.[45, 46] Following cardiopulmonary bypass, iv GTN is often used to treat residual ischaemia, reduce preload and afterload, and treat coronary artery spasm. Combined with a vasopressor so as to increase coronary perfusion pressure, it can be used to treat coronary air embolism. GTN can also be combined with an inotropic drug such as dobutamine for treating left ventricular dysfunction.[47, 48] The above indications may also apply during the postoperative period.

Lell et al. recently studied the prophylactic effects of GTN on regional wall-motion abnormalities, ST segment changes and the incidences of myocardial infarction, cardiac failure, and mortality in 30 patients undergoing coronary artery bypass.[49] Patients received continuous infusions of either saline or GTN (1 μg/kg/min low dose, 2 μg/kg/min high dose) beginning during anaesthesia and continuing for 4 hours postoperatively. The occurrence of wall-motion abnormalities as detected by transoesophageal echocardiography was 38 events in the saline group. Significantly fewer events were recorded in the low dose and high dose GTN groups (20 events and 15 events, respectively) compared to controls. There were no significant differences between the control and GTN groups in respect of the incidence of Holter ST segment events or the incidence of myocardial infarction, cardiac failure, or cardiac death. In this study, GTN reduced the incidence of echocardiographic wall-motion abnormalities in a dose-dependent manner while having no significant effect on other parameters examined.

Acadesine is a purine nucleoside analogue that has been shown in animals to reduce myocardial ischaemic injury by selectively increasing the availability of adenosine in ischaemic tissues. Leung *et al.* investigated whether perioperative use of this acadesine could modify the incidence and severity of perioperative myocardial ischaemia in patients undergoing CABG surgery. One hundred and sixteen patients were randomised to receive one of three continuous intravenous dosing regimens (placebo or one of two doses of acadesine). Before drug administration in the preoperative period (baseline), the incidence and severity of ECG ischaemia did not differ among the three groups. During pre-bypass, the incidence of ECG ischaemia was similar in all three groups. The incidence of ischaemia using transoesophageal echocardiography was numerically lower in the two acadesine groups than in the control group, but this was not statistically significant. During post-bypass, the incidence of ECG and transoesophageal echocardiography was similar in incidence in all groups. Whether acadesine can definitely decrease the frequency of myocardial infarction and the extent of myocardial injury remains to be determined.

Preliminary studies with clonidine suggest that α_2-agonists may be useful to maintain stable haemodynamics in patients undergoing CABG with sufentanil anaesthesia.[50] The new α_2-agonists mivazerol and dexmedetomidine have still to be evaluated to demonstrate their efficacy in reducing myocardial ischaemia and injury in patients undergoing myocardial revascularisation.

Recent attention has focused on calcium-channel antagonists for use during anaesthesia for the prevention and treatment of perioperative myocardial ischaemia, coronary artery spasm, hypertensive episodes, and arrhythmias due to anaesthetic or surgical causes. These agents collectively relax arterial smooth muscle, with little effect on most venous beds. Despite similarities, the calcium antagonists differ in their actions and haemodynamic effects.[51-55] For example, nifedipine acts primarily on vascular smooth muscle, with little effect on the atrioventricular node. In contrast, verapamil[53] acts mainly on the cardiac conduction system and has less effect on vascular smooth muscle and myocardium.

Coronary artery dilatation occurs with calcium-channel blockers, with an increase in total coronary bypass graft flows.[56] Nifedipine and nicardipine are the most potent coronary vasodilators, especially in epicardial vessels, which are prone to vasospasm.[57] Diltiazem is effective in blocking coronary artery vasoconstriction caused by a variety of agents.[58] Calcium-channel blockers may also dilate coronary arteries at their stenotic site, thus reducing the pressure gradient across the coronary lesion. Diltiazem preferentially dilates coronary arteries compared to other peripheral vessels. Animal studies demonstrate that nifedipine, verapamil, and diltiazem increase coronary collateral flow distal to coronary ligation and improve subendocardial flow relative to subepicardial flow.[59, 60]

He et al.[20] examined vasodilator activity first by direct relaxation of precontracted arteries and secondly by pretreating arteries with a relaxing agent to test its inhibition by a constrictor agent. Both approaches have direct clinical applications – relaxing a vessel already in spasm and the prevention of spasm by prophylactic pretreatment. Nifedipine, verapamil, and diltiazem all caused full relaxation, but nifedipine was 15 times more potent than the other calcium antagonists. In contrast, the pretreatment of vessels with GTN failed to alter subsequent contraction to thromboxane or potassium, while nifedipine pretreatment abolished the subsequent contraction to potassium and reduced sensitivity of the internal mammary artery to thromboxane. In an intraoperative study, Cooper[61] confirmed the potential beneficial effects of nifedipine and GTN in relieving internal mammary artery vasospasm. In this study, under controlled haemodynamic conditions free flow was measured before pharmacological intervention and after the pedicle had been sprayed with one of the following agents. Saline produced a small increase in flow from a median of 23 ml/min to 38 ml/min, whereas a significant increase occurred with papaverine from 25 to 43 ml/min. Nifedipine and GTN both increased free flow almost threefold, from 23 to 71 ml/min and from 23 to 62 ml/min respectively. Therefore, these drugs may be recommended to prevent and relieve intraoperative spasm of the internal mammary artery.

Nifedipine is not sufficiently stable to permit formulation in a parenteral form. It has been used experimentally as an iv infusion. Therefore, it must be administered intraoperatively by either the sublingual or intranasal route. In hypertensive emergencies, sublingual nifedipine does not produce a fast enough response to be useful therapy during CABG. Nicardipine is a short-acting dihydropyridine calcium antagonist similar to nifedipine, but possesses a tertiary amine structure in the ester side chain. Unlike other available dihydropyridines, nicardipine is a stable parenteral solution, and, therefore, can be administered intravenously. It has a highly specific mode of action, which includes coronary antispasm and vasodilatory effects, and systemic vasodilatation.[62] Other important haemodynamic effects include reduction in blood pressure and systemic vascular resistance, and an increase in cardiac output. Recent studies have shown that nicardipine produces minimal myocardial depression and significant improvement in diastolic function in patients with ischaemic heart disease.[63, 64]

Nicardipine's rapid onset time and short duration of action make it an attractive drug for the perioperative management of hypertension or myocardial ischaemia. It has been administered to patients in whom haemodynamic control was necessary during either non-cardiac vascular or CABG surgery. During CABG, van Wezel et al.[65] demonstrated that nicardipine was preferable to sodium nitroprusside for controlling intra-operative hypertension and myocardial ischaemia. In their study, a 3–12 µg/kg/min infusion of nicardipine was compared to a 1–3 µg/kg/min infusion of sodium nitroprusside. Both drugs were found to be equally effective in controlling blood pressure; however, there was a 24% incidence of ST segment depression in the sodium nitroprusside group versus 9% in the nicardipine group. The authors concluded that nicardipine offered significant advantages over sodium nitroprusside due to its coronary vasodilatory activity, reduction of coronary artery spasm and production of myocardial protection. Nicardipine has also been shown to be useful for the treatment of postoperative hypertension and this could eventually become its primary indication. The availability of this stable intravenous calcium antagonist is a major advance over previously available drugs in this therapeutic category. In the future, other dihydrophyridine derivatives, such as nimodipine, nisoldipine, nitrendipine, and isradipine, may also offer therapeutic advantages over the present agents.[66]

Use of inotropes after myocardial revascularisation

Vasoactive agents are needed frequently in patients undergoing myocar-dial revascularisation, and postoperative spasm of arterial grafts can cause morbidity and mortality after myocardial revascularisation. Using pulsed Doppler microprobes, implanted on saphenous vein bypass grafts, Beloucif et al.[67] studied the effects of dobutamine (5 and 10 µg/kg/min) 6 h after cardiac surgery. Mean coronary bypass graft flows increased during inotropic stimulation from $61·8 \pm 19·2$ to $81·1 \pm 21·8$ ml/min. Systolic coronary bypass graft flows were held constant because the increase in systolic arterial pressure contributed to the maintenance of coronary perfusion pressure in systole. Diastolic coronary bypass graft flow incrased more than did diastolic arterial pressure and was related to the rate–pressure product taken as an index of myocardial oxygen consumption. Although dobutamine probably has little effect on native coronary arteries or arterial grafts, this drug does not seem to have deleterious effects on the coronary circulation and may be used safely when indicated in patients undergoing myocardial revascularisation.

In recent years, phosphodiesterase inhibitors have been investigated using *in vivo* canine experimental models, and studies on human internal mammary artery.[68-70] Experimental studies in dogs demonstrated that milrinone induces a 33% increase in internal mammary blood flow.[69] Using *in vitro* human artery rings, Salmenpera *et al.* confirmed the potential vasodilatory effect of amrinone on the internal mammary artery.[70] The most striking results were described by Izzat *et al.*[68] who investigated the effect of five agents on internal mammary artery free flow in 50 patients in whom the left internal mammary artery was used for myocardial revascularisation. The increase in free flow expressed as a percentage of initial flow was greater for enoximone (94%±24%) than for saline (18%±11%), dobutamine (40%±27%), and glyceryl trinitate (52%±36%). Therefore, the systemic use of phosphodiesterase inhibitors as inotropic agents with the ability to prevent and treat postoperative spasm of the internal mammary artery may be recommended. However, the dosage must be carefully and progressively titrated to avoid simultaneous use of vasoconstrictors.

Conclusions

While it would seem logical that the focus should be on the pre-bypass period, as the heart has been 'revascularised' after cardiopulmonary bypass, recent studies have shown that there is a higher incidence of ischaemia after rather than before cardiopulmonary bypass. This implies careful monitoring of the patient by the anaesthesiologist during the intraoperative period and throughout the entire intensive care stay.

Graft spasm of the internal mammary artery is a potentially lethal early postoperative phenomenon that must be treated aggressively. The appearance of angina or marked ECG abnormalities may be evaluated by coronary angiography and treated with intracoronary infusions of GTN. For acute, refractory haemodynamic collapse during the immediate postoperative period, we recommend immediate reoperation to assess the nature of the event and its appropriate treatment.

The human internal mammary artery contracts strongly to stimulation by thromboxane-A_2 and α-adrenoreceptor agonists. GTN will rapidly and fully relax a precontracted internal mammary artery, but this dilator agent is a very weak inhibior if applied before the constrictor stimulus. Calcium-channel blocking drugs have a slow onset time but will fully relax a precontracted internal mammary artery. Pretreatment with calcium-channel blockers is very effective in prophylaxis of arterial graft spasm. In potassium-precontracted arteries, nifedipine, verapamil, and diltiazem all cause full relaxation, but nifedipine is 15 times more potent than the other calcium antagonists. Nicardipine is a short-acting dihydropyridine calcium antagonist similar to nifedipine, stable as a parenteral solution, and, therefore, easily administered intravenously. It has a highly specific mode of action, which includes coronary antispasm and vasodilatory effects, and systemic vasodilatation.

1 Wynands JE, Sheridan CA, Kelkar K. Coronary artery disease and anaesthesia (experience in 120 patients for revascularization of the heart). *Can Anaesth Soc J* 1967;14:382–98.
2 Mangano DT. Perioperative cardiac morbidity. *Anesthesiology* 1990;72:153–84.
3 Knight AA, Hollenberg M, London MJ *et al*. Perioperative myocardial ischemia: importance of the preoperative ischemic pattern. *Anesthesiology* 1988;68:681–8.
4 Kotter GS, Kotrly KJ, Kalbfleisch JH, Vucins EJ, Kampine JP. Myocardial ischemia during cardiovascular surgery as detected by an ST segment trend montoring system. *J Cardiothorac Anesth* 1987;1:190–9.
5 Leung JM, O'Kelly B, Browner WS, Tubau J, Hollenber M, Mangano DT. Prognostic importance of postbypass region wall-motion abnormalities in patients undergoing coronary artery bypass graft surgery. SPI Research Group. *Anesthesiology* 1989;71:16–25.
6 Slogoff S, Keats AS. Does chronic treatment with calcium entry blocking drugs reduce perioperative myocardial ischemia? *Anesthesiology* 1988;68:676–80.
7 Slogoff S, Keats AS. Randomized trial of primary anesthetic agents on outcome of coronary artery bypass operations. *Anesthesiology* 1989;70:179–88.
8 Tuman KJ, McCarthy RJ, Spiess BD, Da Valle M, Dabir R, Ivankovich AD. Does choice of anesthetic agent significantly affect outcome after coronary artery surgery? *Anesthesiology* 1989;70:189–98.
9 Nishida H, Hirota J, Yamaki F *et al*. Extensive use of arterial grafts for coronary artery bypass grafting in Japanese patients. *Cardiovasc Surg* 1994;2:93–6.
10 Buxton AE, Goldberg S, Harken A, Hirshfield J, jr, Kastor JA. Coronary-artery spasm immediately after myocardial revascularization: recognition and management. *N Engl J Med* 1981;304:1249–53.
11 Mangano DT, Siliciano D, Hollenberg M *et al*. Postoperative myocardial ischemia. Therapeutic trials using intensive analgesia following surgery. The Study of Perioperative Ischemia (SPI) Research Group. *Anesthesiology* 1992–76:342–53.
12 Girard D, Shulman BJ, Thys DM, Mindich BP, Mikula SK, Kaplan JA. The safety and efficacy of esmolol during myocardial revasalurization. *Anesthesiology* 1986;65:157–64.
13 Harrison L, Ralley FE, Wynands JE *et al*. The role of an ultra short-acting adrenergic blocker (esmolol) in patients undergoing coronary artery bypass surgery. *Anesthesiology* 1987;66:413–18.
14 Buffington CW. Hemodynamic determinants of ischemic myocardial dysfunction in the presence of coronary stenosis in dogs. *Anesthesiology* 1985;63:651–62.
15 Urban MK, Gordon MA, Harris SN, O'Connor T, Barash PG. Intraoperative hemodynamic changes are not good indicators of myocardial ischemia. *Anesth Analg* 1993;76:942–9.
16 Skarvan K, Graedel E, Hasse J, Stulz P, Pfisterer M. Coronary artery spasms after coronary artery bypass surgery. *Anesthesiology* 1984;61:323–7.
17 Black AJ, Mews GC. Coronary artery spasm after coronary bypass grafting. *Am J Cardiol* 1984;54:670–1.
18 Sarabu MR, McClung JA, Fass A, Reed GE. Early postoperative spasm in left internal mammary artery bypass grafts. *Ann Thorac Surg* 1987;44:199–200.
19 Kitamura S, Morita R, Kawachi K *et al*. Different responses of coronary artery and internal mammary artery bypass grafts to ergonovine and nitroglycerin in variant angina. *Ann Thorac Surg* 1989;47:756–60.
20 He GW, Rosenfeldt FL, Buxton BF, Angus JA. Reactivity of human isolated internal mammary artery to constrictor and dilator agents. Implications for treatment of internal mammary artery spasm. *Circulation* 1989;80(Suppl I):141–50.
21 He GW, Buxton B, Rosenfeldt FL, Wilson AC, Angus JA. Weak beta-adrenoceptor-mediated relaxation in the human internal mammary artery. *J Thorac Cardiovasc Surg*

1989;97:259–66.

22 Dignan RJ, Yeh T jr, Dyke CM *et al.* Reactivity of gastroepiploic and internal mammary arteries. Relevance to coronary artery bypass grafting. *J Thorac Cardiovasc Surg* 1992;**103**:166–22.

23 Yang Z, Siebenmann R, Studer M, Egloff L, Luscher TF. Similar endothelium-dependent relaxation, but enhanced contractility, of the right gastroepiploic artery as compared with the internal mammary artery. *J Thorac Cardiovasc Surg* 1992;**104**:459–64.

24 Ochiai M, Ohno M, Taguchi J *et al.* Responses of human gastroepiploic arteries to vasoactive substances: comparison with responses of internal mammary arteries and saphenous veins. *J Thorac Cardiovasc Surg* 1992;**104**:453–8.

25 Furuse A, Klopp EH, Brawley RK, Gott VL. Hemodynamics of aorta-to-coronary artery bypass. Experimental and analytical studies. *Ann Thorac Surg* 1972;**14**:282–93.

26 Carpentier A, Guermonprez JL, Deloche A, Frechette C, Du Bost C. The aorta-to-coronary radial artery bypass graft. A technique avoiding pathological changes in grafts. *Ann Thorac Surg* 1973;**16**:111–21.

27 Acar C, Jebara VA, Porghese M *et al.* Revival of the radial artery for coronary artery bypass grafting. *Ann Thorac Surg* 1992;**54**:652–9.

28 Chardigny C, Jebara VA, Acar C *et al.* Vasoreactivity of the radial artery. Comparison with the internal mammary and gastroepiploic arteries with implications for coronary artery surgery. *Circulation* 1993;**88**(Suppl II):115–27.

29 He GW, Yang CQ. Use of verapamil and nitroglycerin solution in preparation of radial artery for coronary grafting. *Ann Thorac Surg* 1996;**61**:610–14.

30 He GW, Rosenfeldt FL, Angus JA. Pharmacological relaxation of the saphenous vein during harvesting for coronary artery bypass grafting. *Ann Thorac Surg* 1993;**55**:1210–17.

31 Weinstein JS, Grossman W, Weintraub RM, Thurer RL, Johnson RG, Morgan KG. Differences in alpha-adrenergic responsiveness between human internal mammary arteries and saphenous veins. *Circulation* 1989;**79**:1264–70.

32 Marcus ML, Wilson RF, White CW. Methods of measurement of myocardial blood flow in patients: a critical review. *Circulation* 1987;**76**:245–53.

33 Rutishauser W, Simon H, Stucky JP, Schad N, Noseda G, Wellauer J. Evaluation of Roentgen cinedensitometry for flow measurement in models and in the intact circulation. *Circulation* 1967;**36**:951–63.

34 Rumberger JA, Feiring AJ, Lipton MJ, Higgins CB, Ell SR, Marcus ML. Use of ultrafast computed tomography to quantitate regional myocardial perfusion: a preliminary report. *J Am Coll Cardiol* 1987;**9**:59–69.

35 Kajiya F, Tsujioka K, Ogasawara Y *et al.* Analysis of flow characteristics in poststenotic regions of the human coronary artery during bypass graft surgery. *Circulation* 1987;**76**:1092–100.

36 Payen D, Bousseau D, Laborde F *et al.* Comparison of perioperative and postoperative phasic blood flow in aortocoronary venous bypass grafts by means of pulsed Doppler echocardiography with implantable microprobes. *Circulation* 1986;**74**(Suppl III): 61–7.

37 Wilson RF, Laughlin DE, Ackell PH *et al.* Transluminal, subselective measurement of coronary artery blood flow velocity and vasodilator reserve in man. *Circulation* 1985;**72**:82–92.

38 Simon R, Amende I, Oelert H, Hertzer R, Borst HG, Lichtlen PR, Blood velocity, flow and dimensions of aortocoronary venous bypass grafts in the postoperative state. *Circulation* 1982;**66**(Suppl I):34–9.

39. Grondin CM, Lepage G, Castonguay YR, Meere C, Grondin P. Aortocoronary bypass graft. Initial blood flow through the graft, and early postoperative patency. *Circulation* 1971;**44**:815–19.

40 Simon AC, Levenson JA, Levy BY, Bouthier JE, Peronneau PP, Safar ME. Effect of nitroglycerin on peripheral large arteries in hypertension. *Br J Clin Pharmacol* 1982;**14**:241–6.

41 McGregor M. Pathogenesis of angina pectoris and role of nitrates in relief of myocardial ischemia. *Am J Med* 1983;**74**:21–7.

42 Abrams J. Hemodynamic effects of nitroglycerin and long-acting nitrates. *Am Heart J* 1985;**110**:216–24.

43 Conti CR, Feldman RL, Pepine CJ, Hill JA, Conti JB. Effect of glyceryl trinitrate on

coronary and systemic hemodynamics in man. *Am J Med* 1983;74:28–32.

44 Cohen MV, Downey JM, Sonnenblick EH, Kairk ES. The effects of nitroglycerin on coronary collaterals and myocardial contractility. *J Clin Invest* 1973;52:2836–47.

45 Hill JA, Feldman RL, Pepine CJ, Conti CR. Randomized double-blind comparison of nifedipine and isosorbide dinitrate in patients with coronary arterial spasm. *Am J Cardiol* 1982;49:431–8.

46 Conti CR. Use of nitrates in unstable angina pectoris. *Am J Cardiol* 1987;60:31H–34H.

47 Fujita M, Yamanishi K, Hirai T *et al.* Significance of collateral circulation in reversible left ventricular asynergy by nitroglycerin in patients with relatively recent myocardial infarction. *Am Heart J* 1990;120:521–8.

48 Jugdutt BI, Warnica JW. Intravenous nitroglycerin therapy to limit myocardial infarct size, expansion, and complications. Effect of timing, dosage, and infarct location. *Circulation* 1988;78:906–19.

49 Lell W, Johnson P, Plagenhoef J *et al.* The effect of prophylactic nitroglycerin infusion on the incidence of region wall-motion abnormalities and ST segment changes in patients undergoing coronary artery bypass surgery *J Card Surg* 1993;8:228–31.

50 Howie MB, Hiestand DC, Jopling MW, Romanelli VA, Kelly WB, McSweeney TD. Effect of oral clonidine premedication on anesthetic requirement, hormonal response, hemodynamics and recovery in coronary artery bypass graft surgery patients. *J. Clin Anesth* 1996;8:264–72.

51 Griffin RM, Dimich I, Jurado R, Kaplan JA. Haemodynamic effects of diltiazem during fentanyl-nitrous oxide anaesthesia. An *in vivo* study in the dog. *Br J Anaesth* 1988;60:655–9.

52 Kaplan JA. The role of nicardipine during anesthesia and surgery. *Clin Ther* 1989;11:84–93.

53 Kates RA, Kaplan JA. Cardiovascular responses to verapamil during coronary artery bypass gaft surgery. *Anesth Analg* 1983;62:821–6.

54 Lambert CR, Hill JA, Nichols WW, Feldman RL, Pepine CJ. Coronary and systemic hemodynamic effects of nicardipine. *Am J Cardiol* 1985;55:652–6.

55 Turlapaty P, Vary R, Kaplan JA. Nicardipine, a new intravenous calcium antagonist: a review of its pharmacology, pharmacokinetics, and perioperative applications. *J Cardiothorac Anesth* 1989;3:344–55.

56 Mizgala HF. The calcium channel blockers: pharmacology and clinical applications. *Can Anaesth Soc J* 1983;30:5–10.

57 Henry PD. Comparative pharmacology of calcium antagonists: nifedipine, verapamil and diltiazem. *Am J Cardiol* 1980;46:1047–58.

58 Brown BG, Bolson EL, Dodge HT. Dynamic mechanisms in human coronary stenosis. *Circulation* 1984;70:917–22.

59 da Luz PL, Monteiro de Barros LF, Leite JJ, Pileggi F, Decourt LV. Effect of verapamil on regional coronary and myocardial perfusion during acute coronary occlusion. *Am J Cardiol* 1980;45:269–75.

60 Henry PD, Shuchleib R, Clark RE, Perez JE. Effect of nifedipine on myocardial ischemia: analysis of collateral flow, pulsatile heat and regional muscle shortening. *Am J Cardiol* 1979;44:817–24.

61 Cooper GJ, Wilkinson GA, Angelini GD. Overcoming perioperative spasm of the internal mammary artery: which is the best vasodilator? *J Thorac Cardiovasc Surg* 1992;104:465–8.

62 Pepine CJ. Intravenous nicardipine: cardiovascular effects and clinical relevance. *Clin Ther* 1988;10:316–25.

63 Pepine CJ, Lambert CR. Effects of nicardipine on coronary blood flow. *Am Heart J* 1988;116:248–54.

64 Pepine CJ, Lambert CR. Usefulness of nicardipine for angina pectoris. *Am J Cardiol* 1987;59:13–19.

65 van Wezel HB, Koolen JJ, Visser CA *et al.* The efficacy of nicardipine and nitroprusside in preventing poststernotomy hypertension. *J Cardiothorac Anesth* 1989;3:700–6.

66 Hynynen M, Siltanen T, Sahlman A, Pohjasvaara T, Muck W, Kaste M. Continuous infusion of nimodipine during coronary artery surgery: haemodynamic and pharmacokinetic study. *Br J Anaesth* 1995;74:526–33.

67 Beloucif S, Laborde F, Beloucif L, Piwnica A, Payen D. Determinants of systolic and

175

diastolic flow in coronary bypass grafts with inotropic stimulation. *Anesthesiology* 1990;**73**:1127–35.

68 Izzat MB, West RR, Ragoonanan C, Angelini GN. Effect of systemic vasodilators on internal mammary artery flow. Implications for postoperative treatment after myocardial revascularization. *J Thorac Cardiovasc Surg* 1994;**108**:82–5.

69 Gitter R, Anderson JM, Jett GK. Influence of milrinone and norepinephrine on blood flow in canine internal mammary artery grafts. *Ann Thorac Surg* 1996;**61**:1367–71.

70 Salmenpera M, Levy JH. The *in vitro* effects of phodiesterase inhibitors on the human internal mammary artery. *Anesth Analg* 1996;**82**:954–7.

9: Treatment of perioperative left ventricular dysfunction

JOACHIM BOLDT

Treatment of left ventricular dysfunction in the perioperative period represents a never-ending challenge. Acute left ventricular dysfunction is mostly termed as 'acute heart failure', although right ventricular failure may also lead to haemodynamic catastrophe.

Heart failure is characterised by reduced organ perfusion associated with central fluid accumulation.[1] The common denominator of heart failure – independent of its origin – is the inability of the myocardium to match the load imposed on it. The most predominant haemodynamic consequence of abnormalities of left ventricular function is a low output syndrome (LOS). This syndrome of circulatory dysfunction secondary to impaired left heart function is also termed **congestive heart failure**.[2] Pathophysiologically, various mechanisms are involved in the development of heart failure: changes in heart rate (bradycardic or tachycardic arrhythmias), alterations in loading (pre- and afterload), and impairment of myocardial contractility. When talking about 'heart failure', a complex pathophysiological picture is outlined. Myocardial failure can best be characterised by the heart's limited ability to sustain adequate organ perfusion and to provide the tissue with substrates. Aetiologically, it is necessary to distinguish between congenital and acquired heart disease, between left and right ventricular dysfunction and between abnormalities of diastolic (the ability of the heart to relax and fill) and systolic (the ability of the heart to contract) function abnormalities.

Pathogenesis of perioperative heart failure

Left ventricular failure in the perioperative period may occur with or without depression of myocardial contractility. Acute hypertension, extreme tachyarrhythmia, and bradyarrhythmia are reasons for development of acute heart failure in this situation. Ischaemic heart disease is the

177

Classification of heart failure

- **Systolic dysfunction (abnormal emptying)**
  1 Reduced contractile function
      myocardial ischaemia
      dilated cardiomyopathy
  2 Increased afterload
      systemic hypertension
      aortic stenosis
  3 Structural abnormalities
      ventricular septal defect
      aortic/mitral regurgitation

- **Diastolic dysfunction (elevated filling pressure)**
  1 Systolic dysfunction
  2 External compression
      tamponade
      cor pulmonale
      constrictive pericarditis
  3 Decreased distensibility
      hypertropic cardiomyopathies
      ageing
      restrictive cardiomyopathies
  4 Obstruction to filling
      mitral stenosis

Modified from Little and Applegate, 1993[2]

---

most common underlying disease for deterioration in myocardial contractility leading to left ventricular failure.

As surgical technique and anaesthetic management have significantly improved, more critically ill patients have become increasingly acceptable candidates for all kinds of surgery. Many of these patients have a complex medical history and multisystem diseases. Myocardial infarction and reduced ventricular performance are no longer exclusion criteria for performing anaesthesia and surgery. The mechanisms by which acute left ventricular dysfunction is induced in the perioperative period are many. Combined effects of anaesthetic drugs, ablation of sympathetic outflow, and onset of positive pressure ventilation can precipitate rapid haemodynamic deterioration. Since sympathetic nervous system activity is an important physiological and pathophysiological regulator of cardiac muscle contractility, induction of anaesthesia presents a specific situation in which haemodynamic catastrophe may be engendered.

Patients undergoing cardiac surgery are at a particularly increased risk for developing low-output failure since myocardial ischaemic arrest – often coupled with pre-existing cardiac dysfunction – is associated with myocardial dysfunction. Although several (pharmacological) approaches are used to limit ischaemia-related myocardial tissue damage,[3-6] perioperative

178

myocardial ischaemia is still common in cardiac surgery patients. Post-bypass myocardial dysfunction involves depression of both global ventricular and regional performance. The incomplete recovery of regional contraction of previously hypo- or dyskinetic segments contributes to depression of overall global performance. Thus, in the post-bypass period, cardiovascular dynamics are influenced mainly by the post-ischaemic state of the myocardium and pharmacological support is often necessary to generate an adequate cardiac output in this situation.[7]

Monitoring of perioperative left ventricular dysfunction

Using various classes of substances acting on the cardiovascular system, assessment of their influence on ventricular function in humans is problematic. It is often difficult to separate the changes of pre- and afterload from a direct positive inotropic effect. Mostly, (direct) positive inotropic effects are deduced from measurements of arterial pressure, atrial and ventricular filling pressures, and cardiac output,[8] which are easily available in the clinical setting. Some of these indicators relate to the function of the heart as a pump, while others relate to its function as a muscle. Changes of myocardial contractility cannot definitely be concluded from these variables. Transoesophageal echocardiography (TOE) is an established technique for assessing left ventricular function.[9] It is, however, expensive, requires skilled physicians familiar with the technique, and can be used only in selected patients.

Therapy of low output syndrome

In spite of marked improvements in surgical and anaesthetic techniques, some patients still develop acute heart failure in the perioperative period. Besides sufficient volume therapy and correction of metabolic and electrolyte disorders, pharmacological support is often necessary to guarantee stable haemodynamics. The complexity of the pathogenesis of left ventricular dysfunction offers a range of opportunities for pharmacological interventions. Tailoring pharmacological support to the specific haemodynamic disorder is crucial in this situation.

While heart failure starts with myocardial dysfunction, many of the manifestations of low output syndrome result from peripheral circulatory derangements.[10] As the heart fails to meet the metabolic demand, various compensatory neuroendocrine mechanisms are activated. Vasoconstriction, mediated by the sympathetic and renin–angiotensin systems (RAS), increases (right and left) ventricular afterload thereby maintaining or aggravating the haemodynamic abnormality.

The objectives in this situation are to improve overall cardiac function and to provide optimal organ perfusion. Left ventricular performance depends on systolic pump function, active relaxation, passive diastolic

Classification of drugs acting in the cardiovascular system

- **Vasopressors**
  Phenylephrine
  Methoxamine

- **Inotropic vasopressors**
  Ephedrine
  Noradrenaline
  Adrenaline
  Dopamine (high dose)

- **Vasodilators**
  Calcium-channel blockers
  Glyceryl trinitrate (GTN)
  Sodium nitroprusside (SNP)
  Angiotensin converting enzyme (ACE) inhibitors
  Hydralazine
  Adenosine

- **Inotropic vasodilators**
  Dopamine (low dose)
  Dobutamine
  Dopexamine
  Phosphodiesterase (PDE) inhibitors
  Isoprenaline

- **Inotropic depressors**
  Beta-blockers (vascular: vasoconstriction)
  Calcium-channel blockers (vascular: vasodilatation)

actions, and vascular loading conditions. Thus, besides stimulating myocardial contractility with positive inotropes, any effective therapy in this situation also aims at reducing vascular resistance (Figure 9.1).

When treating patients with acute myocardial dysfunction, three major aspects have to be taken into account:

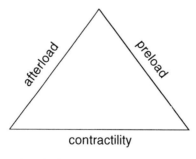

Fig 9.1 Therapeutic triangle for treating cardiac failure in the perioperative period

- The failing myocardium has a residual functional reserve.
- The reserve can be activated when appropriately stimulated.
- The higher level of function can be maintained.

Successful therapy of acute heart failure is directed to improve the reduced myocardial contractility, reduce vascular resistance and improve circulation at the microcirculatory level. In the perioperative period, acute improvement of cardiac performance most often requires positive inotropic stimulation. However, when treating acute low output syndrome secondary to heart failure, it is of major importance to distinguish between patients without a cardiac history and patients in whom chronic myocardial dysfunction is of long standing. In these patients down-regulation of β_1-adrenergic receptors may limit success of 'standard' catecholamine therapy.[11]

Apart from administering positive inotropes to increase myocardial contractility, arteriolar and venous vasodilators to reduce afterload – associated with a favourable reduction in ventricular wall stress – are useful therapeutic strategies in this situation.

Extensive and complex surgical procedures are associated with considerable perioperative haemodynamic and pulmonary complications.[12] A substantial body of evidence supports the concept that deterioration in regional microperfusion (for example, splanchnic perfusion), may be of particular importance for postoperative complications or even for the patient's outcome.[13, 14] Thus, inadequate systemic perfusion and significant reduction in microcirculatory flow are accepted to be important triggers for development of multiple organ dysfunction syndrome (MODS).[15] The ideal pharmacological agent in this situation should improve myocardial function without producing adverse effects, and particularly without resulting in an increased myocardial oxygen debt.

Classification of inotropic drugs

- **cAMP-dependent substances**
  Beta-receptor agonists
  PDE inhibitors (amrinone, enoximone, milrinone)
  activators of adenylate cyclase (forskolin)

- **cAMP-independent substances**
  sodium/potassium pump inhibitors (digitalis glycosides)
  calcium
  Ca^{++}-channel agonists/sensitisers
  Alpha-receptor agonists

- **Drugs that act through metabolic or endocrine pathways**
  tri-iodothyronine

Although this chapter mostly concentrates on treatment of left ventricular dysfunction, other possible pathogenic factors that contribute to the development or maintenance of acute heart failure should never be neglected.

Positive inotropes

Most therapeutic aproaches to the treatment of acute low output failure perioperatively are based on the use of catecholamines. They are still a mainstay for inotropic therapy. Their effects depend on stimulation of various myocardial and vascular receptors (Tables 9.1, 9.2). Most catecholamines are powerful positive inotropic agents, but are associated with marked chronotropic effects with resulting increased myocardial oxygen demand. However, this may be hazardous in patients with ischaemic heart disease. In addition to effects on the myocardium, most of these substances possess negative effects on ventricular loading via arteriolar and venous vasoconstriction, and on myocardial oxygen balance (Table 9.3).

One of the core issues in the controversy surrounding the treatment of acute left ventricular dysfunction is the choice of the ideal inotropic substance. Dobutamine and dopamine are often recommended as first-line catecholamines,[16] whereas adrenaline is indicated for resuscitation and anaphylactic shock.[16] Results in the literature, however, are not conclusive.[17, 18]

Noradrenaline is the physiological mediator of sympathetic nervous system β-stimulation of the heart. It possesses potent α-adrenergic activity, and thus is a potent vasoconstrictor. Because of its (unwanted) increase in wall stress, noradrenaline is usually not given as a cardiac inotrope,[19] and its use is limited to treating reduced blood pressure caused by severely reduced systemic vascular resistance. There is a growing consensus that haemody-

Table 9.1 Adrenergic receptors

Receptor	Location	Action
α_1	Postsynaptic – vascular smooth muscle	Vasoconstriction
α_2	Presynaptic	Inhibits noradrenaline release (negative feedback)
	Postsynaptic – smooth muscle	Vasoconstriction
β_1	Postsynaptic – heart	Positive inotropy and chronotropy Increased automaticity Increased conduction velocity
β_2	Postsynatpic – vascular smooth muscle	Vasodilatation
	– bronchial smooth muscle	Bronchodilatation
	– uterine smooth muscle	Uterine atony
DA1	Postsynaptic – renal, mesenteric vascular	Vasodilatation (splanchnic bed)
	– smooth muscle, coronary?	
DA2	Presynaptic	Inhibition of noradrenaline Release

Table 9.2 Actions of catecholamines

Substance	Receptors					Dose dependence	Comments
	α_1	α_2	β_1	β_2	DA1/DA2	$\alpha, \beta,$ DA	
Isoprenaline			+++++	++++++	0/0	0	
Phenylephrine	+++++		0	0	0/0	++	Primarily vasoconstriction
Adrenaline	+++++	++++	++	0	0/0	++++	
Noradrenaline	+++++	+++	0	0	0/0	+++	Vasoconstriction
Methoxamine	+++++	++	0	0	0/0	++	Vasoconstriction only
Ephedrine	++		+++	++	0/0	++	Direct and indirect
Dopamine	+/+++++		+++++	++	+++/?	+++++	Intropism > chronotropism
Dobutamine	0/+		+++++	++	0/0	+	Splanchnic perfusion ↑
Dopexamine	0	0	+	+++	+++/++	0	

183

Table 9.3   Typical cardiovascular effects of inotropic drugs

	MAP	HR	PAP	PCWP	CO	SVR	M_vO_2
Isoprenaline	↓	↑↑↑	↓	↓	↑	↓	↑↑
Adrenaline	↑	↑↑	↑	↑	↑↑	↑	↑
Noradrenaline	↑↑↑	↔/↓	↑	↑	↑↔↓	↑↑↑	↑↑
Dopamine	↑	↑	↑	↑	↑	↑↓	↑
Dobutamine	↑	↑	↑↔	↑	↑	↑↓	↑
Dopexamine	↓	↑	↓	↓	↑	↓	↑(↔)
PDE inhibitors	↓↔	↑↔	↓	↓↓	↑	↓↓	↓(↔)

namics in patients with sepsis are influenced not only by peripheral vasodilatation but also by alterations in myocardial (right and left ventricular) function. Thus, in these patients, noradrenaline is often used successfully to stabilise haemodynamics.

Adrenaline is one of the most powerful cardiotonic agents available. It is predominantly a β_1- and β_2-agonist with dose-dependent α_1-activation. Tachycardia and increased vascular resistance with increasing doses are the unwanted side effects, which may limit the use of this substance, particularly in patients with chronic congestive heart failure. In acute perioperative low output syndrome, however, its powerful positive inotropic effects may be life-saving. Furthermore, adrenaline is by far the least expensive positive inotropic substance.

Dobutamine, a structural modification of isoprenaline, acts primarily on β_1-adrenergic myocardial receptors which increase contractility. It also induces vasodilatation secondary to (direct) β_2-adrenergic stimulation, but dobutamine also possesses (mild) α-adrenergic actions.[20] Dobutamine is administered at infusion rates of 2–5 µg/kg/min, titrated upward to 20 µg/kg/min as needed to increase cardiac output. In patients treated chronically with β-adrenoceptor blockers and who receive dobutamine for inotropic support, the expected improvement in pump function may be attenuated.[20, 21] Because the unblocked α-receptors are activated more than the blocked β_2-receptors, the unfavourable vasoconstrictive response to dobutamine may be unmasked in β-blocked patients. When dobutamine was introduced to replace adrenaline as a positive inotrope, significantly less increase in heart rate was purported to be one of the advantages of dobutamine. However, enthusiastic initial reports that dobutamine's inotropic effect is not associated with an increase in heart rate have been refuted.[22] In a study from Vanoverschelde et al.,[23] dobutamine was used in healthy volunteers to assess its effects on contractility and myocardial oxygen consumption. Changes of (relative) load-independent measures of ventricular function, such as the maximal slope of the pressure-volume loop (E_{max}) and the ratio of end-systolic stress to end-systolic volume index (Ess/Esv), indicated a true positive inotropic effect. Oxygen consumption, however, was greater than expected and left ventricular efficiency was decreased. In an animal study, Wynsen et al.[24] used ultrasonic crystals to measure ventricular function and documented that, in the presence of severe coronary artery stenosis, increasing doses of dobutamine may be associated with deleterious effects on coronary blood flow and function of the ischaemic area. Thus, in patients with severe left ventricular dysfunction secondary to myocardial ischaemia, the use of dobutamine is not without problems and it is strongly recommended that haemodynamic parameters are monitored continuously in this situation.

Dopamine, a precursor of adrenaline and noradrenaline is valuable because of its ability to stimulate dopaminergic receptors in the renal vasculature, thus improving renal blood flow and enhancing urine output ('renal dose': 3 μg/kg/min). There are, however, no convincing studies proving that dopamine is able to prevent acute renal failure in the critically ill to a greater extent than other catecholamines (for example, dobutamine).[25] The haemodynamic effects of dopamine are dose-dependent. Only doses <5 μg/kg/min are associated with beneficial effects on renal vasculature, whereas infusion rates up to 10 μg/kg/min result in predominantly β-adrenergic stimulation and doses above 10 μg/kg/min result in predominantly α-adrenergic effects with (often unwanted) peripheral vasoconstriction and impaired tissue perfusion. Thus, dopamine is preferred to dobutamine, when restoration of blood pressure is the immediate goal of therapy.[26]

The usefulness of dopamine as a positive inotrope in patients with left ventricular dysfunction must be considered carefully. Van Tright et al.[27] used implanted ultrasonic dimension crystals in cardiac surgery patients with normal cardiac output. In comparison to equal doses of dobutamine, dopamine did not increase myocardial muscle shortening, but it increased peak left ventricular wall stress unfavourably.

Dopexamine hydrochloride is a newer catecholamine which acts on dopaminergic (DA1) and β_2-adrenergic receptors.[28–31] It does not have α-receptor stimulating effects. A (mild) positive inotropic effect is mediated by (slight) β_1-adrenoceptor stimulation and via inhibition of neuronal re-uptake of endogenous noradrenaline.[30, 31] In addition to its systemic vasodilator effects, it appears to possess beneficial actions on splanchnic perfusion.[32, 33] Dose-related increases in cardiac index and heart rate, and reductions in systolic and pulmonary vascular resistances, have been reported, with infusion rates ranging from 1 to 6 μg/kg/min.[29] Important side effects of dopexamine are the increase in heart rate secondary to inhibition of uptake of noradrenaline by sympathetic nerves and the decrease in blood pressure secondary to its vasodilator properties. Maintaining sufficient circulating volume by fluid infusion is the best way to avoid a critical increase in heart rate or decrease in blood pressure in this situation.

The use of dopexamine in the critically ill has not been fully evaluated.

185

Jaski et al. [28] compared the effects of dobutamine (5 and 10 µg/kg/min) and dopexamine (2 and 4 µg/kg/min) in NYHA III patients using micro-manometers placed in the left ventricle to measure dP/dt. A greater increase in dP/dt occurred with dobutamine than with dopexamine, indicating a greater inotropic effect with dobutamine. In patients with chronic congestive heart failure, haemodynamic effects of dopexamine and dobutamine were compared by Baumann et al. [34] Both substances increased cardiac index and produced systemic vasodilatation. Dopexamine was found to be a more potent vasodilator and increased urine output to a greater extent than dobutamine.

Does an ideal catecholamine exist?

Controversies surrounding the role of positive inotropic agents in the treatment of perioperative left ventricular dysfunction still exist. The use of catecholamines is a two-edged sword that effectively may increase contractility, but reduce oxygen supply and increase oxygen demands. It is also a matter of debate as to whether strong isotropes such as adrenaline should be used when treating acute left ventricular dysfunction or whether weaker, "gentler"[17] drugs such as dopamine, dobutamine or dopexamine should be recommended as the therapy of choice (Table 9.4). It is not feasible to compare the results from all studies: the patient population, underlying diseases, additional therapeutic protocols, and even doses of the different substances, often vary widely. Profound knowledge of the pharmacokinetics, pharmacodynamics and side effects of the different substances is fundamental to determine which agent is the drug of choice in each situation.

Alternatives to catecholamine therapy

In recent years, progress in research has continued to shed new light on the physiology and pharmacology of the cardiovascular system. In patients suffering from chronic heart failure, the β_1-adrenoceptor population is reduced and the normal ratio of β_1- to β_2-adrenoceptors is altered

Table 9.4 Comparison of actions of dopamine, dobutamine, and dopexamine

Receptor	Dopamine	Dobutamine	Dopexamine	Effect
β_2	(+)	++	+++	Peripheral vasodilatation
β_1	++	+++	(+)	Increased myocardial contractility
Uptake-1 inhibition	++	+	+++	Indirect β_1 stimulation
DA1	+++	0	++	Renal, splanchnic and hepatic vasodilatation
DA2	++	0	+	Vasodilatation
α	+++	++	0	Vasoconstriction

significantly.[35] Thus in patients with pre-existing severe heart failure, the positive inotropic response to β-sympathomimetic agents is diminished owing to a desensitisation of myocardial β-adrenergic receptors ("down-regulation" phenomenon).[11] The degree of down-regulation is related directly to the severity of ventricular dysfunction. Fowler et al.[11] investigated patients with mild to moderate, or severe, ventricular dysfunction and found reductions of 38 and 57%, respectively. Patients with a left ventricular ejection fraction (LVEF) of less than 30% (severe heart failure) or less than 50% (moderate heart failure) were given graded sequential infusions of dobutamine. Patients with severe cardiac dysfunction showed a marked impairment of the expected response in dP/dt_{max} and stroke work index. This proves that reduction in myocardial β-receptor density and/or function is related to the severity of heart failure, and can be associated with specific impairment of the β-receptor-mediated contractile response to dobutamine.

However, not only pre-existing heart failure may cause β-receptor down-regulation. Advancing age may also be associated with a decreased sensitivity to β-sympathomimetic substances (i.e. isoprenaline).[36] In a study of patients undergoing non-cardiac surgical procedures under general anesthesia, Marty et al.[37] demonstrated that adrenergic activation (induced by surgical stress) may result in a decrease in agonist affinity of β-receptors and thus in altered β-adrenergic responsiveness. This is of particular importance in patients with pre-existing reduced affinity or density of β-receptors, i.e. in patients suffering from chronic heart failure, who are undergoing surgical operations. Treatment with catecholamines is also known to induce desensitisation of β-adrenergic receptors, which results in hyporesponsiveness to further stimulation by sympathomimetic agents. This down-regulation phenomenon developed within 72 hours of initiation of an infusion of dobutamine.[38]

Particular problems arise in patients on long-term β-blocker therapy. In these patients, catecholamines often fail sufficiently to improve pump function when necessary. Substances with a mechanism of action located at a site 'distal' to the β-adrenergic receptor may be useful to treat inotropic abnormalities effectively (Figure 9.2).[21]

The β-receptor down-regulation phenomenon is not the only reason for the insufficient response to catecholamine therapy in patients with heart failure. Stimulation of β-receptors activates the G-regulatory protein, a G-stimulatory (G_s) or a G-inhibitory (G_i) protein, which stimulates or inhibits adenylate cyclase activity and which influences cAMP production and contractility. Changes in β-receptor numbers do not necessarily lead to an enhanced responsiveness. Beta-receptors activate adenylate cyclase by nucleotide regulatory proteins (G_s or G_i), which act as transducers either of a stimulatory or inhibitory signal through the subreceptor complex. Signal transducing G_s-protein concentrations decrease dramatically with myocar-

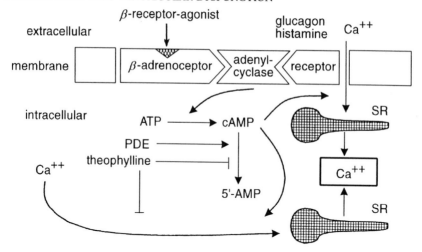

Fig 9.2 Mechanisms of positive inotropic drugs. PDE, phosphodiesterase; SR, sarcoplasmic reticulum

dial ischaemia.[39] Thus the reduced β-adrenergic-stimulated adenylate cyclase activity after an ischaemic event may also be secondary to a loss in G_s-protein and not only to changes in the β-receptor sensitivity.

Phosphodiesterase (PDE) inhibitors

The pharmacological profile of PDE inhibitors is characterised by an increase in the force of contraction as well as by a relaxation of vascular smooth muscle.[40] This results in peripheral vasodilatation, causing end-diastolic wall stress (='preload') and systolic wall stress (='afterload') to be reduced.[41–43] The term "inodilator" was coined to describe the dual haemodynamic properties of this class of compounds. Amrinone, enox-

---

Actions of phosphodiesterase (PDE) III inhibitors

- **Cardiac**
  Positive inotropy
  Positive lusitropy

- **Vascular**
  Peripheral vasodilatation (arterial *and* venous side)
    preload reduction
    afterload reduction
  Decrease in pulmonary vascular resistance

- **Coronary vessels**
  Vasodilatation: increase in myocardial perfusion

Table 9.5   Phosphodiesterase III inhibitors for treatment of low output syndrome

	Loading dose	Maintenance dose
Amrinone	0·5–1·0 mg/kg (iv bolus within 5 min)	5–10 μg/kg min
Enoximone	0·25–0·75 mg/kg (iv bolus within 5 min)	2·5–10 μg/kg/min
Milrinone	50 μg/kg (iv bolus within 5 min)	0·375–0·75 μg/kg/min

imone, and milrinone are the PDE III inhibitors available in most countries[44, 45] (Table 9.5).

The inotropic and vasodilator properties of PDE III inhibitors have been demonstrated in many *in vitro* and *in vivo* preparations. With enoximone, for instance, the slope of the peak isovolumetric pressure–volume relationship shifts to the left, which indicates enhanced contractility.[46] Improvements in other indices of contractility (left ventricular dP/dt_{max}, ratio of peak systolic pressure to end-systolic volume) also show that intropy increases with this PDE III inhibitor in the clinical setting. In animal experiments using enoximone and close control of loading conditions, contractility increased by approximately 66%, whereas systemic vascular resistance (SVR) fell by 30 to 50%.[46]

PDE III inhibitors also act beneficially on the diastolic properties, including compliance, relaxation, and filling.[47–49] They facilitate the relaxation phase of the myocardial contractile cycle. This 'lusitropic' action of PDE inhibitors is also mediated by the increase in intracellular cAMP levels, which is necessary for energy-dependent relaxation.[48] Furthermore, the vascular effects of vasodilatation may induce a secondary increase in sympathetic tone, causing the rate of relaxation to be increased as a result of stimulation of cAMP production. Finally, venodilatation leads to a decrease in right ventricular volume which contributes to a downward displacement of the left ventricular pressure–volume relationship via ventricular interdependence.

When treating patients with reduced myocardial performance, it is imperative to use drugs that will improve ventricular function without jeopardizing an ischaemic myocardium. Myocardial oxygen consumption (MVO_2) reflects the sum of both energy-saving (arterial and venous) vasodilatation and energy-consuming (positive inotropic) effects. Administration of PDE III inhibitors results in an improvement in myocardial performance whereas MVO_2 is unchanged or even decreased.[44, 50] The expected increase in MVO_2 – secondary to the increase in myocardial contractility – may be compensated for by decreases in ventricular preload and afterload. PDE III inhibitors may even cause a reduction in MVO_2 (amrinone: ranging from −20 to −30%; enoximone: −18%).[51, 52] A lack of lactate production[42] suggests that anaerobic metabolism is not induced by PDE III inhibitors.[52] In contrast, the improvement in haemodynamics induced by dobutamine is associated with an increase in myocardial oxygen consumption (ranging from $+30$ to $+40\%$).[53] Potential anti-ischaemic effects have been postulated for some PDE III inhibitors, for example after administration of enoximone.[54] In patients in whom ventricular pacing was performed, enoximone increased the anginal threshold while left ventricular stroke work index (LVSWI) was maintained. The question of whether this effect was due only to a reduction in wall stress secondary to vascular vasodilatation was studied by Schlepper and colleagues.[55] After intracoronary administration of enoximone (0·075 mg/kg) into a stenosed coronary vascular bed, no systemic haemodynamic effects were observed and serum concentrations were below the therapeutic concentration. However, anti-ischaemic actions were similar to those after systemic administration of this PDE III inhibitor. It was concluded that pacing stimulation was unable to elicit ischaemic patterns in the enoximone-treated patients. Regional coronary vascular resistance was reduced by PDE III inhibitors, leading to increased coronary perfusion.[53, 56]

The beneficial effects of PDE III inhibitors appear to be augmented when β-receptor agonists are given simultaneously (Figure 9.3):[57] by complementary action, PDE III inhibitors prevent the destruction of

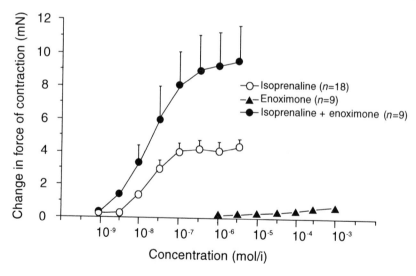

Fig 9.3 Cumulative concentration–response curves for the effects of the PDE III inhibitor enoximone, isoprenaline, and calcium on force of contraction in right ventricular trabeculae from failing human hearts. The absolute values of the positive inotropic effects of isoprenaline were reduced in the failing hearts (compared to non-failing hearts). In the presence of enoximone, the reduced efficacy of isoprenaline in the failing heart was restored and was similar to that of the non-failing heart. (After Bethke *et al.*, 1992[57])

cAMP whereas catecholamines stimulate cAMP production. A synergistic inotropic interaction between catecholamines and PDE III inhibitors is expected particularly in patients with severe, pre-existing heart failure.[58] These patients often show enhanced β-adrenergic stimulation secondary to elevated levels of circulating catecholamines. The combined action of PDE III inhibitors and endogenous catecholamines may explain the drugs significant cardiostimulatory effects in low output syndrome in various situations.

Negative effects of positive inotropes

Dysrhythmias

Patients suffering from heart failure often have a history of dysrhythmias. Catecholamine substances are associated with an increased risk of arrhythmias (Table 9.6).[59] The potential arrhythmogenic activity of PDE III inhibitors is also mediated by the increase in intracellular cAMP levels. The PDE inhibitor enoximone causes a shortened basic sinus cycle length and reduced sinus node recovery time and sinoatrial conduction, whereas atrioventricular atrial refractoriness decreases, resulting in positive chronotropic and dromotropic effects.[60] Amrinone and milrinone show similar electrophysiological actions.[61] Apart from these actions on myocardial automaticity, conduction and refractoriness, the increase in heart rate

---

Possible indications for phosphodiesterase (PDE) III inhibitors (single use or in combination with catecholamines)

- **Non-surgical patients**
  Acute myocardial infarction
  Low output syndrome in patients with chronic congestive heart failure
  Right ventricular dysfunction due to pulmonary hypertension
  Cardiac depression secondary to negative inotropic substances (β-blockers, calcium-channel blockers)

- **Surgical patients**
  Non-cardiac surgery
      low output syndrome in cardiac patients in the perioperative period
  Cardiac surgery
      patients awaiting heart transplantation ("bridging")
      haemodynamic insufficiency prior to CPB
      weaning from CPB
      paediatric cardiac surgery (with high pulmonary vascular resistance)

- **Intensive care patients**
  Myocardial failure in the postoperative period
  Haemodynamic support during aggressive ventilation

Table 9.6   Proarrhythmic potential of intravenous inotropes

Agent	Sinus bradycardia	Sinus tachycardia	Supraventricular arrhythmias	Ventricular arrhythmias
Isoprenaline	−	+ + + +	+	+ + +
Adrenaline	−	+ + +	+	+ + +
Noradrenaline	+	−	−	(+)
Dopamine	−	+ + +	+	+ + +
Dobutamine	−	+ +	+	+ +
PDE inhibitors	−	+	+	+ +

appears to be caused probably by an indirect vasodilatation-mediated increase in sympathetic tone. Since patients with long-lasting, chronic heart failure often have serious arrhythmias, it is difficult to decide whether arrhythmias are definitely caused by the proarrhythmic drug effects secondary to cAMP elevation (for example after administration of catecholamines or PDE inhibitors).

Regional perfusion

In the pathophysiology and pharmacology of low output syndrome secondary to left ventricular dysfunction, regional blood flow and the distribution of cardiac output are important areas for therapeutic interventions. An increase in cardiac output does not always result in an improvement in nutritive organ perfusion. Many of the haemodynamic problems in this situation are due to reduced blood flow to various organs, which promotes further deterioration in microcirculatory blood flow. The microcirculatory profile of drugs with cardiovascular effects is not well documented. In the clinical setting it is difficult to assess blood flow at the microcirculatory level correctly. Catecholamines may improve cardiac output dramatically, but effective nutritive regional perfusion may even deteriorate. Dopexamine is the only catecholaminergic substance which shows convincing beneficial effects on splanchnic perfusion.[62] Leier et al.[63] found that the PDE III inhibitor enoximone (1 mg/kg given orally) significantly increased cardiac output (by approximately 18%) and hepatic-splanchnic blood flow (by approximately 15%), while renal blood flow was reduced (by approximately 13%). Increasing the dose (2 mg/kg orally) caused a similar increase in cardiac output, whereas hepatic blood flow decreased (by approximately 9%) and renal flow even increased slightly (by 1%).

Changes in microcirculatory perfusion depend crucially on the dose and method of administration. The underlying disease is also of importance when considering microcirculatory changes. Patients with chronic congestive heart failure and patients with acute low output syndrome in the post-cardiopulmonary bypass period respond differently. Modification of regional perfusion remains a much-debated issue and further work must be undertaken to evaluate fully the influence of the various positive inotropic agents on the microcirculation.

Vasodilators

Vasodilating drugs are used widely to treat patients with severe (*chronic congestive*) heart failure.[64] The strategy of using vasodilators is based on the principle that 'unloading' the failing left ventricle results in a substantial reduction in filling pressure and an increase in cardiac output with little or no change in blood pressure. The principle of using venodilators is to shift blood from the central blood compartment to the periphery, reducing end-diastolic volume and pressure. A reduction in ventricular dimension results in a lower wall force which is also of particular importance in patients with ischaemic heart disease. The use of arterial vasodilators is aimed to increase cardiac output without a decrease in arterial pressure. In hypertensive patients and in patients with elevated systemic vascular resistance, arterial vasodilators are of benefit. A reduction in systemic vascular resistance reduces myocardial oxygen demand, from which patients with underlying coronary artery disease may benefit.

Sodium nitroprusside (SNP) and *glyceryl trinitrate (GTN)* are the vasodilating substances in patients with heart failure. Arterial vasodilatation, resulting in reduced left ventricular afterload and wall stress (SNP) or increased venous pooling (GTN), leading in turn to reduced preload, may increase ventricular efficacy and improve myocardial oxygen balance. The beneficial use of SNP has been reported in patients suffering from myocardial infarction and persistent left ventricular pump dysfunction.[65, 66] The infusion rate starts at 10–15 μg/min and is gradually titrated upwards to achieve the desired effects on haemodynamics. It possesses effects on both after- and preload with no direct effects on the myocardium. Cardiac output improves while blood pressure changes only slightly because the decrease in systemic vascular resistance is usually offset by the increase in forward flow. SNP should not be used when blood pressure is low, although it may be helpful when cardiac output is low secondary to a massive increase in vascular resistance.

Since some angiotensin converting enzyme (ACE) inhibitors are available as iv preparations (for example enalaprilat), this class of compounds may enlarge our armamentarium of vasodilators. The haemodynamic properties (namely reduction in pre- and afterload without affecting heart rate) of these substances are related mainly to the blocking of the conversion of angiotensin I to angiotensin II in plasma and tissues.[67] In addition, ACE inhibitors appear to be involved in effects which are independent of the systemic renin angiotensin system (RAS) and which may also contribute to the reduction in blood pressure. These mechanisms include the local RAS, the sympathetic nervous system, kinins, and prostaglandins.[68, 69]

The decision to use vasodilators in patients with acute left ventricular dysfunction depends on the availability of extensive haemodynamic monitoring. Low blood pressure (systolic blood pressure <90 mmHg) usually mandates therapy with a positive inotrope or a potent vasoconstrictor. Additional or exclusive use of an arteriolar or venous capacitance vasodilator may be indicated when systemic vascular resistance or left ventricular filling pressure (PCWP) is elevated. In patients with perioperative left ventricular dysfunction, both positive inotropes to increase myocardial contractility and vasodilators to improve myocardial performance are sometimes indicated.

Mechanical assist devices

In spite of optimal pharmacological management using inotropes and afterload-reducing drugs, haemodynamic catastrophes secondary to left ventricular dysfunction cannot always be treated successfully. In this situation, mechanical assist devices can be life-saving and must be considered. These systems have been used mostly in cardiac surgery patients during and after weaning from cardiopulmonary bypass or in patients awaiting heart transplantation. In both cases mechanical assistance represents temporary ventricular support.

The rationale for the use of circulatory support systems is either to provide general support to the systemic and pulmonary circulation ensuring all vital organs (including the heart) receive an adequate blood flow, or to decrease myocardial work and oxygen demand, thus enabling repair and metabolic recovery of damaged muscle cells. Indications for the use of mechanical assist devices include patients with:

- cardiac index <1.8 l/min/m^2
- left atrial pressure >20–25 mmHg
- right atrial pressure <15 mmHg
- systolic blood pressure <90 mmHg
- urine output <20 ml/h

in spite of optimal conventional pharmacological therapy.

The Intra-Aortic Balloon Pump (IABP) has been widely accepted because of its easy use. Implantation of other mechanical left-ventricular assist devices (LVADs) requires a technically demanding surgical procedure which is not always available and which some of these critically ill patients could not tolerate. These are devices for temporary cardiocirculatory

---

Issues in the treatment of left ventricular dysfunction

- Myocardial consumption
- Proarrhythmic effects
- Effects on nutrient blood flow
- Effects on morbidity and mortality
- Risk–benefit analyses
- Cost-effectiveness

---

support; they should only be considered if myocardial dysfunction is potentially reversible or in patients awaiting heart transplantation.

Practical therapeutic concepts

Left ventricular dysfunction in the perioperative period requires a step-by-step therapeutic approach taking various aspects into account. Volume and rhythm normalisation are as important as improvement in oxygen transport by blood transfusion in anaemic patients, or treatment with oxygen. Extensive haemodynamic monitoring is necessary in this situation to assess mean arterial pressure (MAP), filling pressures (CVP, PCWP), cardiac output (CO) and systemic peripheral vascular resistance (SVR) by invasive monitoring using a pulmonary artery catheter. This is of fundamental importance to distinguish between the need for positive inotropes, for lowering pre- or afterload or for increasing perfusion pressure by vasoconstrictors. In patients with acute deterioration of ventricular function without pre-existing heart disease, catecholamines are usually effective. They are positive inotropic drugs with a short half-life, acting on myocardial β-adrenoceptors. Whether synthetic, costly catecholamines such as dobutamine or dopamine offer any advantage over 'natural', low-priced adrenaline is doubtful. Most of the side effects of catecholamines, such as an increase in heart rate (dobutamine, adrenaline) or an increase in afterload (adrenaline, dopamine) are dose-dependent and can be controlled by dose titration and intensive haemodynamic monitoring.

In patients with pre-existing chronic heart disease, patients in whom haemodynamics have deteriorated in spite of optimal catecholamine therapy, and patients in whom β-adrenoceptor numbers and function may be altered, inotropes that bypass the β-receptor may be of advantage. Early use of PDE III inhibitors has to be considered. Combining catecholamines with PDE III inhibitors appears to be promising in this situation.

Vasoactive substances that influence pre- or afterload provide an important therapeutic approach in patients with chronic congestive heart

195

failure rather than acute left ventricular dysfunction in the perioperative period. Nevertheless, they are valuable to reduce left ventricular wall stress and also to improve coronary blood flow when left ventricular dysfunction occurs acutely.

Conclusions

Acute left ventricular dysfunction leading to haemodynamic catastrophes in the perioperative period may have several causes. Knowledge of pre-existing cardiac diseases and fundamental haemodynamic principles are prerequisites for selecting appropriate therapeutic regimens. Adequate monitoring also plays a pivotal role in managing patients with low output syndrome in this situation.

Pharmacological intervention aims to influence the most important aspects of low output failure in cardiac surgery: cardiac output, heart rate, contractility, and vascular resistance. A variety of pharmacological and mechanical therapeutic interventions have been evolved for treatment of 'low output' syndrome in this situation. There is an endless list of biochemical abnormalities including alterations in β-receptor density, cardiac innervation, mitochondrial respiration, deficiency in cAMP generation, G-protein abnormalities, impaired calcium sequestration and others, which may limit our therapeutic approaches in managing acute left ventricular dysfunction in the perioperative period. Various pharmacological techniques to modulate cardiovascular function can be used, including β-receptor agonists, mixed adrenergic agonists, and non-adrenergic inotropes such as phosphodiesterase inhibitors. Standard "natural" and synthetic catecholamines have been the mainstay of circulatory support in this situation for several years.

Our knowledge of cardiac function on all levels has been widened considerably in recent years. The observation of β-receptor down-regulation in patients with pre-existing heart failure has led to the development of substances that act independently of the β-receptor. PDE III inhibitors may be an alternative approach to treat heart failure in the perioperative period. They should not be used as a 'last try' in patients with catecholamine-refractory derangement. The risks associated with increasing the dose of catecholamines may lead to earlier use of PDE III inhibitors. By complementary action, PDE III inhibitors inhibit the destruction of cAMP whereas catecholamines stimulate cAMP production. With this combination, additive or synergistic inotropic effects can be achieved. New substances stimulating β_2-receptors or increasing the sensitivity of the contractile proteins to calcium may improve therapy in perioperative heart failure. Since current evidence suggests that extrapolation from animal models to the critically ill must be made with caution, clinical studies are required to determine the true role of the various classes of substances on myocardial function, microcirculatory blood flow and outcome.[21] The anaesthesiologist must be prepared to administer pharmacological cardiovascular support and be aware of the pathophysiological haemodynamic changes in the perioperative period.

1 Rettig GF, Bette L. Current therapy of acute heart failure. *Cardiovasc Drugs Ther* 1988;2:401–6.
2 Little WC, Applegate RJ. Congestive heart failure: systolic and diastolic function. *J Cardiothorac Vasc Anesth* 1993;7(Suppl 2):2–5.
3 Davies ME, Jones CJH, Feneck RO, Walesby RK. The effects of intravenous nitroglycerin and isosorbide dinitrate on hemodynamics and myocardial metabolism. *J Cardiothorac Vasc Anesth* 1989;3:712–19.
4 Seitelberger R, Zwölfer W, Binder T, Huber S, Peschi F, Spatt J *et al.* Infusion of nifedipine after coronary bypass grafting decreases the incidence of early postoperative myocardial ischemia. *Ann Thorac Surg* 1990;49:61–8.
5 Bolling SF, Groh MA, Mattson AM, Gringae RA, Gallagher K. Acadesine (AICA-Riboside) improves postischemic cardiac recovery. *Ann Thorac Surg* 1992;54:93–9.
6 Dorman BH, Zucker JR, Verrier ED, Gartman DM, Slachman FN. Clonidine improves perioperative myocardial ischemia, reduces anesthetic requirement, and alters hemodynamic parameters in patients undergoing coronary artery bypass surgery. *J Cardiothorac Vasc Anesth* 1992;6:344–59.
7 Breisblatt WM, Stein KL, Wolfe CJ. Acute myocardial dysfunction and recovery: a common occurrence after coronary bypass surgery. *J Am Col Cardiol* 1990;15:1261–9.
8 Merin RC. Positive inotropic drugs and ventricular function. In: Warltier DC, ed. *Ventricular function.* Baltimore: Williams & Wilkins, 1995; 181–212.
9 Leung JM, Schiller NB, Mangano DT. Assessment of left ventricular function using two-dimensional transesophageal echocardiography. In: DeBruijn NP, Clements FM, eds. *Intraoperative use of echocardiography.* Philadelphia: Lippincott, 1991;59–75.
10 Rutman HI, LeJemtel TH, Sonnenblick EH. Newer cardiotonic agents: implications for patients with heart failure and ischemic heart disease. *J Cardiothorac Anesth* 1987;1:59–70.
11 Fowler MB, Laser JA, Hopkins GL, Minobe W, Bristow MR. Assessment of the beta-adrenergic receptor pathway in the intact failing human heart: progressive receptor down-regulation and subsensitivity to agonist response. *Circulation* 1986;74:1290–302.
12 Shoemaker WC, Appel PL, Kram HB. Prospective trial of supranormal values of survivors as therapeutic goals in high-risk surgical patients. *Chest* 1988;94:1176–86.
13 Mythen MG, Webb AR. The role of gut mucosal hypoperfusion in the pathogenesis of postoperative organ dysfunction. *Intensive Care Med* 1994;20:203–9.
14 Fiddian-Green RG. Gastric intramucosal pH, tissue oxygenation and acid-base balance. *Br J Anaesth* 1995;74:591–606.
15 Kirkpatrik CJ, Klosterhalfen B, Hauptmann S. The role of the endothelium in multiple organ failure. In: Vincent JL, ed. *Yearbook of intensive care and emergency medicine*, Berlin: Springer, 1992:14–24.
16 Löllgen H. Use of catecholamines in therapy of acute heart failure – efficacy and limitations. *Intensivmed* 1991;28(Suppl 1):21–32.
17 Tinker J. Strong inotropes (ie, epinephrine) should be drugs of first choice during emergence from cardiopulmonary bypass. *J Cardiothorac Anesth* 1987;3:256–8.
18 Kapur PA. Con: Epinephrine and norepinephrine are the inotropes of choice: an opposing view. *J Cardiothorac Anesth* 1987;3:259–62.
19 Levy JH. Support of the perioperative failing heart with preexisting ventricular dysfunction: currently available supports. *J Cardiothorac Vasc Anesth* 1993;7(Suppl 2):46–51.
20 Tarnow J, Komar K. Altered haemodynamic response to dobutamine in relation to the degree of preoperative β-adrenoceptor blockade. *Anesthesiology* 1988;68:912–19.
21 Boldt J, Kling D, Zickmann B, Dapper F, Hempelmann G. Haemodynamic effects of the PDE-inhibitor enoximone in comparison to dobutamine in esmolol-treated cardiac

surgery patients. *Br J Anaesth* 1990;**64**:611–16.

22 Butterworth JF, Prielipp RC, Royster RL, Spray B, Kon ND, Wallenhaput SL *et al.* Dobutamine increases heart rate more than epinephrine in patients recovering from aortocoronary bypass surgery. *J Cardiothorac Vasc Anesth* 1992;**6**:535–41.

23 Vanoverschelde JJ, Wijns W, Essamri B, Bol A, Robert A, Labar D *et al.* Hemodynamic and mechanical determinants of myocardial O_2 consumption in normal heart: effects of dobutamine. *Am J Physiol* 1993;**265**:H1884–H1892.

24 Wynsen JC, O'Brien PD, Warltier DC. Zatebradine, a specific bradycardiac agent, enhances the positive inotropic actions of dobutamine in ischemic myocardium. *J Am Coll Cardiol* 1994;**23**:233–41.

25 Wenstone R, Campbell JM, Booker PD, McKay R. Renal function after cardiopulmonary bypass in children: comparison of dopamine with dobutamine. *Br J Anaesth* 1991;**67**:591–4.

26 Francis GS, Sharma B, Hodges M. Comparison hemodynamics effects of dopamine and dobutamine in patients with acute cardiogenic circulatory collapse. *Am Heart J* 1982;**103**:995–1000.

27 van Tright P, Spray TL, Pasque, MK, Peyton RB, Pellom GL, Wechsler AS. The comparative effects of dopamine and dobutamine on ventricular mechanics after coronary artery bypass grafting: a pressure-dimension analysis. *Circulation* 1984;**70**(Suppl 1):112–17.

28 Jaski BE, Peters C. Inotropic, vascular, and neuroendocrine effects of dopexamine hydrochloride and comparison with dobutamine. *Am J Cardiol* 1988;**62**:63C–67C.

29 Goldberg LI. Dopamine and new dopamine analogs: receptors and clinical applications. *J Clin Anesth* 1988;**1**:66–74.

30 Mitchell PD, Smith GW, Wells E, West PA. Inhibition of uptake-1 by dopexamine hydrochloride. *Br J Pharmacol* 1987;**92**:265–70.

31 Brown RA, Dixon J, Farmer JB *et al.* Dopexamine: a novel agonist at peripheral dopamine receptors and beta-2-adrenoceptors. *Br J Pharmacol* 1985;**85**:599–608.

32 Biro GP, Douglas JR, Keon WJ, Taichman GC. Changes in regional blood flow distribution induced by infusions of dopexamine hydrochloride or dobutamine in anesthetized dogs. *Am J Cardiol* 1988;**62**:30C–36C.

33 Fitton A, Benfield P. Dopexamie hydrochloride. A review of its pharmacodynamic and pharmacokinetic properties and therapeutic potential in acute cardiac insufficiency. *Drugs* 1990;**39**:308–30.

34 Baumann G, Felix SB, Filcek SA. Usefulness of dopexamine hydrochloride versus dobutamine in chronic congestive heart failure: effects on hemodynamics and urine output. *Am J Cardiol* 1990;**65**:748–54.

35 Bristow MR, Ginsburg R, Minobe W, Cubiceiotti RS, Sageman WS. Decreased catecholamine sensitivity and beta-adrenergic receptor density in failing human hearts. *N Engl J Med* 1978;**299**:1373–7.

36 Tenero DM, Bottorff MB, Burlew BS, Williams JB, Lalonde RL. Altered beta-adrenergic sensitivity and protein binding to 1-propanolol in the elderly. *J Cardiovasc Pharmacol* 1990;**16**:702–07.

37 Marty J, Nimier M, Rocchiccioli C, Manz J, Luscombe F, Henzel D *et al.* Beta-adrenergic receptor function is acutely altered in surgical patients. *Anesth Analg* 1990;**71**:1–8.

38 Unverfert DV, Blaunford M, Kates RE, Leier CV. Tolerance to dobutamine after a 72-hour continuous infusion. *Am J Med* 1980;**69**:262–6.

39 Maisel AS, Motulsky HJ, Ziegler MG, Insel PA. Ischemia and agonist induced changes in α- β-adrenergic receptor traffic in guinea pig hearts. *Am J Physiol* 1987;**253**:H1159–H1167.

40 Scholz H. Inotropic drugs and their mechanism of action. *J Am Coll Cardiol* 1984;**4**:389–97.

41 Allaf DE, D'Orio V, Carlier J. The new inotropic phosphodiesterase inhibitors. *Arch Int Physiol Biochem* 1984;**92**:69–79.

42 Weber KT, Gill SK, Janicki JS, Maskin CS, Jain MC. Newer positive inotropic agents in the treatment of chronic cardiac failure. *Drugs* 1987;**33**:503–19.

43 Dage RC, Roebel LE, Hsieh CP, Weiner DL, Woodward JK. Cardiovascular properties of a new cardiotonic agent: MDL 17,043. *J Cardiovasc Pharmacol* 1988;**4**:500–8.

44 Skoyles JR, Sherry KM. Pharmacology, mechanisms of action and uses of selective phosphodiesterase inhibitors. *Br J Anaesth* 1992;**68**:293–302.

45 Mager G, Klocke RK, Kux A, Hopp HW, Hilger HH. Phosphodiesterase III inhibition or adrenoceptor stimulation: milrinone as an alternative to dobutamine in the treatment of severe heart failure. *Am Heart J* 1991;**121**:1974–83.

46 Janicki JS, Shroff SG, Weber KR. Physiologic response to the inotropic and vasodilator properties of enoximone. *Am J Cardiol* 1987;**60**:15C–118C.

47 Grayson RF, Marino P, Kass DA. The effects of amrinone on indices of left ventricular diastolic function assessed by volume (inductance) catheter. *Anesthesiology* 1988;**69**:A103.

48 Levy JH, Bailey JM. Amrinone: pharmacokinetics and pharmacodynamics. *J Cardiothorac Anesth* 1989;**3**:10–14.

49 Smith VE, Katz AM. Inotropic and lusitropic abnormalities as the basis for heart failure. *Heart Failure* 1988;**3**:55–6.

50 Baim DS. Effect of phosphodiesterase inhibition on myocardial oxygen consumption and coronary blood flow. *Am J Cardiol* 1989;**63**:23A–26A.

51 Benotti JR, Grossman W, Braunwald E, Carabello BA. Effects of amrinone on myocardial energy metabolism and hemodynamics in patients with severe congestive heart failure due to coronary artery disease. *Circulation* 1980;**62**:28–34.

52 Chatterjee K. Phosphodiesterase inhibitors: alterations in systemic and coronary hemodynamics. *Bas Res Cardiol* 1989;**84**(Suppl 1):213–24.

53 Bendersky R, Chatterjee K, Parmley WW, Brundage BH, Ports TA. Dobutamine in chronic ischemic heart failure: alterations in left ventricular function and coronary hemodynamics. *Am J Cardiol* 1981;**48**:554–6.

54 Thormann J, Kremer P, Mitrovic V. Effects of enoximone in coronary artery disease: increased pump function, improved ventricular wall motion and abolition of pacing induced myocardial ischemia. *J Appl Cardiol* 1989;**4**:152–67.

55 Schlepper M, Thorman J, Mitrovic V. Cardiovascular effects of forskolin and phosphodiesterase-III inhibitors. *Bas Res Cardiol* 1989;**84**(Suppl 1):197–212.

56 Amin KA, Shah PK, Hulse S, Shellock FG, Swan HC. Myocardial metabolic and haemodynamic effects of intravenous MDL 17,043, a new cardiotonic drug, in patients with chronic severe heart failure. *Am Heart J* 1984;**108**:1285–92.

57 Bethke T, Eschenhagen T, Klimkiewicz A *et al*. Phosphodiesterase inhibition by enoximone in preparations from nonfailing and failing human hearts. *Arzn Forsch/Drug Res* 1992;**41**(I):437–45.

58 Francis GS. Development of arrhythmias in the patient with congestive heart failure: pathophysiology, prevalence and prognosis. *Am J Cardiol* 1986;**57**:3B–7B.

59 Katz AM. Potential deleterious effects of inotropic agents in the therapy of chronic heart failure. *Circulation* 1986;**73**(Suppl III):III184–III188.

60 Pop T, Treese N, Cremer GM, Haegele KD, Meyer J. Electrophysiological effects of intravenous MDL 17.043. *Int J Cardiol* 1986;**12**:223–232.

61 Nacarelli GV, Gray EL, Dougherty AH, Hanna JE, Goldstein RA. Amrinone: acute electrophysiologic and hemodynamic effects in patients with congestive heart failure. *Am J Cardiol* 1984;**54**:600–4.

62 Biro GP, Douglas JR, Keon WJ, Taichman GC. Changes in regional blood flow distribution induced by infusions of dopexamine hydrochloride or dobutamine in anesthetized dogs. *Am J Cardiol* 1988;**62**:30C–36C.

63 Leier CV. Regional blood flow response to vasodilators and inotropes in congestive heart failure. *Am J Cardiol* 1988;**62**:86E–93E.

64 Furberg CD, Yusuf S. Effect of vasodilators in chronic congestive heart failure. *Am J Cardiol* 1985;**55**:1110–13.

65 Franciosa JA, Limas CJ, Guiha NH, Rodriguera E, Cohn JN. Improved left ventricular function during nitroprusside infusion in acute myocardial infarction. *Lancet* 1972;**i**:650–4.

66 Cohn JN, Franciosa JA, Francis GS *et al*. Effect of short-term infusion of sodium nitroprusside on mortality rate in acute myocardial infarction complicated by left ventricular failure. *N Engl J Med* 1982;**306**:1129–35.

67 Edwards CR, Padfield PL. Angiotensin-converting enzyme inhibitors. Past, present and bright future. *Lancet* 1985;**i**:30–4.

68 Johnston CI, Jackson B, Cubela R, Arnolda L. Mechanism for hypotensive action of angiotensin converting enzyme inhibitors. *Clin Exp Hypertens* 1984;6:551–61.
69 Dzau VJ. Circulating versus local renin–angiotensin in cardiovascular homeostasis. *Circulation* 1988;77(Suppl I):104–13.

10: Treatment of perioperative arrhythmias

HELFRIED METZLER

Preoperative arrhythmias

The presence of preoperative cardiac arrhythmias requires a differentiated approach. Usually, frequent ventricular ectopic beats or atrial arrhythmias are found only in patients with cardiac disease, most often coronary artery disease or left ventricular dysfunction.[1] The arrhythmias may be the 'sensitive marker' of a serious underlying cardiac disease. In this case, arrhythmias are proven outcome predictors, which tend to correlate with perioperative cardiac complications and add quantitatively to the risk index.[1, 2] Patients with frequent premature ventricular contractions (PVCs) undergoing non-cardiac surgery have a high probability of intraoperative arrhythmias and hypotension.[3] Therefore, careful and meticulous evaluation and, if possible, treatment of the underlying cardiac disease is the major goal in the management of these patients and not the symptomatic treatment of the arrhythmia *per se*.

In addition, non-cardiac causes and triggers for arrhythmias must be assessed and treated. These include:

- Hypokalaemia
- Hypomagnesaemia
- Drug side effects (digoxin, lithium antidepressants, phenothiazines)
- Pain, hypoxaemia, anxiety
- Catecholamines (exogenous and endogenous)
- Hyperthyroidism.

If **asymptomatic arrhythmias** are found in patients without evidence of cardiac disease, there is no additional risk, and the arrhythmia should not be treated.[4-6] Only patients with **symptomatic preoperative arrhythmias**, compromising cardiovascular status, should be treated by antiarrhythmic drugs preoperatively. Depending on the urgency of the surgical procedure, antiarrhythmics are given either intravenously or orally. Elective surgery should be postponed for several days.

Patients receiving an antiarrhythmic drug regimen should be evaluated carefully in terms of cause, duration, dosage of the antiarrhythic drug therapy and preceding cardiac complications, preferably by a cardiologist. If drug treatment is justified, therapy should be continued intravenously throughout the perioperative period with tailored dosage.

Intraoperative arrhythmias

Intraoperatively, the reported incidence of cardiac arrhythmias is 13–84%.[1, 7] The incidence of serious arrhythmias is low, ranging from 0·6 to 6%. One of the best approaches to the intraoperative management of arrhythmias is to follow J. Atlee's fundamental substrate + trigger concept of the two intraoperative main sources of arrhythmias[8] (Figure 10.1).

Substrate

Various cardiac structural diseases are the sources of different types of arrhythmias. The type and severity of the arrhythmias are usually determined by the existing cardiac disease:

- Coronary artery disease
- Hypertension
- Left ventricular and right ventricular dysfunction
- Congestive heart failure
- Cardiomyopathy
- The 'aged heart'
- Myocarditis
- Congenital arrhythmias.

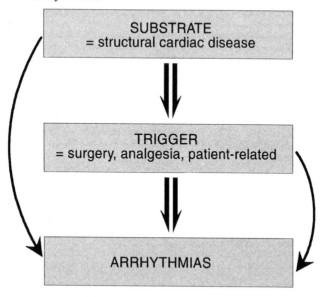

Fig 10.1 Substrate and trigger: dependent and independent mechanisms in the genesis of intraoperative arrhythmias

Patients with structural cardiac disease present either with arrhythmias in the preoperative period – and intraoperative arrhythmias are simply the continuation of the preoperative pattern – or preoperative arrhythmias are not present and the appearance of new arrhythmias may be caused either by the aggravation of the underlying disease or by triggering mechanisms.

Triggers

In contrast to the relatively 'simple' scenario of cardiological patients, the perioperative period initiates and produces numerous triggers for cardiac arrhythmias. The most frequent triggers are:

- Autonomic imbalance
- Surgical stimulation
- Anaesthetic drug effects
- Electrolyte imbalance
- Acid–base imbalance
- Complications such as, hypovolaemia, etc.

A clear, logical approach to the treatment of intraoperative arrhythmias follows three steps:

Step 1 If the underlying mechanism is activation or worsening of a structural cardiac disease, try to treat primarily this probable cause (example: transient myocardial ischaemia in coronary artery disease).

Step 2 If there is a relevant trigger mechanism, try to eliminate or at least minimise it (example: probable trigger surgical stimulation → stop stimulation for some minutes).

Step 3 In most circumstances appropriate assessment and treatment of these two mechanisms is effective. Antiarrhythmic drug treatment is indicated only as the last step, if:

- there is a sudden life-threatening arrhythmia;
- step 1 and 2 management is ineffective.

One of the most frequent mistakes in the perioperative management of arrhythmias is the uncritical, primary treatment of arrhythmias with an antiarrhythmic drug before correcting the underlying causative factors.

Lessons from cardiology

The perspectives of cardiologists and anaesthesiologists differ substantially. Cardiologists focus on long-term prognosis and sudden cardiac death,[9, 10] whereas anaesthesiologists and intensivists are usually confronted with the need to treat arrhythmias compromising cardiocirculatory stability. Despite these differences, many concepts and strategies can be transferred from cardiology to the specific perioperative scenario, improving anaesthesiologists' pathophysiological knowledge:

- The proarrhythmogenic effect:
  antiarrhythmic drugs have the potential to exacerbate rather than suppress arrhythmias.[11]
- Arrhythmias and increased cardiac sympathetic activity:
  in patients with depressed ventricular function, reflex cardiac sympathetic activation may contribute to the genesis of major ventricular arrhythmias.[12]
- The role of β-blockers:
  Beta-blocker therapy after myocardial infarction has been shown to reduce the incidence of reinfarction and associated mortality. Beta-adrenergic blockers may also be of benefit in congestive heart failure by reducing sympathetic nervous activity and restoration of the β-receptor population.[9, 13–15]

Currently available drugs and their classification

For many years, all antiarrhythmic drugs were traditionally categorised according to the Vaughan Williams classification. It represented an empirical classification according to the most important antiarrhythmic property of a drug. More recently, our knowledge of electrophysiological mechanisms has widened, and the drawbacks of the Vaughan Williams

---

The Vaughan Williams classification of antiarrhythmic drugs

- **Class 1** Drugs with direct membrane action (Na^+ channel blockade)
  - Class 1A Depress phase 0, slow conduction prolong repolarisation
    procainamide, quinidine, disopyramide
  - Class 1B Little effect on phase 0 in normal tissue, depress phase 0 in abnormal fibres, shorten repolarisation *lignocaine, mexiletine, tocainide*
  - Class 1C Markedly depress phase 0, markedly slow conduction, slight effect on repolarization
    encainide, flecainide, propafenone

- **Class 2** Sympatholytic drugs
  Antagonism of sympathetic nervous system
  esmolol, metoprolol

- **Class 3** Drugs that prolong repolarisation
  Increased refractoriness
  amiodarone, bretylium, sotalol

- **Class 4** Calcium-channel blocking drugs
  verapamil

---

classification have become increasingly apparent.[16-18]

- Most antiarrhythmic drugs have more than one mechanism of action (typical example: amiodarone).
- The Vaughan Williams classification is 'hybrid' (classes 1 and 4 refer to a block of specific ion channels, class 2 to autonomic receptors and class 3 denotes a change in an electrophysiological parameter).
- The classification is incomplete and does not include α-blockers, adenosine, digitalis, etc.
- The classification describes essentially antiarrhythmic effects by blocking channels and currents and not the possibility of activation.

In view of this unsatisfactory situation, a Task Force of the Working Group on Arrhythmias of the European Society of Cardiology revised the logistic approach following a multidimensional concept[16] (Figure 10.2). This new, so-called 'Sicilian Gambit' (named from the meeting place of the Task Force in Sicily), reflects our expanding knowledge and aims rather to open avenues for thought and investigation rather than to be a simple compendium.[17, 18] At present, therefore, there is no methodical way to list the available antiarrhythmic drugs. In this chapter, the drugs – primarily the newer ones and those most often used perioperatively – will be discussed in alphabetical order.

Adenosine

Adenosine appears to be a useful drug in the treatment of supraventricular tachycardia (SVT), as well as for differential diagnosis. It has a class 1 recommendation for the treatment of paroxysmal SVT in adults.[19]

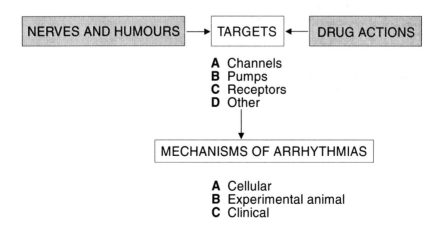

Fig 10.2 Elements of drug activation and their relationship to modulating factors and arrhythmias

Because of its short half-life, the adverse side effects are usually transient.

The recommended initial iv dose is 3–6 mg.

Ajmalin

This is a class 1A antiarrhythmic drug, effective for the treatment of Wolff–Parkinson–White (WPW) syndrome.

The recommended initial iv dose is 25–50 mg.

Amiodarone

Amiodarone's antiarrhythmic mechanisms include, in addition to class 3 effects, sodium and calcium-channel blockade, as well as β-adrenergic blockade. Amiodarone appears to be one of the most effective drugs of the newer generation for the treatment of severe, life-threatening ventricular and supraventricular arrhythmias, even when other drugs are ineffective.[20] Many cardiological trials have demonstrated a favourable trend for amiodarone both after myocardial infarction and in congestive heart failure patients.[21-26] Its usefulness is complicatd by the frequent development of adverse side efects. The most severe is pulmonary toxicity, with an overall incidence of 5–10%.[27-30] Amiodarone-induced pulmonary toxicity may appear as:

- a subacute or chronic disease resembling an infectious pneumonitis

  or

- an acute process resembling in some extreme cases adult respiratory distress syndrome (ARDS).

The mechanism of amiodarone-induced pulmonary toxicity is not completely understood. Because of the risk, amiodarone should be used in the perioperative scenario only in severe arrhythmias and not prophylactically.

The recommended initial iv dose is 2·5–5 mg/kg.

Bretylium

This is a class 3 agent, usually used in cases where life-threatening ventricular arrhythmias do not respond to lignocaine therapy.

The recommended initial iv dose is 5–10 mg/kg.

Esmolol

Because of its short duration of action, esmolol is currently the β-blocker of choice for the perioperative period.

The recommended initial iv dose is 100 μg/kg.

Lignocaine

Lignocaine is a class 1B drug. It is still the first-line drug for the treatment of ventriculr arrhythmias. There has been some confusion about the applications of lignocaine.[31, 32] Meta-analysis of the effects of lignocaine on in-hospital mortality among patients with acute myocardial infarction has suggested that despite the reduction in ventricular fibrillation the risk of death increased (statistically insignificantly) in patients treated with lignocaine. Canine experiments have shown that lignocaine can increase the likelihood of inducing sustained ventricular tachycardia after myocardial infarction and can increase defibrillation energy requirements, especially in the presence of acidosis. In the light of these findings, the prophylactic use of lignocaine may be questioned, whereas, for the definitive treatment of severe ventricular arrhythmias, lignocaine is still the drug of choice.

The recommended initial iv dose is 50–100 mg.

Magnesium

Magnesium is a crucial co-factor in more than 300 intracellular enzyme processes. The important role of magnesium is well established. Most of the recent trials relate to cardiological patients (ISIS-4, LIMIT-2, etc.)[33–35] and investigate protection of the ischaemic myocardium, modulation of reperfusion injury and the relationship between hypomagnesaemia and arrhytthmias in acute myocardial infarction.[36]

For the perioperative setting, the following facts should be kept in mind:[37–40]

- Owing to the underlying disease (diuretic therapy, stress, exogenous catecholamines), hypomagnesaemia is frequent in surgical patients.
- Only 0·3–1% of total magnesium is pooled extracellularly. Plasma concentrations do not reflect the intracellular status.
- Hypokalaemia is often associated with hypomagnesaemia. After isolated potassium substitution, hypomagnesaemia still persists.
- Magnesium is the agent of choice for the treatment of torsades de pointes, polymorphic ventricular tachycardia, and digitalis toxicity.
- In all other arrhythmias, magnesium may be used as an adjunct to antiarrhythmic drug therapy, even if the serum magnesium concentration is normal.

There is no established dose recommendation. We recommend to start with 1·5–3 mmol as a bolus, followed by 6–12 mmol infusion.

Mexiletine

Mexiletine is comparable to lignocaine, but its negative inotropic effects are less pronounced. Given orally, mexiletine causes adverse gastro-intestinal side effects.

The recommended initial iv dose is 100–250 mg.

Procainamide

This is a class 1A agent with a significant proarrhythmogenic potential.

Propafenone

This class 1C drug has additional β-blocker and calcium antagonistic effects. It is an effective drug for the treatment of supraventricular and ventricular arrhythmias.

The recommended initial iv dose is 1 mg/kg.

Sotalol

This drug has class 2 and 3 effects and is used for the treatment of supraventricular and ventricular arrhythmias.

The recommended initial iv dose is 20 mg.

Verapamil

Verapamil is a class 4 agent. It is an effective antiarrhythmic calcium antagonist for the treatment of paroxysmal supraventricular tachycardia, atrial fibrillation or flutter.

The recommended initial iv dose is 5–10 mg.

Emergency treatment of tachyarrhythmias

Experience suggests that the clinician, confronted with sudden severe arrhythmias, is not forced to make an instant decision about the many different forms of atrial and ventricular arrhythmias, but should follow a simple algorithm of treatment which includes two key steps (Figures 10.3, 10.4).

- **Step 1** Differentiation between a narrow and broad QRS complex.
- **Step 2** Differentiation between regular and irregular RR intervals.

Always keep in mind the possibility of digitalis toxicity.

Be careful with carotid sinus massage in elderly atherosclerotic patients and patients with a history of cerebral emboli.

Digitalis and verapamil are absolutely contraindicated in arrhythmias with a broad QRS complex. In addition, verapamil is contraindicated in WPW syndrome and poor left ventricular (LV) function. Differential diagnosis of arrhythmias with a broad QRS complex and regular RR interval is sometimes difficult, even for an expert; therefore, assume the more critical cause, ie an arrhythmia of ventricular origin.

In torsades de pointes, avoid antiarrhythmic drugs; they may have produced the ventricular tachycardia.

Drug treatment of bradycardic arrhythmias

In contrast to tachyarrhythmia, there has been little change in the perioperative treatment of bradyarrhythmias, other than the fact that

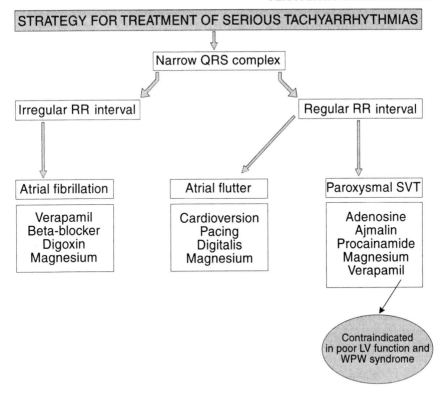

Fig 10.3   Algorithm for the treatment of serious tachyarrhythmias with narrow QRS complex

improved transient pacing equipment favours the use of mechanical stimulation in many circumstances.

- **Anticholinergic drugs**
  Atropine, ipratropium bromide
- Beta-sympathomimetic drugs
Orciprenaline, isoprenaline

According to the recommendation of the advanced cardiac life support committee of the European Resuscitation Council[41] regarding the management of peri-arrest arrhythmias, atropine, in a dose of 0·5 mg to a maximum of 3 mg is the drug of choice in life-threatening bradycardia. If ineffective, follow with a β-sympathomimetic drug. External or transvenous pacing equipment should always be available.

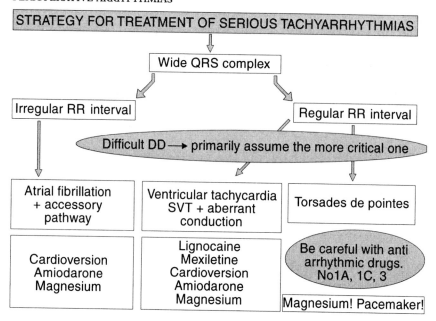

Fig 10.4   Algorithm for the treatment of serious tachyarrhythmias with broad QRS complex

1 Mangano DT. Perioperative cardiac morbidity. *Anesthesiology* 1990;**72**:153–84.
2 Goldman L. Cardiac risk in noncardiac surgery: *Anesth Analg* 1995;**80**:810–20.
3 Forrest JB, Rehder K, Cahalan MK, Goldsmith CH. Multicenter study of general anesthesia. III. Predictors of severe perioperative adverse. *Anesthesiology* 1992;**76**:3–15.
4 Kennedy HL, Whitlock JA, Sprague MK, Kennedy LJ, Buckingham TA, Goldberg RJ. Long-term follow-up of asymptomatic healthy subjects with frequent and complex ventricular ectopy. *N Engl J Med* 1985;**312**:193–7.
5 O'Kelly B, Browner WS, Massie B, Tubau J, Ngo L, Mangano DT. Ventricular arrhythmias in patients undergoing noncardiac surgery. The Study of Perioperative Ischemia Research Group. *JAMA* 1992;**268**:217–21.
6 Smith RC, Leung JM, Keith FM, Merrick S, Mangano DT. Ventricular dysrhythmias in patients undergoing coronary artery bypass graft surgery: incidence, characteristics, and prognostic importance. Study of Perioperative Ischemia (SPI) Research Group. *Am Heart J* 1992;**123**:73–81.
7 Atlee JL, IIIrd, Bosnjak ZJ. Mechanisms for cardiac dysrhythmias during anesthesia. *Anesthesiology* 1990;**72**:347–74.
8 Atlee JL, IIIrd. *Arrhythmias and pacemakers. Practical management for anesthesia and critical care medicine.* Philadelphia: W.B. Saunders, 1996.
9 Pitt B. The role of beta-adrenergic blocking agents in preventing sudden cardiac death. *Circulation* 1992;**85**:107–11.
10 Stevenson WG, Middlekauff HR, Saxon LA. Management of arrhythmias in heart failure. *Curr Opin Cardiol* 1993;**8**:419–28.
11 Roden DM. Risks and benefits of antiarrhythmic therapy. *N Engl J Med* 1994;**331**:785–91.
12 Meredith IT, Broughton A, Jennings GL, Esler MD. Evidence of a selective increase in cardiac sympathetic activity in patients with sustained ventricular arrhythmias. *N Engl J Med* 1991;**325**:618–24.
13 Armstrong PW, Gordon WM. Medical advances in the treatment of congestive heart failure. *Circulation* 1993;**88**:2941–52.

14 Brand DA, Newcomer LN, Freiburger A. Cardiologists' practices compared with practice guidelines: use of beta-blockade after acute myocardial infarction. *J Am Cell Cardiol* 1995;**26**:1432–9.

15 Doughty RN, MacMahon S, Sharpe N. Beta-blockers in heart failure: promising or proved? *J Am Coll Cardiol* 1994;**23**:814–21.

16 The 'Sicilian Gambit'. A new approach to the classification of antiarrhythmic drugs based on their actions on arrhythmogenic mechanisms. The Task Force of the Working Group on Arrhythmias of the European Society of Cardiology. *Eur Heart J* 1991;**12**:1112–31.

17 Breithardt G, Borggrefe M, Camm J, Borggrefe M, ed. *Antiarrhythmic drugs. Mechanisms of antiarrhytyhmic and proarrhythmic actions.* New York: Springer, 1995.

18 Katritsis D, Camm AJ. Antiarrhythmic drug classifications and the clinician: a gambit in the land of chaos. *Clin Cardiol* 1994;**17**:143–8.

19 Emergency cardiac care committee and subcommittee, American Heart Association. Guidelines for cardiopulmonary resuscitation and emergency cardiac care. *JAMA* 1992;**268**:2171–295.

20 Scheinman MM, Levine JH, Cannom DS. Dose-ranging study of intravenous amiodarone in patients with life-threatening ventricular tachyarrhythmias. *Circulation* 1995;**92**:3264–72.

21 Cairns JA, Connolly SJ, Roberts R, Gent M. Canadian Amiodarone Myocardial Infarction Arrhythmia Trial (CAMIAT): rationale and protocol. CAMIAT Investigators. *Am J Cardiol* 1993;**72**:87F–94F.

22 Cairns JA, Connolly SJ, Gent M, Roberts R. Post-myocardial infarction mortality in patients with ventricular premature depolarizations. Canadian Amiodarone Myocardial Infarction Arrhythmia Trial Pilot Study. *Circulation* 1991;**84**:550–7.

23 Ceremuzynski L, Kleczar E, Krzeminska Pakula M *et al.* Effect of amiodarone on mortality after myocardial infarction: a double-blind, placebo-controlled, pilot study. *J Am Coll Cardiol* 1992;**20**:1056–62.

24 Doval HC, Nul DR, Grancelli HO, Perrone SV, Bortman GR, Curiel R. Randomised trial of low-dose amiodarone in severe congestive heart failure. Grupo de Estudio de la Sobrevida en la Insuficiencia Cardiaca en Argentina (GESICA). *Lancet* 1994;**344**:493–8.

25 Nademanee K, Singh BN, Stevenson WG, Weiss JN. Amiodarone and post-MI patients. *Circulation* 1993;**88**:764–74.

26 Pfisterer ME, Kiowski W, Brunner H, Bruckhardt D, Burkart F. Long-term benefit of 1-year amiodarone treatment for persistent complex ventricular arrhythmias after myocardial infarction. *Circulation* 1993;**87**:309–11.

27 Dusman RE, Stanton MS, Miles WM *et al.* Clinical features of amiodarone-induced pulmonary toxicity. *Circulation* 1990;**82**:51–9.

28 Greenspon AJ, Kidwell GA, Hurley W, Mannion J. Amiodarone-related postoperative adult respiratory distress syndrome. *Circulation* 1991;**84**:1407–15.

29 Retz JL, Martin WJ, IInd. Amiodarone pulmonary toxicity. *Intens Care Med* 1992;**18**:388–90.

30 Van Mieghem W, Coolen L, Malysse I, Lacquet LM, Deneffe GJ, Demedts MG. Amiodarone and the development of ARDS after lung surgery. *Chest* 1994;**105**:1642–5.

31 Discher TJ, Kumar P. Pro: antiarrhythmic drugs should be used to suppress ventricular ectopy in the perioperative period. *J. Cardiothorac Vasc Anesth* 1994;**8**:699–700.

32 Miller SM, Mayer RC. Con: Antiarrhythmic drugs should not be used to suppress ventricular ectopy in the perioperative period. *J Cardiothorac Vasc Anesth* 1994;**8**:701–3.

33 ISIS-4 (Fourth International Study of Infarct Survival) Collaborative Group. ISIS-4: a randomised factorial trial assessing early oral captopril, oral mononitrate, and intravenous magnesium sulphate in 58,050 patients with suspected acute myocardial infarction. *Lancet* 1995;**345**:669–85.

34 Moran JL, Gallagher J, Peake SL. Parenteral magnesium sulfate versus amiodarone in the therapy of atrial tachyarrhythmias: a prospective, randomized study. *Crit Care Med* 1995;**23**:1816–1995.

35 Woods KL, Fletcher S, Roffe C, Haider Y. Intravenous magnesium sulphate in suspected acute myocardial infarction: results of the second Leicester Intravenous Magnesium Intervention Trial (LIMIT-2). *Lancet* 1992;**339**:1553–8.

36 Antmann EM. Magnesium in acute MI. Timing is critical. *Circulation* 1995;**92**:2367–71.

37 Aglio LS, Stanford GG, Maddi R, Boyd JL, IIIrd, Nussbaum S, Chernow B. Hypomagnesemia is common following cardiac surgery. *J Cardiothorac Vasc Anesth* 1991;5:201–8.

38 Birch RF, Lake CL. Pro: Magnesium is a valuable therapy in the cardiac surgical patient. *J Cardiothorac Vasc Anesth* 1991;5:518–21.

39 Gettes LS. Electrolyte abnormalities underlying lethal and ventricular arrhythmias. *Circulation* 1992;85:170–6.

40 Tzivoni D, Keren A. Suppression of ventricular arrhythmias by magnesium. *Am J Cardiol* 1990;65:1397–9.

41 Chamberlain D, Vincent R, Baskett P *et al*. Management of periarrest arrhythmias. A statement for the Advanced Cardiac Life Support Committee of the European Resuscitation Council, 1994. *Resuscitation* 1994;28:151–9.

11: Treatment of pulmonary hypertension

JOSE OTAVIO AULER JR, PEDRO POSO RUIZ-NETO

Pulmonary hypertension is defined as when mean pulmonary artery pressure is higher than 25 mmHg at rest, or 30 mmHg upon exercise, with a cardiac output less than 5 1/min.[1] Acute pulmonary hypertension or its re-exacerbation represents an important cause of acute heart failure during anaesthsia and postoperative care. It is a frequent haemodynamic feature of acute lung injury, commonly associated with sepsis, severe trauma, and multiple blood transfusion, as well as after cardiopulmonary bypass. Furthermore, previous pulmonary hypertension can arise in patients with chronic lung disease, prolonged left heart failure, and congenital heart disease. Primary pulmonary hypertension may also be exacerbated during and after major surgery or after insults to the lungs. The proposed mechanism of this acute increase in pulmonary arterial blood pressure or its re-exacerbation seems to be a disarrangement of the control mechanism of vascular smooth muscle tone, due to injury of the pulmonary vascular endothelium resulting in exaggerated pulmonary vasoconstriction. This chapter provides a review of the pathophysiology of pulmonary hypertension and outlines both conventional forms of treatment and new therapeutic approaches in this area.

Factors influencing vascular pulmonary tone

Vascular pulmonary tone is maintained by the action of vasoconstrictor and vasodilator influences on pulmonary vascular smooth muscle cells present in the precapillary resistance vessels.

Autonomic control

Both sympathetic and parasympathetic pathways are present in the pulmonary circulation, with the former, although not as important as the systemic vasculature, being more strongly represented than the latter. The vasoconstrictor noradrenaline and the vasodilator isoprenaline act on α- and β-sympathetic receptors, respectively. The range of vessels affected by

213

this control consists of those with a diameter of 30 μm and more. Acetylcholine is the mediator of the parasympathetic endings and its effect is vasodilatation. Some studies have described the effects of acetylcholine as due to the release of nitric oxide locally from the vascular endothelium (see below).

Oxygen and carbon dioxide

Hypoxia has a vasoconstriction effect on the pulmonary circulation, converse to its effect on the systemic vascular tone. Both the pulmonary arterial and the alveolar partial tensions of oxygen play a role in this mechanism.[2,3] Some investigations showing the effect of both alveolar P_{O_2} (P_{AO_2}) and mixed venous P_{O_2} (P_{VO_2}) over the vasoconstrictor response, have demonstrated a non-linear relationship. Thus the relationship between hypoxia in alveolar and mixed venous blood and the stimulus to pulmonary vasoconstriction is described as:

$$P \text{ (stimulus) } O_2 = P_{VO_2}^{0.375} \times P_{AO_2}^{0.626}$$

Regional vasoconstriction is a beneficial defence mechanism as it diverts blood flow from alveolar regions where there is low oxygen tension or insufficient alveolar ventilation. This helps to keep the ventilation/perfusion relationship as normal as possible, avoiding the onset of shunting. On the other hand, in clinical conditions where there is chronic alveolar hypoxia, this defence mechanism could lead to a high pulmonary pressure affecting right ventricular function. Administration of oxygen may correct this situation temporarily.[4] The vessels affected by this mechanism are those with a diameter of 1 mm or less. Although no definitive explanation has been given for the vasoconstriction reflex, many substances have been associated with it. Previous investigations have highlighted the leukotriene metabolites of the 5-lipoxygenase pathway of arachidonic acid as a key substance in controlling the hypoxic vasoconstriction reflex.[5] Thus, in hypoxic conditions, the constricting effects of the leukotrienes (B4, C4, and D4) would counterbalance the vasodilating actions of prostaglandins, notably prostacyclin.[6,7] Hypoxic pulmonary vasoconstriction can occur in the isolated lung, thus being independent of sympathetic innervation.[1] Warren et al.[8] and Brenner et al.[9] proved from animal studies that when a hypoxic condition was established, cultured pulmonary endothelial cells responded by reducing the production of endothelium-derived relaxing factor (EDRF). As will be discussed later in this chapter, there is evidence that inhibiting the action of EDRF increases vasoconstriction during alveolar hypoxaemia, a situation that can be reversed by the inhalation of nitric oxide (NO).

It seems that the integrity of the vascular endothelium is important in establishing hypoxic vasoconstriction, although some discordance may exist in the literature.[10,11] NO has been shown to be a potent vasodilator of the pulmonary circulation without causing a decrease in the systemic blood pressure[12] (see below). Hypercapnia has less effect on the pulmonary circulation than hypoxia, but the increase in CO_2 may perhaps reinforce the hypoxic vasoconstriction.[13]

Pulmonary endothelial mediators

Endothelial cells synthase and many active substances which are believed to help in maintaining the patency of the vessels and the fluidity of the blood. The list of substances linked to these functions is long and includes large molecules such as interleukin, fibronectin, heparin sulphate, tissue plasminogen activator and smaller substances like EDRF, platelet-activating factor, and endothelin-1.[14]

Acetylcholine has been proved to be helpful in evaluating the status of the pulmonary vascular tone. After acetylcholine injection, the fall in pulmonary blood pressure is greater and the degree of vasomotor tone in the pulmonary circulation is increased.[15]

Some studies have also indicated that histamine can be involved in regulating pulmonary vascular tone.[16, 17] The existence of H_1- and H_2-receptors in the pulmonary circulation has been described, and this can explain both the vasoconstrictor and vasodilator effects of histamine in the lungs. Alpha-receptors are stimulated by adrenaline and dopamine, causing an increase in pulmonary vascular resistance. Isoprenaline, a primary β-receptor stimulant, causes a fall in pulmonary pressure, and the same effect has been demonstrated for aminophylline, bradykinin, prostaglandin PGE_1, prostacyclin, and ganglionic-blocking agents. Other substances that increase pulmonary pressure are serotinin, thromboxane-A_2, and the prostaglandin $PGF_{2\alpha}$ and PGE_2.

Endothelium-derived relaxing factor (EDRF)

The long list of chemical substances described above notwithstanding, it seems likely that the core mechanism involved in regulating vascular pulmonary tone relates to a specific endothelial factor defined as EDRF. A study by Furchgott and Zawadzki in 1980 using simple strips of artery first described the obligatory role of the endothelium in vascular relaxation induced by acetylcholine.[15] Stimulation of muscarinic M_2-receptors on endothelial cells promotes the release of a substance called endothelium-derived relaxing factor. This substance is a non-prostanoid, labile humoral molecule with a half-life of 3–50 seconds, released from the vascular endothelium after a variety of stimuli. Later, NO was identified as the endothelium-derived relaxing factor; it relaxes the vascular smooth muscle and inhibits platelet aggregation and adhesion. NO is synthesised from the terminal guanidine nitrogen atom of L-arginine.[18, 19] This substrate is specific to the reaction since a number of analogues including its D-enantiomer are inactive. The production of NO also depends on the presence of calcium and calmodulin.[20, 21] Production of NO has been

215

demonstrated in endothelial cells, macrophages, and nervous tissue, where the enzyme nitric oxide synthetase has been identified.[22] An analogue of L-arginine, L-Ng-monomethyl arginine (L-NMMA), is a competitive and enantiomorphically specific inhibitor of NO Production.[23] L-NMMA blocks NO production increasing vascular resistance. NO is a highly diffusible gas and its water and lipid solubility are similar to carbon monoxide and oxygen.[24, 25]

NO exerts its vasodilator effect through the generation of guanosine 3,5'-cyclic monophosphate (cGMP) by activation of soluble guanylyl cyclase. Increase in cGMP decreases the intracellular calcium ion available for smooth muscle contraction. Hypoxia induced impairment of guanylyl cyclase in segments of proximal pulmonary arteries of rats breathing low O_2 tension room air over 2–7 days. It was observed that in this condition the guanylyl cyclase malfunction may contribute to the predominance of pulmonary vasoconstriction through activation of the hypoxia reflex.[26]

Once in blood circulation, NO is rapidly inactivated by binding to haemoglobin; because of its great affinity, the reaction is almost 300 times faster than with carbon monoxide,[27] thus restricting the vasodilatory action to the vicinity of the site of its generation. NO action can be abolished by superoxide ions and potentiated by superoxide dismutase.[14]

The action of NO involves the mechanisms of muscle relaxation, so one might expect that it involves the inhibition of the release of calcium into the contracting smooth muscle cell by shutting down the calcium channels and not allowing intracellular increased calcium or by releasing cytoplasmic bounded calcium. All these mechanisms will establish a balance toward vasodilatation. It is well known that potassium channels can act on calcium channel tone, by controlling the cell membrane depolarisation. In a depolarised state, calcium channels are opened and calcium increases in the cytosol, establishing adequate conditions for vasoconstriction.[28, 29] It has been postulated that potassium channels could work as a receptor for O_2 partial tension in the pulmonary circulation. Hypoxic contraction of the pulmonary artery can be inhibited by the potassium-channel opener cromakalin and enhanced by the potassium-channel blocker glibencla-mide.[1] Thus, when an alveolar unit is experiencing hypoxia, the potassium receptors in adjacent vessels would change their conformation and ion permeability, decreasing the intracellular concentration of this ion and, as a final pathway, increasing the concentration of calcium. This would provide the substrate for the vascular smooth muscle cell to contract in seeking to reestablish the ventilation/perfusion relationship in the hypoxic area. A mechanism involving the action of the potassium channels might help to explain why the pulmonary circulation responds in a different way to hypoxia when compared to the systemic circulation. As suggested by Peacock[1] on vasodilators in pulmonary hypertension, the pharmacological manipulation of the potassium channel at the level of the pulmonary circulation may provide the best chance of developing a selective pulmonary vasodilator.

Atrial natriuretic factor

Atrial natriuretic factor (ANF) is a peptide secreted by auricular cardiac cells. ANF is a diuretic, a natriuretic, and a vasodilator that inhibits the renin angiotensin aldosterone system. ANF is extracted and metabolised by receptors largely distributed in the lungs during its intravascular transit. Being a potent vasodilator, this peptide contributes to right ventricular performance by decreasing afterload. ANF also probably acts by modifying pulmonary capillary permeability. Hypoxia and hypercapnia are involved in increased secretion of ANF, levels of which are elevated in pulmonary arterial hypertension and chronic respiratory insufficiency.[30]

Physical factors

Physical stimuli such as increased shear stress on endothelial cells can also provoke EDRF release.[31–34] This may be caused by changes in membrane conformation induced by the shear stress. Besides the release of EDRF, prostacyclin can also be released. Both can be involved in a defence mechanism of the endothelium, protecting it against mechanical injury.

The pulmonary circulation has an extraordinary capacity to adapt to an increase in blood flow. This can be well observed in the acute increase of blood flow that follows a pneumonectomy. The remaining pulmonary parenchyma almost immediately combines with compensatory physical mechanisms to receive the total cardiac output that was being divided through both lungs minutes before clamping of the pulmonary artery. Rare episodes of cardiac arrhythmia have been described during the immediate postoperative period, probably due to the overdistension of the right atrium. Most patients, however, seem able within hours to manage the situation of high blood flow in the single lung. It appears pulmonary resistance is reduced at higher flow rates, implying an increase in the total cross-sectional area of the pulmonary vascular bed. The mechanism is explained by the recruitment of new capillaries and distension of the existing vessels.

The transmural pressure in the pulmonary circulation depends on alveolar pressure and it can also play a role in the pulmonary circulation. The elements of the vasculature more affected by these factors are the capillaries, due to their spatial intimacy with the alveolar walls. Increasing the intrathoracic mean pressure can produce alveolar pressure values high enough to decrease the capillary diameter, increasing pulmonary resistance in patients prone to develop pulmonary hypertension and those requiring positive-pressure mechanical ventilation.

Pathophysiology of pulmonary hypertension

Pulmonary hypertension results from many causes: left cardiac failure, increased pulmonary blood flow, proximal vascular obstruction or decrease of the distal vascular bed, such as loss of vessels narrowing of their luminal diameter, or endoluminal obstruction. Apart from passive haemodynamic responses, active processes contribute to pulmonary hypertension by vasomotricity and remodelling of the vascular wall. The biopathology of vasomotor mediators, as well as of endothelial and smooth muscle interactions, will be discussed next. The pulmonary vascular bed is characterised to be a high flow, low pressure circuit with great capacity to accommodate increase in blood flow. In pulmonary hypertensive states this capacity is lost, causing elevation in pulmonary artery pressure. Pulmonary hypertension is defined as when mean pulmonary artery pressure exceeds 20 mmHg and may be caused by increased resistance at one of several locations in the pulmonary circulation. According to the level of the pulmonary wedge pressure, pulmonary hypertension could be classified as precapillary hypertension when the resistance is located in the arteries and arterioles, and postcapillary hypertension when the resistance is caused by some restriction to pulmonary blood flow. There are four principal causes of precapillary pulmonary hypertension:

1   *Alveolar hypoxia*, which may be caused by chronic obstructive pulmonary disease, acute lung injury, interstitial lung diseases, kyphoscoliosis, morbid obesity, and neuromuscular disorders. Prolonged hypoxia induces vasoconstriction, destruction, narrowing of the pulmonary vessels characterised by abnormal deposition of increased amounts of collagen and elastin within the adventia, medial smooth muscle cell hypertrophy, and hyperplasia as well as neomuscularisation.[35, 36] The cellular mechanisms reponsible for hypoxia-induced vascular remodelling are not completely elucidated, but studies have hypothesised they are similar to what happens in embryonic tissue interactions: one tissue causes an effect on the adjacent tissue. These mutual interchanges are related to a variety of mediators, including growth factors, basement membrane components, and metalloproteases, ultimately resulting in the generation of new composite tissue. Modern knowledge of pulmonary vascular remodelling results from research that submits cultured vascular cells to a low concentration of oxygen. These endothelium cells release mediators that seem to affect the behaviour of smooth muscle cells. At the same time, proliferation factors predominate over growth inhibitor factors, causing multiplication of endothelial cells, fibroblasts, and smooth muscle cells. The endothelium has been shown to be essential for the cellular changes produced in response to hypoxia. The vascular tone modulation depends, in normal states, on a balance between endothelium-derived relaxing and contracting fac-

tors.[37] This fact was demonstrated in isolated pulmonary artery segments assayed the contractility of the vascular rings and by cGMP levels. In this investigation hypoxia was shown to inhibit the basal production of EDRF and its agonist-stimulated release.[38] The chemical mediator responsible for EDRF activity is mainly nitric oxide, which causes smooth muscle cell dilatation by activating guanylyl cyclase and increasing intracellular cGMP levels. From *in vitro* data, McQuillan *et al.*[39] have shown that hypoxic pulmonary and non-pulmonary endothelial cells secrete decreased amounts of NO due to decreased expression of the endothelial nitric oxide synthase gene.[39] Thus, hypoxia is believed to suppress NO release in pulmonary artery vessels.

Endothelin, a 21-amino acid peptide, is a potent mediator involved with systemic and pulmonary circulation; its production is increased mainly in diseases of the vasculature. Endothelin is synthesised by endothelial cells and has intense vasoconstrictor effects in the pulmonary circulation. The basal production of endothelin is regulated by epinephrine, angiotensin II, arginine vasopressin, growth factor, β-thrombin, interleukin-1, and hypoxia. In vascular smooth muscle, endothelin binds to a specific receptor, which activates phospholipase C, leads to the formation of inositol triphosphate, diacylglycerol, and increased intracellular calcium. This justifies the contention that that calcium antagonists inhibit endothelin-induced contractions in certain, but not all, blood vessels. The pulmonary circulation plays an important role in the metabolism of endothelin, as the lungs take over important amounts of the peptide during its passage through these territories.[40]

2   *Vascular disorders*, such as primary pulmonary hypertension and autoimmune tissue diseases, include scleroderma, rheumatoid arthritis, systemic lupus erythematosus, and dermatomyositis. The mechanisms responsible for the development of primary pulmonary hypertension still remain completely unexplained. Plexogenic arterio-pathy is the most common form of this disease which promotes narrowing and destruction of pulmonary arteries and is characterised by vascular lesions consisting of neo-intimal fibrosis proliferation, plexiform lesions and necrotising arteritis.[41]

3   *Massive acute and chronic recurrent pulmonary embolism* appears to cause pulmonary hypertension by capacitance decrease in the vascular bed as well as through clot release of vasoconstrictor substances.[42]

4   *Congenital left-to-right intracardiac and extracardiac shunts* may also cause pulmonary hypertension due to exhaustion of the capacitance reserve, medial hypertrophy and intimal hyperplasia of pulmonary arteries, and reflexed vasoconstriction in response to passive distension of the muscular pulmonary arteries.[43]

5   *Pulmonary arterial hypertension* has been observed in sepsis and the *adult respiratory distress syndrome*.[44] It has been seen both in experimental

219

animal and human sepsis, even before development of the adult respiratory distress syndrome. Several mechanisms have been proposed for the association of pulmonary arterial hypertension with sepsis and the adult respiratory distress syndrome; obstruction of the pulmonary microcirculation with microthrombi composed of platelets and leucocytes, and active pulmonary vasoconstriction induced by the autonomous nervous system, hypoxia or vasoactive mediators. Some of these mediators, in particular serotonin and arachidonic acid metabolites, have been the subject of substantial research aimed to help in therapeutic manipulation. Since pulmonary arterial hypertension imposes an increased afterload to the right ventricle and appears to be a major factor in the outcome of sepsis, its treatment may be expected to produce a better result.[44]

Postcapillary pulmonary hypertension is commonly caused by some restriction to pulmonary venous blood flow as observed in cor triatriatum, mitral stenosis, atrial myxoma or elevation in left ventricular end-diastolic pressure caused by cardiomyopathies, constrictive pericarditis, and aortic stenosis. The mechanisms in this type of hypertension are due to a passive backward pressure elevation causing mild to moderate pulmonary hypertension. However, one-third of these patients may develop severe pulmonary hypertension due to medial hypertrophy and intimal hyperplasia of the pulmonary arteries.

In summary, there are several mechanisms involved in the pathophysiology of pulmonary hypertension. A wide variety of acute and chronic respiratory system disorders and cardiocirculatory diseases are the principal causes. The main mechanisms included are alveolar hypoxia, excessive distension of the pulmonary vascular bed, and capacity-decreasing or inflammatory process of the vessels. The sustained elevation in pulmonary artery pressure is probably mediated through two principal mechanisms at the vascular level: sustained vasospasm and vascular structural remodelling, which association causes luminal narrowing and vessel obliteration which reduce cross-sectional vascular area sufficiently for the development of pulmonary hypertension.

Right ventricle (RV)

The RV is responsible for accepting venous return and pumping it to the pulmonary circulation, and under normal conditions the work pressure required by the RV to maintain cardiac output is discrete. The thin-walled right ventricle is two times as distensible as the left ventricle during diastole, and during systole its stroke volume is twice as sensitive to the level of impedance. Conditions that result in a right ventricular pressure overload, acute or chronic, are the most frequent causes of RV dysfunction. Under normal conditions, any elevation in afterload is followed by an important reduction in right ventricular ejection fraction.[45] In this way, right ventricular performance could be maintained until mean pulmonary artery pressure is 40 mmHg or greater. Previous studies have described the incapacity of the right ventricle to support an acute increase in pulmonary vascular resistance.[46, 47] During progressive pulmonary artery pressure elevation there is compensatory right ventricular hypertrophy. The RV stroke work increases in order to counteract the elevated pulmonary resistance that occurs in association with the vascular disease. The decline in RV stroke work is generally manifested by a fall in RV stroke volume rather than a fall in RV systolic pressure. Acute pulmonary hypertension caused by further elevation in this pressure may impair the cardiac function, even in the hypertrophied right ventricle.[41] The mechanisms of acute reduction in RV ejection fraction include both depression of RV systolic function and alterations in ventricular interdependence, which indirectly affect LV function. The most common causes of RV pressure overload include adult respiratory distress syndrome, mechanical ventilation, pulmonary embolism, acute hypoxia, and re-exacerbation of pre-existent pulmonary hypertension. The haemodynamic consequences of acute RV dysfunction are hypotension and low cardiac output. It can be verified by increases in central venous and pulmonary pressures, RV ejection fraction decrease, enlargement of right chambers and septal displacement to the left. In experimental models of acute pulmonary emboli the ventricular septum is usually displaced and flattened into the left ventricular chamber.[48] This and other studies have shown that the principal mechanism of ventricular dysfunction correlated with any acute increase in RV afterload is a deviation in ventricular interaction leading to a reduction in LV preload secondary to a great increase in RV volumes. The management of RV dysfunction remains controversial. The strategies are based mainly on the mechanisms behind RV dysfunction. Volume loading is recommended only when pulmonary vascular resistance (PVR) and RV contractility are normal. In normal high-compliant RV, the rationale of volume expansion is by means of maximal fibre stetching to obtain increase in contractility. Catecholamines have been demonstrated to be effective when RV dysfunction is associated with decreased contractile status. When increase in PVR is associated with reduction of RV contractility, use of a pharmacological agent that combines inotropic and vasodilator properties is preferable. Vasoconstrictors such as noradrenaline have a role in situations in which RV dysfunction occurs primarily as a decreased coronary perfusion pressure. Vasodilators are precisely indicated when the aim is to reduce PVR and transpulmonary gradient. However, there are conflicting data concerning the usefulness of common vasodilator agents: systemic hypotension, increase of right ventricular end-diastolic volume, decrease of RV perfusion, and worsening of hypoxaemia consequent to attenuation of vasoconstriction reflex, could be seen in the attempt to reduce PVR employing traditional vasodilators. For instance, nitroglycerin and sodium nitroprusside, when utilised in COPD patients, may decrease PVR and right ventricular end-diastolic volume resulting in significant decrease in cardiac index.[49] Other agents, such as prostaglandins, nitric oxide and phosphodiesterase inhibitors, will be discussed in the section on pharmacological agents below. In addition to pharmacological treatment, mechanical devices have also been successfully employed to support a severely compromised right ventricle.

Methods of treatment

In the past few years there has been a renewal of interest in control of the pulmonary vascular system and the effectiveness of pharmacological manipulation of the pulmonary circulation. As discussed previously, understanding of the pathophysiology and consequences of pulmonary hypertension is required when considering pharmacological treatment. Information concerning the potential benefits and toxicities of drug therapy for primary and secondary hypertension is essential, taking into account the use of specific agents for individual diseases.[50]

The physiological role of the endothelium has been extensively investigated, but the role of new vasoactive substances, and their neural influence on the pulmonary vasculature, has still to be clarified, as has their control of the matching of ventilation to perfusion. Even in normal conditions some aspects of these regulatory processes are unclear, and consequently much more investigation is required in the circumstances of lung injury.

Oxygen

Oxygen therapy is central to the management of different situations associated with alveolar hypoxia. Along with the harmful systemic effects associated with oxygen arterial content deprivation, modifications in the haemodynamics of the pulmonary circulation are also important. The modulation of pulmonary vascular tone during hypoxaemic states has received much attention in the literature and the rightful position of oxygen as therapy still needs to be clarified.

The arterioles in the pulmonary vascular bed seem morphologically common; however, these vessels are the most responsive system of any organ in addition to being responsible for changes in oxygen levels. In the presence of acute hypoxia, arteriolar vasoconstriction causes a marked elevation in pulmonary vascular resistance. Sustained hypoxia causes multiplication and migration of the smooth muscle cells and over-accumulation of extracellular matrix in the arteriolar wall, a process termed vascular remodelling. Such alterations as vascular tone abnormalities and cellular hyperplasia characterise diseases including pulmonary fibrosis, idiopathic pulmonary hypertension, and persistent pulmonary hypertension of the newborn (PPHN). In these and other situations hypoxia is

222

believed to be a triggering factor for the remodelling process. To demonstrate this point, *in vivo* intrauterine oxygen deprivation in animals has promoted pulmonary hypertension in their newborns characterised by pulmonary vascular smooth muscle cell vasoconstriction and hyperplasia.[51]

Along with the decreased NO production that contributes to pulmonary hypertensive states associated with hypoxaemia, increased production of vasoconstrictors by the endothelial cells was also observed. One of these agents is endothelin, a potent vasoconstrictive substance that can be detected in high levels in plasma and lung endothelial cells in patients with pulmonary hypertension.[52, 53]

Hypoxic pulmonary vasoconstriction (HPV) is an adjustment reflex responsible for matching ventilation to perfusion, thus HPV contributes to the efficiency of gas exchange by reducing blood flow to lung regions with low Va/Q ratios. On the other hand, excessive generalised HPV is a frequent determinant in the pulmonary hypertension associated with acute and chronic pulmonary disorders. This reflex is unique to the pulmonary circulation and has continuously been studied since it was first described by von Euler in cats.[54, 55] The understanding of HPV is important because of its involvement in pulmonary hypertension in patients with hypoxic lung disease. It is interesting to note that HPV, even being a reflex, does not rely on substantial sympathetic innervation of the pulmonary vasculature because it occurs in the denerved lung and in the isolated pulmonary vascular ring. However, it does seem to depend mainly on endothelial control, for the following reasons:

1   chronic hypoxia impairs the release of nitric oxide;[56]
2   inhaled nitric oxide reverses acute hypoxic pulmonary vasoconstriction;[57]
3   nitric oxide synthase inhibitors seem to increase hypoxic pulmonary vasoconstriction.[58]

In addition, these studies have all suggested that a reduction in nitric oxide release caused either by damage to the endothelium or by inhibition of nitric oxide synthesis modulates the vascular response to hypoxia. Other vasoconstrictor factors, such as endothelin-1 released by the endothelium, could also play an important role in the vasoconstrictive response to hypoxia. A further mechanism recently described for vascular control has proposed potassium channels as a sensor for hypoxia in pulmonary vascular smooth muscle membrane cells by controlling the state of depolarisation of the membrane.[28, 59, 60]

Aside from the role identified for potassium channels as a sensor for hypoxia in pulmonary vascular smooth muscle cells,[28] much research has been addressed to the search for a specific receptor for hypoxia and for some humoral mechanism that could be the transducer which sends signals to the vascular smooth muscle to contract. Several questions have been raised concerning the vessel size in response to hypoxia. It has been clearly shown that the stimulus for HPV may be a simple function of both mixed venous and alveolar oxygen tension.[61, 62] The location of the hypoxic constriction was identified in small arteries and cells in the proximity of the vascular smooth muscle, like mast cells[73] and endothelial cells,[71] which might act as hypoxia sensors. This fact has been demonstrated and subsequently confirmed independently.[63, 64] Thus, oxygen tension across the wall of the small arteries could be the stimulus, given that the endothelial cells are encircled by alveolar gas on the outside and by mixed venous blood on the inside. The diffusion oxygen gradient and the individual vascular smooth muscle cells respond to the local oxygen tension. On the other hand, studies have suggested that arteries of different sizes could respond to variation of oxygen tension in a manner identical to the small arteries.[65, 66] Since HPV could only be demonstrated in small arteries *in vivo*, and the large arteries do not invariably respond, the constriction in these vessels is probably determined by the systemic arterial oxygen tension.[66] The classic observation that ventilation with hypoxic gas mixtures caused pulmonary vasoconstriction, led to the concept that the stimulus for HPV may in fact be alveolar oxygen tension. One explanation for large artery vasoconstriction could be hypoxic blood present in the vasa vasorum originating from bronchial arteries.[65] In contrast, neurogenic pathways have been offered to explain the difference in constrictive mechanisms between large and small arteries.[67] In summary, neurogenic mechanisms permit the large arteries to react only during systemic hypoxaemia, and showing less sensitivity than small vessels, which respond well to local variations of oxygen concentration.

Chronic hypoxia is postulated to promote structural changes in the pulmonary vessels, including hypertrophy of the muscular media and muscularisation of the arterioles as well as fibrosis of the intima. One careful study has suggested alveolar hypoxia to be the main determinant of pulmonary vasoconstriction in healthy conditions and in chronic respiratory diseases.[68] There are some controversies about the effectiveness of long-term oxygen therapy in patients with chronic lung disease concerning the response of pulmonary circulation to this agent. Oxygen seems to reduce, and occasionally modify the progression of pulmonary hypertension, which very infrequently returns to normal levels. Probably the structural changes of pulmonary arteries are not changed by the oxygen therapy, but prolonged oxygen is associated with haemodynamic improvement and a reduction in episodes of right heart failure.[69] On the other hand, increase in the fraction of inspired oxygen has been shown to be a potent pulmonary vasodilator on vascular territory in children with pulmonary blood hyperflow[70] as well as in animals under experimental investigation, these effects being more pronounced in neonate compared to adult animals.[71] Acute elevation of PVR and PAP has also been described in patients with different causes of respiratory failure and in animal models of acute lung injury.[72, 73] PVR has been increased in the earlier stage of ARDS, even after the correction of arterial hypoxaemia. In lung injury there is a probable reduction in NO release secondary to the resulting endothelial damage in pulmonary hypertension. However, controversy persists about the responsibility for maintenance of pulmonary vascular tone in healthy pulmonary circulation during conditions of normoxia. Leeman et al.[74] examined the effects of NO on pulmonary vasomotor tonus modulation in dogs during hyperoxia, normoxia, and hypoxia. Utilising a system to maintain the cardiac output and pulmonary pressure constant, the authors showed that no inhibitor significantly affected the pulmonary driving pressure during hyperoxia and normoxia, thus suggesting that endogenous NO is not involved with low basal vascular tonus.[74] Moreover, the lungs from rats in normoxic conditions, examined by immunohistochemistry, showed that the expression of NO synthase was encountered in the endothelium of large pulmonary arteries but not in the endothelium of small pulmonary resistance vessels.[75] In conclusion, what the role of NO might be in low basal pulmonary vascular tonus remains open to discussion. Many studies fairly suggest that hypoxia stimulates NO release, which then modulates hypoxic vasoconstriction. Thus, inhibitors of NO synthase have been shown to magnify the vascular response to hypoxia under various experimental conditions including in vivo animals.[74, 76–78] Recently an increase of NO synthesis was demonstrated[75–77] in cultures of endothelial cells submitted to hypoxic conditions; thus in oxygen deprivation, NO seems to exert an important role in vascular tone modulation.

In summary, during alveolar hypoxia there is a probable detriment in NO synthesis or activity, and hypoxic vasoconstriction may result from a reduced NO dilating effect. As observed in acute hypoxia, during chronic pulmonary hypertension experimental data have shown a reduced response of the endothelium-dependent relaxation factor. A possible mechanism to explain the impairment of L-arginine–NO pathway during chronic hypoxia could arise from modified NO synthase or guanylate cyclase function.[79, 80] However, some contradictory results have shown that chronic pulmonary hypertension does not depend on an NO-deficient state.[81–83] This inconsistency between data may suggest that the main problem is due to the diversity of the animal models used. We conclude, therefore, that oxygen plays an important role in pulmonary vascular tonus. In addition, NO is continuously released in the pulmonary circulation and is associated with endothelium-dependent vasodilatation. Therefore, some points involving NO still remain open to discussion. First, the contribution of continuous NO to low pulmonary vascular tone remains to be totally clarified. The second point involves acute and chronic hypoxia, NO and hypoxic pulmonary vasoconstriction. One could speculate that hypoxaemia exerts an inhibitory effect on NO synthesis, thus enhancing the vasoconstriction and shunting blood from collapsed areas to ventilated ones. The contrary view is that oxygen deprivation increases NO production and the vasoconstrictive reflex could be attenuated. In this way NO could be acting in favour of the ventilation–perfusion matching mechanism. Considering these points, the basis of the treatment of pulmonary hypertension secondary to acute or chronic alveolar hypoxia should be reviewed. More studies are required to address the use of oxygen along with NO inhalation in situations of severe hypoxaemia when accompanied by pulmonary hypertension. More needs to be learned about the cellular and molecular adaptation to hypoxia in man, but the future may soon bring novel approaches to the treatment of patients with chronic obstructive lung disease and secondary pulmonary hypertension, as well as those with respiratory failure.[84]

Conventional Therapy

Besides pharmacological support, a general approach to the control of pulmonary hypertension includes sedation, adequate ventilation, and acid–base equilibrium. During the postoperative period, profound sedation has been shown to control exacerbation of pulmonary hypertension effectively in response to tracheal and other painful stimuli.[85] Hypoxia and acidosis may induce and exacerbate pulmonary arterial reactivity. Oxygen may be an effective vasodilator, mainly when hypertension is due to hypoxic stimulation of the precapillary arteriolar vasculature.[86] Correction of metabolic acidosis and a mild level of hypocapnia has been demonstrated to prevent re-exacerbation of pulmonary hypertension.

Selective reduction of pulmonary vascular resistance (PVR) continues to be a therapeutic goal for the treatment of pulmonary hypertension, but current therapeutic options remain limited. The reduction in PVR is based on the belief that pulmonary vasoconstriction is an important component of pulmonary hypertension. The ultimate response to vasodilator therapy is reduction of pulmonary artery pressure (PAP) with a rise in cardiac output. The successful pharmacological manipulation of pulmonary vascular control is influenced by such factors as lack of specificity and systemic effects, as well as the choice between a wide variety of drugs that have been employed in the treatment of pulmonary hypertension. The majority of vasodilators are not selective to the pulmonary vasculature; they act also as systemic vasodilators. Many different vasodilator agents have been used to treat virtually all forms of pulmonary arterial hypertension, with that due to pulmonary thromboembolic disease, primary hypertension, chronic obstructive lung disease or pulmonary hypertension associated with connective tissue diseases receiving most attention. The drugs involved in treatment of pulmonary hypertension include α-adrenergic blocking agents, β-agonists, direct vasodilators, calcium-channel blockers, angiotensin converting enzyme inhibitors, serotonin antagonists, prostaglandins, and parasympathycomimetic agents. Intravenous or oral vasodilators may be used to treat any form of pulmonary hypertension. Although there are arguments against pharmacotherapy to control pulmonary hypertension associated with chronic respiratory diseases, especially COPD, the main argument in favour is that acute increase in PAP in the presence of hypoxaemia may contribute to the development of right heart failure.[68]

The population of patients with primary pulmonary hypertension is a heterogeneous one, both clinically and histologically. As the aetiological mechanisms are unknown, therapy is directed towards the consequences of the pulmonary vascular process. The long-term use of conventional therapy to control severe primary pulmonary hypertension remains controversial. Oxygen supplementation, the use of digoxin and diuretics for symptomatic heart failure, and anticoagulation may all have a role in treating primary pulmonary hypertension, although vasodilator therapy has been the main area of investigation. In general, vasodilators have failed to selectively reduce PVR and may lead to undesirable effects, mainly systemic hypotension and worsening of oxygenation. Among all the cited drugs, oral calcium-channel blockers, principally nifedipine, as well as continuous intravenous infusion of prostacyclin, have demonstrated the most consistent haemodynamic improvement. Calcium antagonists are of particular importance in the treatment of systemic and pulmonary hypertension because they influence the free cytoplasmic calcium concentration and therefore many pressor mechanisms in the smooth muscle cell. A decline in the vascular resistance is the main haemodynamic effect, and this is more marked with second generation calcium antagonists because they are more vasoselective than the first calcium-channel blockers. Calcium antagonists are effective, safe, and well-tolerated antihypertensive agents that can be associated with the majority of other agents.[87] When medical therapies, especially for primary pulmonary hypertension, are exhausted heart–lung or lung transplantation has increasingly become an option for selected patients.[88] In patients with pulmonary hypertension associated with connective tissue disease, and non-thrombotic forms of secondary pulmonary arterial hypertension, oxygen therapy along with calcium-channel antagonists and prostacyclin seem to be promising.[89] In patients with chronic hypoxic lung disease, there is evidence of important circulatory abnormality, accompanied by pulmonary hypertension. Consequently, there are many studies using a wide variety of vasodilators and in most of them a discrete vasodilator effect has been described, accomplished with an improvement in oxygen delivery. However, no long-term enhancement in pulmonary haemodynamics has been observed. The angiotensin converting enzyme inhibitors may be useful because the oedema that characterises this disease is due in part to renal dysfunction.[1] In the absence of an orally administered selective pulmonary agent, the efforts in chronic hypoxic lung

227

disease should be focused on improving lung function and reversing hypoxia. Furthermore, acute pulmonary hypertension associated with different forms of lung injury or re-exacerbation of pulmonary hypertension, as seen after cardiac surgery in patients with severe diastolic dysfunction, valve diseases or consequent to left-to-right intracardiac shunts, often requires immediate pharmacological support.

Volume expansion

In the presence of the acute right ventricular dysfunction that accompanies pulmonary hypertension, the first step in treatment should be volume expansion. This strategy requires relative preservation of ventricular contractility and reduction of pulmonary vascular resistance. With this approach, the end-diastolic volume increase may augment cardiac output to overcome the increase afterload.[90, 91] However, volume expansion should be carefully monitored because the depressed right ventricle in the presence of an elevated afterload may not adequately manage the volume overload imposed on it. In this situation, it would be better to combine volume expansion with inotropic and vasodilator agents.[92-94]

Pharmacological agents

Intravenous agents

Inotropes

Catecholamines have been shown to be effective in the treatment of severe dysfunction of the right ventricle due to pulmonary hypertension. Studies have reported the efficiency of adrenaline, dobutamine, isoproterenol, and dopamine in improving RV function.[90, 93] Beta-adrenergic agonists may also exert vasodilator as well as positive inotropic effects and effectively argument RV contractility while at the same time promoting a decrease in afterload.[95-97] It is important to note that excessive vasodilatation may lead to right ventricular ischaemia and decreased coronary perfusion.[98]

Vasodilators

Vasodilator agents such as hydrazaline, nitroglycerin, nitrates, and sodium nitroprusside have been employed in the attempt to selectively dilate the pulmonary vasculature. Afterload reduction can enhance cardiac output by decreasing both RV afterload and PVR.[90, 99, 100] However, significant reductions in LV afterload and preload may also occur, resulting in arterial hypotension. As a result, new studies have focused on the ability of agents such as prostaglandins, nitric oxide, and the phosphodiesterase fraction-III inhibitors to more specifically decrease PVR.[100-108]

Prostaglandins

Prostaglandin E_1 is well known to improve arterial oxygenation in hypoxaemic neonates due to pulmonary hyperfusion. This agent has also been reported to be useful as a pulmonary vasodilator in the treatment of pulmonary hypertension in the newborn, in the cases of acute right heart failure and pulmonary hypertension after cardiac surgery and/or heart transplantation. D'Ambra *et al.* demonstrated the potential clinical application of prostaglandins as pulmonary vasodilators.[109] In patients undergoing mitral valve replacement with refractory right heart failure and pulmonary hypertension, PGE_1 was able to dilate the pulmonary vasculature and improve RV function. Systemic hypotension, however is the major factor limiting the clinical use of prostaglandin E_1. In this study, right PGE_1 was associated with a left atrial noradrenaline infusion to counterbalance the systemic hypotension. Okada *et al.*[110] investigated the pharmacological effect of endothelin-receptor antagonists compared to prostaglandin E_1 in an animal model of pulmonary hypertension. Receptor antagonist drugs lowered pulmonary artery and systemic arterial pressures in both pulmonary hypertensive and control animals, with a significantly greater effect on pulmonary artery pressure in pulmonary hypertensive dogs. Prostaglandin E_1 produced a greater decrease in systemic arterial pressure in pulmonary hypertensive rather than in normal beagles despite having the same effect on pulmonary artery pressure in both.[110] In another study of animal models of pulmonary hypertension the haemodynamic effects of PGE_1, isoproterenol, prostacyclin, and nifedipine were evaluated.[106, 107] Although all four drugs decreased PAP and PVR, they had varying systemic effects. Prostaglandin E_1 and isoproterenol demonstrated the greatest pulmonary specificity, significantly increased cardiac output and decreased PVR. Among them prostaglandin E_1 produced the largest decrease in PAP, prostacyclin demonstrated an intermediate action, and nifedipine was the least effective agent in decreasing pulmonary artery pressure.

Prostacyclin

Prostacyclin (PGI_2) is an endoperoxide derivative of arachidonic acid generated in the cyclooxygenase pathway.[111] Its major properties are vascular relaxation, platelet aggregation inhibition, and an apparent ability to attenuate sepsis-induced tissue damage.[112] In severe adult respiratory distress syndrome, increased pulmonary vascular resistance may lead to a progressive right ventricle dysfunction, with a further reduction in left ventricular performance. This may result in a fall in cardiac output and in DO_2, and probably interfere negatively with the survival of these patients. Radermacher *et al.*[113] infused prostacyclin in patients with adult respiratory distress syndrome and reported an improvement in RV function attributed to a significant reduction in pulmonary artery pressure. Although a powerful vasodilator, however, PGI_2, like other agents, is limited by its non-specific vascular actions. In this regard the effects of inhaled nitric oxide and intravenous prostacyclin on pulmonary haemodynamics, blood gases, and ventilation perfusion ratio were compared in patients with adult respiratory distress syndrome. Both agents lowered pulmonary artery pressure to the same extent, but PGI_2 caused a fall in systemic arterial pressure and elevation in cardiac output whereas these same parameters remained unchanged during NO inhalation. In contrast to prostacyclin infusion, NO inhalation promoted a distinct improvement in pulmonary oxygenation.[114] Among the vasodilators employed for the treatment of primary pulmonary hypertension, adenosine and prostacyclin have been shown to reduce PVR in these patients. Patients unresponsive to medical therapy received an infusion of adenosine, haemodynamics were allowed to return to baseline, and thereafter a prostacyclin infusion was begun. Both drugs were titrated to the maximum tolerated dose. Prostacyclin caused a fall in pulmonary vascular resistance and an increase in cardiac output with decreased systemic arterial pressure, but no change in pulmonary arterial pressure. Adenosine and prostacyclin have similar haemodynamic effects and adenosine may be a useful test for the potential of long-term prostacyclin therapy in patients with primary pulmonary hypertension.[115]

Phosphodiesterase III inhibitors

Phosphodiesterase fraction-III inhibitors (PDE-I) are a new class of nonadrenergic cardioactive agents. These compounds combine vasodilatation with positive inotropic effects, being useful in hypertensive pulmonary vascular states, accompanied by right-sided heart failure. In 12 patients with right ventricular failure due to mitral valve stenosis, Hess *et al.* found[116] that amrinone increased cardiac output and decreased pulmonary artery pressure by 30% and 50% respectively. In a second study,[103] the haemodynamic properties of amrinone versus sodium nitroprusside were compared in patients with aortic or mitral valve failure, where both agents lowered systemic vascular resistance equally. Pulmonary vascular resistance decreased significantly (25%) only in the amrinone group. In patients with congestive heart failure, amrinone improved RV systolic performance, predominantly due to afterload reduction, which in the majority of patients, exceeded the results observed with the administration of a pure vasodilator.

Because of their positive inotropic effects and pulmonary vasodilating properties, amrinone and other PDE-I agents appear to be useful for the successful treatment of RV failure caused by pulmonary hypertension.

Alternative methods for therapy

Nitric oxide

As previously stated, nitric oxide is an endogenous mediator of vascular dilatation, neural transmission, defence against microorganisms, and inhibitor of platelet adhesion, and has been identified as endothelin-derived relaxing factor.[117] Endothelium-derived nitric oxide is essential in the maintenance of normal vascular tone in the systemic and pulmonary circulation. EDRF is probably identical to nitric oxide and is released by the vascular endothelium both in the basal unstimulated state and in response to an extended variety of physical and chemical stimuli. The synthesis impairment is associated with the severity of respiratory failure and structural change of vessel walls. The capacity of NO selectively to dilate the pulmonary vasculature without any significant effect on the systemic circulation has been the focus of recent research.[118, 119] In an *in vivo* canine model with fixed cardiac output, Tonz *et al.*[120] examined the effectiveness of inhaled NO as a selective pulmonary vasodilator in acute pulmonary hypertension. Under total right heart bypass, pulmonary hypertension was induced by infusion of the thromboxane analogue. NO was administered at 10 and 40 ppm for 5 minutes followed by breathing of the oxygen mixture without NO. Pump flow was held constant during the experiment and infusion of the thromboxane analogue resulted in an increase in pulmonary vascular resistance and systemic vascular resistance. During inhalation of 10 ppm NO, pulmonary vascular resistance significantly decreased, and further decreased with 40 ppm NO inhalation. Systemic vascular resistance did not change during NO inhalation and there was no increase in intrapulmonary shunting or methaemoglobin levels during its administration. Although the induced pulmonary vasoconstriction was only partially reversed by NO inhalation, this agent acted as a selective pulmonary vasodilator without changing systemic vascular resistance. The haemodynamic results of 17 postoperative cardiac patients who inhaled nitric oxide (20 ppm) can be seen in Figure 11.1, which is derived from unpublished data of our ICU. A significant decrease in pulmonary vascular resistance index was observed, while the systemic vascular resistance remained practically unchanged.

The exciting results of the therapeutic use of inhaled nitric oxide in human pulmonary hypertension due to different causes, including those that occur in the presence of acute respiratory failure, have encouraged the use of this gas as a theapeutic agent. NO has been proved to oppose hypoxic pulmonary vasoconstriction (HPV) in the awake lamb and in volunteers breathing 12% oxygen.[118, 119] Additionally, inhaled NO seems selectively to dilate vessels of ventilated areas of the lung, causing a decrease in intrapulmonary shunt and improving the oxygenation.[121] Pulmonary vascular resistance and pulmonary artery pressure in ARDS patients,[114, 122] persistent pulmonary hypertension of the newborn[123, 124] and severe pulmonary hypertension[125] have all been reduced during NO inhalation. These same effects can also be seen in cardiac surgical patients, including children with congenital cardiopathy, during haemodynamic diagnostic investigation,[126] after paediatric[125] and adult surgical correction,[127-129] as well as during heart and lung transplantation. Selective pulmonary vasodilatation is a desirable effect after heart[130] and lung transplantation[131] to control the severe pulmonary hypertension that may result in right ventricular failure.[130] In our investigation, low doses of inhaled nitric oxide showed beneficial effects on pulmonary haemodynamics in patients submitted to heart transplantation, decreasing pulmonary vascular resistance and transpulmonary gradient, and improving cardiac output.[132]

This recently used therapy may also be an important adjunct in the management of postoperative pulmonary hypertension in the child with congenital heart disease. Miller *et al.* administered low doses of inhaled nitric oxide together with a high inspired oxygen concentration after corrective surgery in infants who were at risk of postoperative pulmonary hypertension because of their congenital heart disease and left-to-right

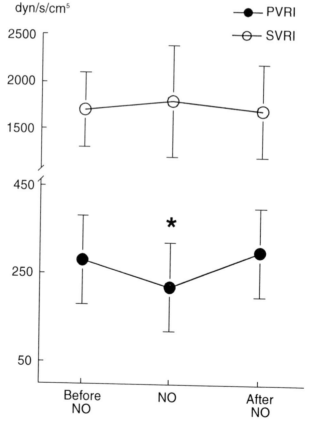

Fig 11.1 Systemic (SVRI) and pulmonary (PVRI) vascular resistance index in response to nitric oxide given postoperatively in 17 cardiac patients. NO, nitric oxide (20 ppm); * significant decrease (P 0·005)

shunt. Inhaled nitric oxide, even in a very low dose (2 ppm), caused selective pulmonary vasodilatation, accompanied by only a 10% fall in the systemic vascular resistance index. A 16% rise in mean cardiac index was also observed.[133] In children with ventricular septal defect (VSD) and moderate pulmonary hypertension, pulmonary vascular resistance was selectively decreased by nitric oxide inhalation. In this study a greater decrease in PVR was seen with oxygen and inhhaled nitric oxide than with either nitric oxide or oxygen alone.[134]

Nitric oxide has been successfully employed in the management of severe persistent pulmonary hypertension of the newborn (PPHN). Manifestations of PPHN often involve dysfunctional pulmonary vasoregulation with suprasystemic pulmonary vascular resistance causing extrapulmonary shunting and/or pulmonary parenchymal disease causing intrapulmonary shunting and systemic haemodynamic worsening. Inhaled NO can cause marked improvement in oxygenation when optimal lung inflation is completed and systemic blood volume and vascular resistance are adequate. Kinsella and Abman[135] have found that the successful application of inhaled NO in PPHN has reduced costs of hospitalisation and duration of hospital stay by approximately 50% and 40%, respectively. These authors concluded that inhaled NO may be an important instrument in the management of severe PPHN when its utilisation is limited to patients with severe extrapulmonary shunting. On the other hand, inhaled NO alone is unlikely to cause sustained increments in oxygenation in neonatal hypoxaemic respiratory failure associated with severe parenchymal lung disease without extrapulmonary shunting.

In patients with ARDS, inhaled nitric oxide (2 ppm) reverses the increased pulmonary resistance induced by permissive hypercapnia, and significantly improves the oxygenation.[136] According to this study, nitric oxide could be an effective combination with hypoventilation during mechanical ventilation in severe ARDS cases. Nitric oxide was also successfully employed to reverse pulmonary hypertension after surgical correction of congenital diaphragmatic hernia[137] and promoted a sustained pulmonary vasodilatation in a child with idiopathic pulmonary hypertension.[138]

Although NO is not yet widely available for routine clinical use, these studies suggest that it will be a desirable supplementary agent in the pharmacological management of RV dysfunction associated with pulmonary hypertension. In patients with pulmonary hypertension due to acute respiratory failure, inhaling a low dose of NO as a pulmonary vasodilator has been shown to induce selective vasodilatation in ventilated lung areas.[136] It achieves this without the inconvenient effects attributed to systemically infused vasodilators, such as systemic vasodilatation and an increase in pulmonary right-to-left shunt with a consecutive decrease in oxygenation.

In conclusion, the use of inhaled NO in animal studies of experimental pulmonary hypertension, as well as in the clinical experience so far reported in newborns, children, and adults indicates that NO could be a promising agent in the treatment of pulmonary hypertension. However, it must be borne in mind that nitric oxide requires special equipment for administration, has a short biological half-life, and may potentially be toxic at certain levels. Considering these points, controlled clinical trials and further studies on potential toxicity are needed before this new therapy can be definitively accepted for routine clinical use.[139]

1 Peacock A. Vasodilators in pulmonary hypertension. *Thorax* 1993;**48**:1196–9.
2 Nunn JF. The pulmonary circulation. In: Nunn JF, ed. *Applied respiratory physiology*, 4th edn. London: Butterworth, 1993:135–55.
3 Marshall BE, Marshall C, Frasch F, Hanson CW. Role of hypoxic pulmonary vasoconstriction in pulmonary gas exchange and blood flow distribution. *Intens Care Med* 1994;**20**:291–7.
4 Timms RM, Khaja FV, Williams GW. Hemodynamic response to oxygen therapy in chronic obstructive pulmonary disease. *Ann Intern Med* 1985;**102**:29–36.
5 Macnee W. Pathophysiology of cor pulmonale in chronic-obstructive pulmonary disease. *Am J Respir Crit Care Med* 1994;**150**:833–52.
6 Leeman M, Neite R, Lejeune P, Melot C. Influence of cyclooxygenase inhibition and leukotriene receptor blockade on pulmonary vascular pressure: cardiac index relationships in hyperoxic and in hypoxic dogs. *Clin Sci* 1987;**72**:717–24.
7 Morganroth MI, Reeves JT, Murphy RC, Voelkel F. Leukotriene synthesis and receptor blockers block hypoxic pulmonary vasoconstriction. *J Appl Physiol* 1984;**56**:1340–6.
8 Warren BA, Maltby NH, McCormack D, Barnes PJ. Pulmonary endothelium-derived relaxing factor impaired in hypoxia. *Clin Sci* 1989;**77**:671–6.
9 Brenner BM, Troy JL, Ballerman BJ. Endothelium-dependent vascular responses. Mediators and mechanisms. *J Clin Invest* 1989;**84**:1373–8.
10 Burke-Wolin T and Wolin MS. Inhibition of cGMP-associated pulmonary arterial relaxation to H_2O_2 and O_2 by ethanol. *Am J Physiol* 1990;**258**:H1267–H1273.
11 Murray TR, Marshall BE and Macarack EJ. Contraction of vascular smooth muscle in cell culture. *J Cell Physiol* 1990;**143**:26–38.
12 Rossaint R, Pison U, Gerlach H, Falke KJ. Inhaled nitric oxide: its effects on pulmonary circulation and airway smooth muscle cells. *Eur Heart J* 1993;1:133–40.
13 Durand J, Leroy-Ladurie M, Ransom-Bitker B. Effects of hypoxia and hypercapnia on the repartition of pulmonary blood flow in supine subjects. *Progr Resp Res* 1970;5:156–65.
14 Epstein FH. Mechanisms of disease. *N Engl J Med* 1990;**323**:27–36.
15 Furchgott RF, Zawadki JV. The obligatory role of endothelial cell in the relaxation of arterial smooth muscle by acetylcholine. *Nature (Lond)* 1980;**288**:373–6.
16 Fishman AP. Pulmonary circulation. In: *Handbook of physiology: the respiratory system. Circulation and non-respiratory function*, vol 1. Bethesda: American Physiological Society, 1985;93–166.
17 Reeves JT, Voelkel NF. Mechanisms of chronic pulmonary hypertension: basic considerations. In: Wagenvoort A, Denolin H, eds. *Pulmonary circulation, advances and controversies*. Amsterdam: Elsevier, 1989:27–39.
18 Moncada S, Palmer RMJ, Higgs EA. Biosynthesis of nitric oxide from L-arginine. A pathway for the regulation of cell function of cell function and communication. *Biochem Pharmacol* 1989;**38**:1709–15.
19 Palmer RMJ, Ferrige AG, Moncada S. Nitric oxide release accounts for the biological activity of endothelium-derived relaxing factor. *Nature (Lond)* 1987;**327**:524–6.
20 Peach MJ, Singer HA, Izzo NJ , Loeb AL. Role of calcium in endothelium-dependent relaxation of arterial smooth muscle. *Am J Cardiol* 1987;**59**:35–43.
21 Weinheimer G, Oswald H. Inhibition of endothelium-dependent smooth muscle relaxation by calmodulin antagonists. *Arch Pharmacol* 1986;**332**:391–7.

22 Bredt DS, Hwang PM, Snyder SH. Localization of nitric oxide synthetase indicating a neural role for nitric oxide. *Nature (Lond)* 1990;**437**:768–70.

23 Rees DD, Palmer RMJ, Hodson HF, Moncada S. A specific inhibitor of nitric oxide formation from L-arginine attenuates endothelium-dependent relaxation. *Br J Pharmacol* 1989;**96**:418–24.

24 Borland CDR, Higenbottam TW. A simultaneous single breath measurement of pulmonary diffusing capacity with nitric oxide and carbon monoxide. *Eur Respir J* 1989;**2**:56–63

25 Centers for Disease Control. Recommendations for occupational safety and health standard. *MMWR* 1988;**37**(Suppl):21.

26 Rodman DM. Chronic hypoxia selectively augments rate pulmonary artery Ca++ and K++ channel mediated relaxation. *Am J Physiol* 1992;**263**:88–94.

27 Doyle MP, Hoekstra JW. Oxidation of nitrogen oxides by bound dioxygen in haemoproteins. *J Inorg Biochem* 1981;**14**:351–8.

28 Rubanyi GM, Vanhoute MP. Hypoxia releases a vasoconstrictor substance from the canine vascular endothelium. *J Physiol (Lond)* 1985;**364**:45–56.

29 Vender RL. The role of endothelial cells in the proliferative response of cultured pulmonary vascular smooth cells to reduced oxygen tension. *In Vitro Cell Dev Biol* 1992;**28**:403–9.

30 Menard O. Facteur atrial natriurétique et poumon. *Rev Mal Respir* 1991;**8**:153–67.

31 Griffith TM, Henderson AH, Edwards OH, Lewis MJ. Isolated perfused rabbit coronary artery and strip preparations: the role of endothelium-derived relaxant factor. *J Physiol* 1984;**351**;13–24.

32 Holtz J, Forstermann U, Pohl U, Giesler M, Bassenge E. Flow-dependent endothelium-mediated dilatation of epicardial coronary arteries in conscious dogs: effects of cyclooxygenase inhibitor. *J Cardiovasc Pharmacol* 1984;**6**:1161–9.

33 Komori K, Suzuki H. Electrical responses of smooth muscle cells during cholinergic vasodilatation in the rabbit saphenous artery. *Circ Res* 1987;**61**:586–93.

34 Rubanyi GM, Romero JC, Vanhoutte PM. Flow-induced release of endothelium-derived relaxing factor. *Am J Physiol* 1986;**250**:1145–9.

35 Rabinovitch M, Gamble W, Nadas AS, Miettinen OS, Reid L. Rat pulmonary circulation after chronic hypoxia: hemodynamic and structural features. *Am J Physiol* 1979;**236**:818–27.

36 Reid L. The pulmonary circulation: remodeling in growth and disease. *Am Rev Respir Dis* 1979;**119**:531–46.

37 Adnot S, Raffestin B, Eddahibi S, Braquet P, Chabrier PE. Loss of endothelium-dependent relaxant activity in the pulmonary circulation of rats exposed to chronic hypoxia. *J Clin Invest* 1991;**87**:155–62.

38 Johns RA, Linden JM, Peach MJ. Endothelium-dependent relaxation and cyclic GMP accumulation in rabbit pulmonary artery are selectively impaired by moderate hypoxia. *Circ Res* 1989;**65**:1508–15.

39 McQuillan LP, Leung GK, Marsden PA, Kostyk SK, Kourembanas S. Hypoxia inhibits expression of endothelial constitutive NOS via transcriptional and post-transcriptional mechanisms. *Am J Physiol* 1994;**36**(5):H1921–H1927.

40 Luscher TF. Endothelin: systemic arterial and pulmonary effects of a new peptide with potent biologic properties. *Am Rev Respir Dis* 1992;**146**:2.

41 Rubin LJ. Pathology and pathophysiology of primary pulmonary hypertension. *Am J Cardiol* 1995;**75**:51A–54A.

42 Willens HJ, Kessler KM. Severe pulmonary hypertension associated with diastolic left ventricular dysfunction. *Chest* 1993;**103**:1877–83.

43 Grossman W, Braunwald E. Pulmonary hypertension. In: Braunwald E, ed. *Heart disease: a textbook of cardiovascular medicine*, 3rd edn. Philadelphia: WB Saunders, 1988:798–9.

44 Leeman M. The pulmonary circulation in acute lung injury: a review of some recent advances. *Intens Care Med* 1991;**17**:254–60.

45 Weber K, Janicki J, Shroff S *et al*. The right ventricle: physiologic and pathophysiologic considerations. *Crit Care Med* 1983;**11**:323–8.

46 Abel FC, Waldhausen JA. Effects of alterations in pulmonary vascular resistance in right ventricular function. *J Thorac Cardiovasc Surg* 1967;**54**:886–94.

47 Morrison D, Sorensen S, Caldwell J, Wright L, Ritchie J, Kennedy W *et al*. The normal right ventricular response to supine exercise. *Chest* 1982;**82**:686–90.

48 Visner MS, Arentzen CE, O'Connor MJ, Virgil Larson E, Anderson RW. Alterations in left ventricular three-dimensional dynamic geometry and systolic function during acute right ventricular hypertension in the conscious dog. *Circulation* 1983;**67**:353–70.

49 Brent BN, Berger HJ, Matthay RA, Mahler D, Pytlik L, Zaret BL. Contrasting acute effects of vasodilators (nitroglycerin, nitroprusside, and hydralazine) on right ventricular performance in patients with chronic obstructive pulmonary disease and pulmonary hypertension: a combined radionuclide-hemodynamic study. *Am J Cardiol* 1983;**51**:1682–9.

50 Brown G. Pharmacologic treatment of primary and secondary pulmonary hypertension. *Pharmacotherapy* 1991;**11**:137–56.

51 Kourembanas S, Bernfield. Hypoxia and endothelial-smooth muscle cell interctions in the lung. *Am J Respir Cell Mol Biol* 1994;**11**:373–4.

52 Rosenberg AA, Kennaugh J, Koppenhafer SL, Loomis M, Chatfield BA, Abman SH. Elevated immunoreactive endothelin-1 levels in newborn infants with persistent pulmonary hypertension. *J Pediatr* 1993;**123**:109–14.

53 Giaid A, Yanagisawa M, Langleben D *et al*. Expression of endothelin-1 in the lungs of patients with pulmonary hypertension, *N Engl J Med* 1993;**328**:1732–9.

54 Von Euler US, Liljestrand G. Observation on the pulmonary arterial blood pressure in the cat. *Acta Physiol Scand* 1946;**12**:301–20.

55 Kourembanas S, Bernfield M. Hypoxia and endothelial-smooth muscle cell interactions in the lung. *Am J Respir* 1994;**11**:373–4.

56 Adnot S, Raffestin B, Eddahibi S, Braquet P, Chabrier PE. Loss of endothelin-dependent relaxant activity in the pulmonary circulation of rats exposed to chronic hypoxia. *J Clin Invest* 1991;**87**:155–62.

57 Frostell C, Fratacci MD, Wain JC, Jones R, Zapol WM. Inhaled nitric oxide, a selective pulmonary vasodilator reversing hypoxic pulmonary vasoconstriction. *Circulation* 1991;**83**:2038–47.

58 Robertson BE, Warrn JB, Nye PC. Inhibition of nitric oxide synthesis potentiates hypoxic vasoconstriction in isolated rat lungs. *Exp Physiol* 1990;**75**:255–7.

59 Voelkel NF. Mechanisms of hypoxic pulmonary vasoconstriction. *Am Rev Respir Dis* 1986;**133**:1186–95.

60 Cutaia M, Rounds S. Hypoxic pulmonary vasoconstriction. *Chest* 1990;**93**:707–18.

61 Marshall C, Marshall BE. Site and sensitivity for stimulation of hypoxic pulmonary vasoconstriction. *J Appl Physiol* 1983;**55**:711–16.

62 Bergofsky EH, Haas F, Porcelli R. Determination of the sensitive vascular sites from which hypoxia and hypercapnia elicit rises in pulmonary arterial pressure. *Fed Proc* 1968;**27**:1420–5.

63 Madden JA, Vadula MS, Kurup VP. Effects of hypoxia and other vasoactive agents on pulmonary and cerebral artery smooth muscle cells. *Am J Physiol* 1992;**263**:384–93.

64 Murray TR, Chen L, Marshall BE, Macarek EJ. Hypoxic contraction of cultured pulmonary vascular smooth muscle cells. *Am J Respir Cell Mol Biol* 1990;**3**:357–465.

65 Heistad DD, Armstrong ML, Amundson S. Blood flow through vasa vasorum in arteries and veins: effects of luminal pressures. *Am J Physiol* 1986;**250**:H434–H442.

66 Marshall BE, Marshall C, Magno M, Lilagan P, Pietra GG. Influence of bronchial arterial PO$_2$ on pulmonary vascular resistance. *J Appl Physiol* 1991;**70**:405–15.

67 Levitsky MG, Newell JC, Dutton RE. Effect on chemoreceptor denervation with pulmonary vascular responses to atelectasis. *Respir Physiol* 1978;**35**:43–51.

68 Weitzenblum E, Kessler R, Oswald M, Fraisse Ph. Medical treatment of pulmonary hypertension in chronic lung disease. *Eur Respir J* 1994;**7**:148–52.

69 Weitzenblum E, Sautegeau A, Ehhart M, Mammosser M, Pelletier A. Long-term oxygen therapy can reverse the progression of pulmonary hypertension in patients with chronic obstructive pulmonary diseases. *Am Rev Respir Dis* 1985;**131**:493–8.

70 Lock JE, Einjig S, Bass JL, Moller JH. Pulmonary vascular response to oxygen and its influence on operative results in children with ventricular septal defects. *Pediatr Cardiol* 1982;**3**:41–6.

71 Custer JR, Hales CA. Influence of alveolar oxygen on pulmonary vasoconstriction in

newborn lambs vs sheep. *Am Rev Respir Dis* 1985;**132**:326–31.

72 Zapol WM, Snider MT. Pulmonary hypertension in severe acute respiratory failure. *N Engl J Med* 1977;**296**:476–80.

73 Jones R, Reid L. Pulmonary vascular changes in adult respiratory distress syndrome. In: Artigas A, (eds). *Adult respiratory distress syndrome*. New York: Churchill Livingstone, 1992:45–9.

74 Leeman M, Zegers de Beyl V, Naeije R. Effects of endogenous nitric oxide on pulmonary vascular tone in intact dogs. *Am J Physiol* 1994;**266**:2343–7.

75 Xue C, Rengasami A, Le Cras TD, Koberna PA, Dailey GC, Johns RA. Distribution of NOS in normoxic vs. hypoxic rat lungs: upregulation of NOS by chronic hypoxia. *Am J Physiol* **267**:667–78.

76 Archer SL, Tolins JP, Raiji L, Weir EK. Hypoxic pulmonary vasoconstriction is enhanced by inhibition of the synthesis of an endothelium-derived relaxing factor. *Biochem Biophys Res Commun* 1989;**164**:1198–205.

77 Wiklund NP, Persson MG, Gustafsson LE, Moncada S, Hedqvist P. Modulatory role of endogenous nitric oxide in pulmonary circulation *in vivo*. *Eur J Phamacol* 1990;**185**:123–4.

78 Liu S, Crawley DE, Barnes PJ, Evans TW. Endothelium-derived relaxing factor inhibits hypoxic pulmonary vasoconstriction in rats. *Am Rev Respir Dis* 1991;**143**:32–7.

79 Eddahibi S, Adnot S, Carville C, Blouquit Y, Raffestin B. L-arginine restores endothelium-dependent relaxation in pulmonary circulation of chronically hypoxic rats. *Am J Physiol* 1992;**72**:194–200.

80 Dinh-Xuan AT, Higgenbottam TW, Clelland CA *et al*. Impairment of endothelium-dependent pulmonary artery relaxation in chronic obstructive lung disease. *N Engl J Med* 1991;**324**:1539–47.

81 Isaacson TC, Hampl V, Weir EK, Nelson DP, Archer SL. Increased endothelium-derived NO in hypertensive pulmonary circulation of chronically hypoxic rats. *J Appl Physiol* 1994;**76**:933–40.

82 Hampl V, Archer SL, Nelson DP, Weir EK. Chronic EDRF inhibition and hypoxia. Effects on pulmonary circulation and systemic blood pressure. *J Appl Physiol* 1993;**75**:1748–57.

83 Orton EC, Reeves JT, Stenmark KR. Pulmonary vasodilation with structurally altered pulmonary vessels and pulmonary hypertension. *J Appl Physiol* 1988;**65**:2459–67.

84 Higenbottam T, Cremona G. Acute and chronic hypoxic pulmonary hypertension. *Eur Respir J* 1993;**8**:1207–12.

85 Hickey P, Hansen D, Wessel D, Lang P, Jonas R, Elixson E. Blunting of stress responses in the pulmonary circulation in infants by fentanyl. *Anesth Analg* 1985;**64**:1137–42.

86 Goetzman B, Sunshine P, Johnson J *et al*. Neonatal hypoxia and the pulmonary vasospasm response to tolazoline. *J Pediatr* 1976;**89**:617–21.

87 Klaus D. The role of calcium antagonists in the treatment of hypertension. *J Cardiovasc Pharmacol* 1992;**20**(Suppl 6):S5–14.

88 Palevsky HI, Fishman AP. The management of primary pulmonary hypertension. *JAMA* 1991;**265**:1014–20.

89 Alpert MA, Concannon MD, Mukerji B, Mukerji V. Pharmacotherapy of chronic pulmonary arterial hypertension: value and limitations. *Angiology* 1994;**45**:667–76.

90 Dell'Italia L, Starling M, Blomhardt R, Lasher JC, O'Rourke R. Comparative effects of volume loading, dobutamine and nitroprusside in patients with predominant RV infarction. *Circulation* 1985;**72**:1327–35.

91 Coma-Canella I, Lopez-Sendon J. Ventricular compliance in ischemic right ventricular dysfunction. *Am J Cardiol* 1980;**45**:555–61.

92 Sharkey SW, Shelley W, Carlyle PF, Rysauy J, Cohn JN. M-mode and two-dimensional echocardiographic analysis of the septum in experimental right ventricular infarction: correlation with hemodynamic alterations. *Am Heart J* 1985;**110**:1210–18.

93 Ghignone M, Girling L, Prewit R. Volume expansion versus norepinephrine in treatment of a low cardiac output complicating an acute increase in right ventricular afterload in dogs. *Anesthesiology* 1984;**60**:132–5.

94 Leir CV, Huss P, Margorien RD, Unverferth SV. Improved exercise capacity and differing arterial and venous tolerance during chronic isosorbide dinitrate therapy for congestive

heart failure. *Circulation* 1983;**67**:817–22.

95 Lejeune P, Naeije R, Leeman M, Mélot C, DellofT, Delcroix M. Effects of dopamine and dobutamine on hyperoxic and hypoxic pulmonary vascular tone in dogs. *Am Rev Respir Dis* 1987;**136**:29–37.

96 Molloy DW. Effects of noradrenaline and isoproterenol on cardiopulmonary function in a canine model of acute pulmonary hypertension. *Chest* 1985;**88**:432–5.

97 Ducas J, Duval D, Dasilva H, Boiteau P, Prewitt RM. Treatment of canine pulmonary hypertension: effects of norepinephrine and isoproterenol on pulmonary vascular pressure-flow characteristics. *Circulation* 1987;**75**:235–41.

98 Mentzer RM, Alegre C, Nolan SP. The effects of dopamine and isoproterenol on the pulmonary circulation. *J Thorac Cardiovasc Surg* 1976;**71**:807–14.

99 Harris P, Heath D. Pulmonary haemodynamics of disease of the mitral valve. In: Harris P, Heath D, eds. *The human pulmonary circulation*, 3rd edn. Edinburgh: Churchill Livingstone, 1986:345–58.

100 Priebe HJ. Efficacy of vasodilator therapy in canine model of acute pulmonary hypertension. *Am J Physiol* 1988;**255**:H1232–H1238.

101 Hickey PR, Hansen DD, Strafford M, Thompson JE, Jonas RE, Mager JE. Pulmonary and systemic hemodynamic effects of nitrous oxide in infants with normal and elevated PVR. *Anesthesiology* 1986;**65**:374–8.

102 Hess W, Arnold B, Veit S. The hemodynamic effect of amirinone in patient with mitral stenosis and pulmonary hypertension. *Eur Heart J* 1986;**7**:800–7.

103 Konstam MA, Salem DN, Isner JM, Zile RM, Kahn CP, Bonin DJ *et al.* Vasodilator effect on right ventricular function in congestive heart failure and pulmonary hypertension: end-systolic pressure-volume relation. *Am J Cardiol* 1984;**54**:132–6.

104 Ziskand Z, Pohoryles L, Mohr R, Smolinsky A, Quang HT, Ruvolo G *et al.* The effect of low-dose intravenous nitroglycerin on pulmonary hypertension immediately after replacement of a stenotic mitral valve. *Circulation* 1985;**72**:II 164–9.

105 Brent BN, Berger HJ, Mathay RA, Mahler D, Pytlik L, Zaret BL. Contrasting acute effects of vasodilators (nitroglycerin, nitroprusside, and hydralazine) on right ventricular performance in patients with chronic obstructive pulmonary disease and pulmonary hypertension: a combined radionuclide-hemodynamic study. *Am J Cardiol* 1983;**51**:1682–9.

106 Prielipp RC, Rosenthal MH, Pearl RG. Vasodilator therapy in vasoconstrictor-induced pulmonary hypertension in sheep. *Anesthesiology* 1988;**68**:552–8.

107 Prielipp RC, Rosenthal MH, Pearl RG. Hemodynamic profiles of prostaglandin E, isoproterenol, prostacyclin and nifedipine in vasoconstrictor-induced pulmonary hypertension in sheep. *Anesth Analg* 1988;**67**:722–9.

108 Lee KY. Effects of hydralazine and nitroprusside on cardiopulmonary function when cardiac output is acutely reduced by increased pulmonary vascular resistance. *Circulation* 1983;**68**:1299–303.

109 D'Ambra M, La Raia P, Philbin DM, Watkins WB, Hilgenberg AS, Buckberg MJ *et al.* Prostaglandin E1 – a new therapy for refractory right heart failure and pulmonary hypertension after mitral valve replacement. *J Thorac Cardiovasc Surg* 1985;**89**:567–72.

110 Okada M, Yamashita C, Okada M, Okada K. Endothelium receptor antagonists in beagle model of pulmonary hypertension: contribution to a possible potential therapy. *J Am Coll Cardiol* 1995;**25**:1213–17.

111 Bunting S, Gryglewski R, Moncada S, Vane JR. Arterial generate from prostaglandin endoperoxides a substance (prostaglandin X) which relaxes strips of mesenteric and coeliac arteries and inhibits platelet aggregation. *Prostaglandins* 1976;**12**:897–913.

112 Bihari DJ, Tinker J. The therapeutic value of vasodilator prostaglandins in multiple organ failure associated with sepsis. *Intens Care Med* 1988;**15**:2–7.

113 Radermacher P, Santak B, Wust HJ, Tarnow J, Falke KJ. Prostacyclin and right ventricular function in patients with pulmonary hypertension associated with ARDS. *Intens Care Med* 1990;**16**:227–32.

114 Rossaint R, Falke KJ, Lopez F, Slama K, Pison U, Zapol WM. Inhaled nitric oxide in adult respiratory distress syndrome. *N Engl J Med* 1993;**328**:399–405.

115 Nootens M, Schrader B, Kaufmann E, Vestal R, Long W, Rich S. Comparative acute effects of adenosine and prostacyclin in primary pulmonary hypertension. *Chest*

1995;**107**:54-7.
116 Hess WJ. Effects of amirone on the right side of the heart. *J Cardiothorac Anesth* 1989;**6**(Suppl):38-44.
117 Cremona G, Dinh Xuan AT, Higenbottam TW. Endothelium derived relaxing factor and pulmonary circulation. *Lung* 1991;**169**:185-202.
118 Frostell C, Blomquist H, Lundberg J, Hendenstierna G, Zapol W. Inhaled nitric oxide dilates human hypoxic pulmonary vasoconstriction without causing systemic vasodilatation. *Anesthesiology* 1991;**75**:A989.
119 Girard C, Lehot J, Clerc J, French P, Estanove S. Inhaled nitric oxide in pulmonary hypertension following mitral valve replacement. *Anesthesiology* 1991;**75**:A984.
120 Tonz M, von Segesser LK, Schilling J, Luscher TF, Noll G, Leskosek B, Turina MI. Treatment of acute pulmonary hypertension with inhaled nitric oxide. *Ann Thorac Surg* 1994;**58**:1031-5.
121 Frostell CG, Fratacci MD, Wain JC, Jones R, Zapol WM. Inhaled nitric oxide: a selective pulmonary vasodilator reversing hypoxic pulmonary vasoconstriction. *Circulation* 1991;**83**:2038-47.
122 Gerlach H, Pappert D, Lewandowski K, Rossaint R, Falke KJ. Long-term inhalation with evaluated low doses of nitric oxide for selective improvement of oxygenation in patients with adult respiratory distress syndrome. *Intens Care Med* 1993;**19**:443-9.
123 Roberts JD, Polaner DM, Lang P, Zapol WM. Inhaled nitric oxide in persistent pulmonary hypertension of the newborn. *Lancet* 1992;**340**:818-19.
124 Pepke-Zaba J, Hogenbottam TW, Dihn-Xuan AT, Stone D, Wallwork J. Inhaled nitric oxide as a cause of selective pulmonary vasodilation in pulmonary hypertension. *Lancet* 1991;**338**:1173-4.
125 Journouis D, Pouard P, Mauriat P, Malhere T, Vouhe P, Safran D. Inhaled nitric oxide as a therapy for pulmonary hypertension after operations for congenital heart defects. *J Thorac Cardiovasc Surg* 1994;**107**:1129-35.
126 Roberts JD, Lang P, Bigatello LM, Vlahakas GJ, Zapol WM. Inhaled nitric oxide in congenital heart disease. *Circulation* 1993;**87**:447-53.
127 Snow DJ, Gray SJ, Ghosh S, Foubert L, Oduro A, Higenboltan TW *et al*. Inhaled nitric oxide in patients with normal and increased pulmonary vascular resistance after cardiac surgery. *Br J Anaesth* 1994;**72**:185-9.
128 Rich GF, Murphy GD Jr, Ross CM, Johns RA. Inhaled nitric oxide: selective pulmonary vasodilatation in cardiac surgical patients. *Anesthesiology* 1993;**78**:1028-35.
129 Girard C, Lehot JJ, Pannetier JC, Filley S, French P, Estanove S. Inhaled nitric oxide after mitral valve replacement in patients with chronic pulmonary artery hypertension. *Anesthesiology* 1992;**77**:880-3.
130 Girard C, Durand PG, Vedrinne C, Panntenier JC, Estanove S, Kalke K. Inhaled nitric oxide for right ventricular failure after heart transplantation. *J Cardiothorac Vasc Anesth* 1993;**7**:481-5.
131 Adatia I, Lillehei C, Arnold JH *et al*. Inhaled nitric oxide in the treatment of postoperative graft dysfunction after lung transplantation. *Ann Thorac Surg* 1994;**57**:1311-18.
132 Auler Jr JOC, Carmona CMJ, Bocchi E, Bacal F, Fiorelli I, Stolf G *et al*. Low doses of inhaled nitric oxide in patients submitted to heart transplantation. *J Heart Lung Transplant* 1996;**5**:443-50.
133 Miller OI, Celermajer DS, Deanfield JE, Macrae DJ. Very low dose inhaled nitric oxide: a selective pulmonary vasodilator after operations for congenital heart disease. *J Thorac Cardiovasc Surg* 1994;**108**:487-94.
134 Day RW, Lynch M, Shaddy RE, Orsmond GS. Pulmonary vasodilatory effects of 12 and 60 parts per million inhaled nitric oxide in children with ventricular septal defect. *Am J Cardiol* 1995;**75**:196-8.
135 Kinsella JP, Abman SHJ. Inhaled nitric oxide in treatment for stabilization and emergency medical transport of critically ill newborns and infants. *Pediatr* 1995;**126**:853-64.
136 Puybasset L, Stewart T, Rouby JJ, Cluzei P, Mourgeon E, Belin MF *et al*. Inhaled nitric oxide reverses the increase in pulmonary vascular resistance induced by permissive hypercapnia in paients with acute respiratory distress syndrome. *Anesthesiology* 1994;**80**:1254-67.

239

137 Frostell CG, Lonnqvist PA, Sonesson SE, Gustafsson LE, Lohr G, Noack G. Near fatal pulmonary hypertension after surgical repair of congenital diaphragmatic hernia. *Anaesthesia* **48**:679–83.

138 Kinsella JP, Toews HW, Henry D, Abman SH. Selective and sustained pulmonary vasodilation with inhalation nitric oxide therapy in a child with idiopathic pulmonary hypertension. *J Pediatr* 1993;**122**:803–6.

139 Giacoia GP. Nitric oxide: an environmental pollutant as a therapeutic agent. *Okla State Med Assoc* 1995;**88**:17–23.

12: Pharmacological treatment of hypoxaemia in patients with acute respiratory distress syndrome

LOUIS PUYBASSET, JEAN-JACQUES ROUBY

Life-threatening hypoxia often complicates the clinical course of patients with ARDS.* Until recently the only therapeutic means of re-establishing a safe level of oxygenation in these patients was mechanical ventilation with a high inspired oxygen concentration and positive end-expiratory pressure. Such an approach could be counterproductive in some patients as high oxygen concentrations and high airway pressures could entail further lung damage due to oxygen toxicity and pulmonary barotrauma. The pharmacological approach which is emerging as an adjunct to the conventional management aims to decrease the need for high oxygen concentrations and high airway pressures, thereby decreasing ventilator-induced lung injury. The objective of most of these newer modalities of therapy is to redistribute the pulmonary blood flow preferentially towards well-ventilated alveoli.

Pathophysiological basis

Ventilation–perfusion mismatch is one of the important hallmarks of ARDS. In the lung, regions with normal ventilation/perfusion (V/Q) ratios coexist along with regions having high or low V/Q ratios. A large proportion of the lung regions which appear to be ventilated on a chest radiograph and computerised thoracic scan is not perfused at all, or is poorly perfused, constituting the alveolar dead space. At the same time, a substantial

---

* The abbreviation ARDS is now taken to mean 'acute' rather than the former term 'adult' respiratory distress syndrome.

proportion of the unventilated zones continues to be perfused due to the failure of hypoxic pulmonary vasoconstriction (HPV), a reflex which tends to limit the pulmonary blood flow perfusing poorly oxygenated alveolar spaces. High tidal volumes and consequently high airway pressures are needed to maintain normal $Paco_2$ in the face of increased alveolar dead space.

Acute pulmonary hypertension is frequently observed in patients with ARDS. It is a result of pulmonary vasoconstriction characterising the early stages of ARDS and anatomical remodelling of the pulmonary vasculature observed in the late stages of the disease. In turn, pulmonary vasoconstriction could be due to the hypoxic pulmonary vasoconstrictor reflex or chemical mediators such as thromboxane-A_2 and platelet activating factor. Anatomical remodelling comprises muscular hypertrophy, microthrombosis, fibrosis, and destruction of pulmonary vessels.

Theoretically, selective constriction of the pulmonary vessels in the unventilated zones or selective dilatation of the vessels in the ventilated zones should decrease the V/Q mismatch. Administration of selective pulmonary vasoconstrictors and vasodilators to achieve the above objective forms the basis of the pharmacological approach to hypoxaemia. These vasoactive drugs should have a predominant effect on the pulmonary circulation and minimal or no effects on systemic circulation. Nitric oxide and prostacyclin in low doses administered by inhalation produce pulmonary vasodilatation in the ventilated lung regions. Almitrine and diclofenac (cyclo-oxygenase inhibitor) act by reinforcing the hypoxic pulmonary vasoconstrictor reflex in the unventilated regions.

Inhaled nitric oxide

In 1987, nitric oxide (NO) was identified to be one of the endothelium-derived relaxing factors.[1,2] It was demonstrated to be released continuously by endothelial cells after activation of the constitutive NO synthase in response to shear stress. Later studies revealed its involvement in a large number of physiological systems such as coagulation, neuronal transmission, and inflammation.

The first description of inhaled NO as a therapeutic agent in humans was published in 1988 as an abstract by Higenbottam's group.[3] Inhaled NO was shown to reduce pulmonary artery presure in seven patients with severe primary pulmonary hypertension, without inducing any systemic effect. This work was published as a full paper in 1991.[4] Inhaled NO-induced selective pulmonary vasodilatation was later confirmed in different experimental models of pulmonary hypertension: injection of an analogue of thromboxane-A_2 or injection of heparin-protamine,[5] hypoxic pulmonary vasoconstriction,[6-9] lipopolysaccharide or streptococcal intravenous infusion[10-13] and oxidant-induced acute lung injury.[14] A sustained improvement in arterial oxygenation along with a reduction in pulmonary arterial pressure in response to NO in patients with adult respiratory distress syndrome was described by Falke's group in 1993,[15] and then confirmed by other studies.[16-19] In addition, pulmonary hypertension secondary to cardiac surgery[20, 21] or chronic obstructive pulmonary disease[22, 23] was shown to be responsive to inhaled NO. Although the beneficial effects of NO on arterial oxygenation and pulmonary pressure have been well demonstrated, the potential pro- or anti-oxidant effects of NO are still a subject of controversy. It is also not clear whether the potent antithrombic effect of inhaled NO is beneficial or detrimental in critically ill patients. The potential benefits on mortality of the long-term administration of NO during acute respiratory failure are presently under investigation in controlled, multicentre human studies.

Administration and monitoring

NO tanks used in the ICU are highly concentrated (200–1000 ppm) in order to limit the reduction in Fio_2 resulting from the administration of NO which is diluted in pure nitrogen. *In concentrations above 200 ppm, NO is cytotoxic. Therefore, it should not be administered directly through an intra-tracheal catheter in contact with the tracheal mucosa.* NO should be diluted in the respiratory circuits before reaching the tracheobronchial tree, in order to obtain the desired concentration in the patient's airways.

NO can be delivered into the respiratory circuit either before or after the ventilator. In the former type of administration, mass flow regulators are necessary to mix precisely NO, air, and oxygen. The main benefit of this technique, initially developed in Northern Europe,[24] is the precision and the stability of the inspiratory NO concentration delivered to the patient.[25] However, it has some drawbacks namely high cost of mass flow regulators, long contact time between NO and oxygen resulting in the generation of NO_2 and requiring the mandatory use of a soda lime absorber on the inspiratory limb, and risk of oxidation of the internal circuits of the ventilator as they are permanently in contact with nitrogen oxides.[26]

NO can also be administered into the inspiratory circuit after the ventilator. In this system, administration of a precise concentration is difficult without monitoring the concentration. At present, there is no equipment capable of delivering exact preset concentrations in the face of changing ventilatory settings. In most centres it is a common practice to administer a continuous flow of NO into the inspiratory limb of the ventilatory circuit (**continuous mode**). A variety of formulae have been used to predict the concentrations received by the patient.[27, 28] They are all based on the assumption that NO delivered continuously into the inspiratory limb is homogeneously mixed with the tidal volume coming from the ventilator and that the NO concentration remains constant during inspiration. One of the commonly used formulae is as follows.

$$NO_{insp} = V_{NO} \times NO_{tank}/MV$$

where NO_{insp} = inspired NO concentration
V_{NO} = flow of NO
NO_{tank} = concentration of NO in the tank
MV = minute volume of the patient

As can be seen from Figure 12.1, however, concentrations predicted by the above formula do not correlate well with the inspiratory concentrations in the trachea measured by chemiluminescence apparatus. In fact, a constant *continuous* flow of NO is administered with a constant *intermittent* flow of gas from the ventilator, and as a result, NO delivered from the cylinder is not uniformly mixed with the tidal volume.[29] NO delivered during the expiratory phase accumulates in the inspiratory limb and is flushed as a bolus into the airways during the subsequent inspiration. Therefore, there is a wide fluctuation of the concentration of NO in the inspiratory limb of the ventilatory circuit during continuous modes of administration (Figure 12.2).

On the contrary, during **sequential mode** administration (a *constant* flow of NO is administered with a *constant* flow coming from the ventilator only during the inspiratory phase), the concentration of NO in the inspiratory limb is fairly stable and the inspired tracheal concentration correlates well with the value predicted by the above formula (Figure 12.1). However, in the trachea, the concentration still exhibits wide fluctuations and the peak intratracheal concentration is always slightly less than that in the inspiratory limb. Both these phenomena probably represent the uptake of NO from the alveoli and the dilution of inspired NO within the anatomical dead space. It is highly likely that, in patients with ARDS, the difference between inspiratory and expiratory tracheal concentrations of NO correlates with the volume of aerated lung tissue available for NO uptake. With a sequential mode of administration, where the NO concentration is constant in the inspiratory limb, inspiratory tracheal concentrations will change if the tidal volume and the inspiratory time settings of the ventilator are modified because the inspiratory flow delivered from the ventilator will change while the inspiratory flow of NO remains constant. As a consequence, if NO is administered after the ventilator to patients on pressure support ventilation, NO concentrations can vary widely from one respiratory cycle to another.

From the above observations it follows that an ideal system for administration of NO into the downstream of the ventilatory circuit should have the following features.

CONTINUOUS ADMINISTRATION

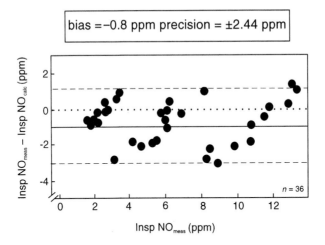

SEQUENTIAL ADMINISTRATION

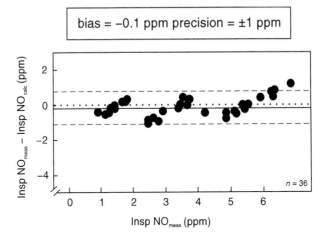

Fig 12.1 Correlation between calculated and monitored inspiratory tracheal NO concentrations. Inspiratory tracheal NO concentrations measured by chemiluminescence apparatus are plotted against the difference between the measured and the calculated inspiratory tracheal NO concentrations (*see text*). The upper panel corresponds to continuous mode of administration and the lower panel, to sequential mode. The dark line in the centre represents the mean difference and the two dotted lines represent mean ± 2 s.d. Only during sequential mode are the calculated values very close to the measured tracheal NO concentrations. (From Mourgeon *et al.*, 1997[29] with permission)

245

1 It should deliver NO only during inspiration.
2 The device should synchronise the flow of NO with the gas flow signal of the ventilator.
3 It should also regulate the flow of NO proportionate to the gas flow delivered by the ventilator, in order to ensure a stable output concentration.

Such a device would ensure a stable and predictable inspired NO concentration in spite of a wide variation of the ventilatory parameters such as minute volume, flow and I:E ratio. At present there is no system that fulfils all of these requirements.

Due to the potential toxicity of NO itself and its oxidative derivative NO_2, it is recommended that NO and NO_2 concentrations are monitored during long-term administration of inhaled NO in patients with acute respiratory failure.[30] Because measurements are performed on gases saturated with water vapour, a humidity absorber must be interposed before the analyser if an infrared technique is used for this purpose.

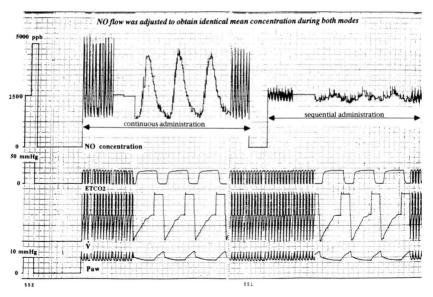

Fig 12.2 Inspired NO concentrations during continuous and sequential modes of administration. NO is administered into the inspiratory limb of the ventilator 120 cm before the Y-piece either in a continuous or sequential mode. NO concentrations are measured by using a fast-response chemiluminescence apparatus (NOX 4000 Sérès, Aix-en-Provence, France). Expired CO_2, respiratory flow, and airway pressure curves are recorded simultaneously. NO concentration fluctuates widely during continuous mode, indicating that NO is not homogeneously mixed with the tidal volume. In contrast, NO concentration in the inspiratory limb is stable during sequential mode, indicating that NO is homogeneously mixed with the tidal volume

Secondly, as NO_2 is absorbed together with water vapour, it cannot be measured by this method. Consequently, only two methods of monitoring appear appropriate: the **chemiluminescence** method and the **electrochemical** method. The electrochemical method is less expensive than chemiluminescence but has some disadvantages: frequent recalibrations are necessary; the electrochemical cells themselves have to be renewed regularly; and the precision of the method is low for NO and NO_2 concentrations below 2 ppm.[31] As far as NO is concerned, an inspiratory concentration of 5 ppm is precisely the optimum concentration to be used in patients,[18, 32] while 2 ppm of NO_2 is far greater than the acceptable threshold in humans. A bronchoconstrictor effect of NO_2 has been described for concentrations of 0·3 ppm[33] and 0·6 ppm[34] and a pro-inflammatory pulmonary effect for a concentration of 2·25 ppm.[35] Thus, the electrochemical method appears to be less appropriate than chemiluminescence for clinical monitoring of NO and NO_2 concentrations during long-term administration of inhaled NO in humans.

The reference method, chemiluminescence, allows measurement of very low NO and NO_2 concentrations with a precision in the range of parts per billion (ppb). Chemiluminescence apparatus designed for measuring atmospheric pollution had a slow response time of around 40 s. The intrinsic response time of chemiluminescence is in the range of a millisecond. The observed response time depends mainly on the sampling flow rate and on the apparatus dead space represented by connecting tubes and internal circuits. Chemiluminescence apparatus designed for medical use should have a fast response time of around 100 ms, allowing accurate measurement of inspired and expired concentrations of NO.[29,32] Such a fast response requires a high sample flow rate of around 1 l/min. As shown in Figure 12.2, inspired and expired NO concentrations can be measured accurately by a fast-response bedside chemiluminescence apparatus. The inspired NO concentration is usually 1·5 times the mean intratracheal NO concentration (Figure 12.3). It is the true concentration reaching the alveoli and should be considered as the effective concentration in terms of therapeutic effects and toxicity.[29,32]

Metabolism and toxicity

Metabolism of inhaled NO in humans

Inhalation of NO at a concentration of 25 ppm in healthy volunteers results in increased methaemoglobin and plasma nitrate concentrations.[36] After traversing the alveolo-capillary barrier, NO can react with oxygen to generate nitrates or can bind to haemoglobin for which it has a very high affinity (1000 times more than CO). If NO binds to oxyhaemoglobin, methaemoglobin is generated together with nitrates; if NO binds to reduced haemoglobin, nitrosylhaemoglobin is generated.[36] Methaemoglobin is detoxified back to haemoglobin by a slow endogenous process and several hours are necessary for it to return to control values after accidental inhalation of high NO concentrations.[37] The concentrations of methaemoglobin increase at inspiratory concentrations above 5 ppm.[32] The upper limit of inspired concentration is 100 ppm of inhaled NO and should not be exceeded in order to maintain methaemoglobin within safe limits. In healthy volunteers, inhalation of 32, 64, 128, and 512 ppm of NO results in methaemoglobin concentrations of 1·04%, 1·75%, 3·75%, and 6·93%.[37] Thus, in normal individuals, inhalation of up to 100 ppm of NO does not result in any significant methaemoglobinemia. Maximum methaemoglobin concentrations are likely to be reached in 3–5 hours after the beginning of inhalation. However, these figures are not applicable to critically ill patients. These patients have higher concentrations of deoxyhaemoglobin, which has a higher tendency to form methaemoglobin. Since foetal haemoglobin is more prone to form methaemoglobin, the above recommendations are also not applicable to neonates. Methaemoglobin is converted to haemoglobin mostly by an NADH-methaemoglobin reductase system (67–95%) and to a small extent by NADPH dehydrogenase, ascorbic acid, and reduced

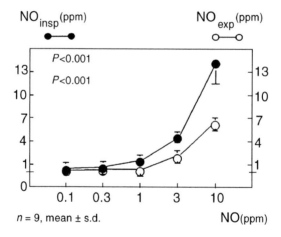

Fig 12.3   Relation between inspiratory (NO_{insp}), expiratory (NO_{exp}) and mean (NO) concentrations of inhaled NO in nine critically ill patients whose lungs were mechanically ventilated. Inhaled NO is administered continuously into the inspiratory limb of the ventilator 120 cm before the Y-piece. Endotracheal gas is aspirated continuously at a flow rate of 1 l/min for chemiluminescence analysis. NO_{insp}, NO_{exp} and NO are measured continuously using a fast-response chemiluminescence apparatus (NOX 4000, Sérès, Aix-en-Provence, France). Inhaled NO is administered at increasing mean concentrations ranging from 0·1 ppm to 10 ppm. NO_{insp} is approximately 1·5 times the FNO. Up to 1 ppm, no detectable nitric oxide is observed during expiration. (From Lu et al., 1995[32] with permission)

glutathione. The time constant for elimination of methaemoglobin is 43–125 minutes in dogs and the figures are probably similar in humans.[37]

Toxicity of inhaled NO

Inhaled NO toxicity can be due to NO itself or to its oxidative derivatives NO_x in addition to the methaemoglobin generated by it. In the presence of high concentrations of oxygen, NO_2 is the principal nitrogen oxide generated. In the presence of water vapour, NO and NO_2 may form nitric acid and nitrous acid, which are known to be toxic.

Toxicity of NO NO released by the macrophages after induction of the inducible NO synthase is a potent cytotoxic agent. NO also has a high mutagenic potential through DNA deamination.[38–41] This property could theoretically increase the incidence of cancer in patients receiving NO for prolonged periods. Therefore, registration of all patients receiving long-term NO inhalation should be implemented. NO toxicity can also be due to peroxynitrite anion synthesised when NO reacts with a superoxide anion:

$$NO + O_2^- \rightarrow ONOO^-$$

This compound is a highly potent oxidant, inducing lipid peroxidation of cell membranes[42] and structural changes of surfactant.[43]

In dogs, NO is lethal at a concentration of 20 000 ppm. Death is caused by high levels of methaemoglobin and non-cardiogenic pulmonary oedema.[44] Inhalation of low concentrations of NO over very long periods has been shown to be apparently free from toxic effects. In mice 10 ppm for 6 months[45] or 2 ppm for 2 years[46] did not induce major pulmonary histological changes. However some recent evidence suggests that even very low concentrations could be toxic. In rats, exposure to NO 0·5 ppm for 9 weeks was associated with focal degeneration of pulmonary interstitial cells, interstitial matrix and connective tissues fibres and formation of fenestrae in the alveolar septa. NO was significantly more potent than NO_2 in the production of these defects, which were similar to those seen in the early stages of emphysema.[47]

In neonates and infants with pulmonary hypertension, inhalation of NO has been reported to reduce the neutrophil respiratory burst (the ability to generate reactive oxygen species), which is essential for neutrophils to kill infective organisms.[48] This effect, which was seen after 24 hours of NO administration, persisted throughout the therapy and lasted up to 4 days after the end of NO inhalation. The clinical importance of this side effect with respect to bacterial infections in patients treated with NO remains to be studied.

Toxicity induced by NO_2 The amount of NO_2 generated by NO in the presence of oxygen depends on the contact time, the $F\text{io}_2$ and the concentration of NO according to the formula:[49]

$$NO_2 = k.t.[Fio_2] \times [NO]^2$$

At an inspiratory NO concentration of 15 ppm and an Fio_2 of 1, the observed NO_2 concentration is above the threshold of 0·3 ppm. In the range of 5–150 ppm, NO_2 increases exponentially with inspiratory NO concentrations. At an inspiratory concentration of 45 ppm, NO_2 concentration reaches 1·7 ppm.[32] Oxidation of NO to NO_2 takes place continuously in the ventilatory breathing system. Administration of NO at the Y-piece of the circuit increases NO levels by 35–60% and NO_2 levels by 110–230% in comparison with administration before the ventilator. Soda lime absorbers remove 60–70% of NO_2 and 7% of NO when they are used in the inspiratory limb of the circuit. Charcoal absorbers reduce NO_2 levels to the same extent as soda lime absorbers, but they reduce NO concentration by 45%.[50]

Inhalation of NO_2 may produce acute lung injury. It can also increase bronchial reactivity and enhance the susceptibility of the lung to viral infections.

(1) Increased alveolo-capillary membrane permeability In dogs, NO_2 inhaled at a concentration of 400 ppm for 1 h induces interstitial and alveolar oedema.[51] Similar results have been described in other species, such as guinea-pigs[52] and rats.[53, 54] In humans, an inflammatory cell response in bronchoalveolar lavage fluid has been observed after inhalation of NO_2 at concentrations as low as 2·25 ppm.[35]

(2) Increased bronchial reactivity NO_2 increases the bronchomotor tone of isolated human bronchi.[55] In asthmatics, inhaled NO_2 at a concentration of 0·3 ppm potentiates exercise-induced bronchospasm.[33] In healthy volunteers, NO_2 can sensitise the airways to air-ozone exposure[34] when inhaled at a concentration of 0·6 ppm and can increase bronchial reactivity when inhaled at a concentration of 1·5 ppm for 3 h.[56]

(3) Increased incidence of lung viral infections Mice inhaling NO_2 have a concentration-dependent increase in the incidence of pneumonia after intratracheal instillation of a normally non-infective viral innoculum. It requires 100 times less virus to induce a pneumonia in mice inhaling 5 ppm of NO_2 than in control animals.[57]

Effects of NO on pulmonary circulation

Mechanisms of inhaled NO-induced pulmonary vasodilatation

NO, either inhaled or produced by the vascular endothelium, relaxes the pulmonary vascular smooth muscle through activation of the soluble guanylate cyclase. In contrast to the other pulmonary vasodilators,[58, 59] inhaled NO has no systemic effect because it is inactivated by fixation to haemoglobin when it reaches the vascular lumen. Because endogenous NO continuously vasorelaxes pulmonary vascular smooth muscle cells,[60] inhaled NO has no effect on the normal, nonconstricted, pulmonary circulation.[61]

In acute lung injury, a large part of the lung parenchyma is no longer accessible to gas. Because NO is administered by inhalation, it can reach only the pulmonary vessels which perfuse the ventilated part of the lung. Therefore, inhaled NO-induced vasodilatation is doubly specific: specific to the pulmonary circulation – inhaled NO has no effect on the systemic circulation – and specific to the pulmonary vessels of the ventilated part of the lung – NO does not reach vessels perfusing the non-ventilated zone. The latter property explains how inhaled NO decreases pulmonary shunt and increases Pao_2 through a redistribution of intrapulmonary blood flow.[15]

During the early phases of ARDS, the main determinant of the decrease in pulmonary vascular resistance index (PVRI) induced by inhaled NO is the basal level of PVRI.[16, 62] *The greater the baseline PVRI, the greater the inhaled NO-induced decrease in PVRI* (Figure 12.4). In the absence of pre-existing constriction of the pulmonary vessels, no decrease in PVRI is observed. The decrease in PVRI induced by NO varies from 0% when PVRI is normal to 50% if PVRI is around 2000 $dyn/s/cm^5/m^2$.

The increased PVRI observed in acute respiratory failure, which in the initial phases, is related mainly to the constrictor effect of circulating inflammatory mediators such as thromboxane-A_2, platelet activating factor or endothelin,[63] becomes partly fixed at a later stage due to irreversible mechanisms such as microthrombosis or increase in vascular thickness

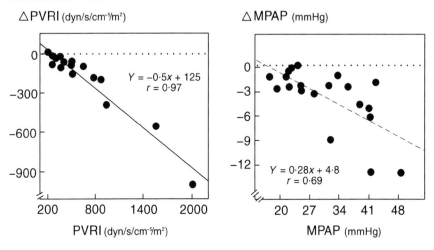

Fig 12.4 Predictive factors of pulmonary vascular effects of inhaled NO. Regression lines between basal pulmonary vascular resistance index (PVRI) and inhaled NO-induced decrease in PVRI (ΔPVRI) and between basal mean pulmonary arterial pressure (MPAP) and inhaled NO-induced decrease in MPAP (ΔMPAP). Each point represents a patient with severe ARDS and inhaled NO was administered to each patient at a mean tracheal concentration of 2 ppm. Both the regressions were significant. (From Puybasset *et al.*, 1995,[62] with permission)

251

secondary to smooth muscle proliferation.[64] The so-called 'NO-responders' are patients with an increase in PVRI related to vasoconstriction (>200 dyn/s/cm^{-5}/m^2). 'NO non-responders' are either patients with normal pulmonary vascular tone or patients with an increase in PVRI related mainly to thrombosis or to anatomical remodelling of the pulmonary vessels. The correlation between the basal level of PVRI and the NO-induced decrease in PVRI observed during the early stages of ARDS[16, 62] has also been documented in pulmonary hypertension complicating cardiac surgery.[20]

The correlation between the decrease in mean pulmonary artery pressure (MPAP) induced by NO and the baseline MPAP, although statistically significant, appears more variable than the correlation between the NO-induced decrease in PVRI and baseline PVRI (Figure 12.4). At least two reasons can be given to explain this. First, pulmonary hypertension can be mainly flow-dependent with a fairly normal PVRI. As a consequence, NO will not reduce MPAP even though the baseline MPAP is elevated. Secondly, the inhalation of NO can increase cardiac output indirectly, for instance, by unloading a failing right ventricle;[17, 65] therefore, despite a decrease in PVRI, MPAP will decrease only slightly or not at all. Such an increase in cardiac output induced by NO is observed in the presence of right heart failure due to acute pulmonary hypertension. Rossaint et al.[66] reported improvement in right ventricular function in ARDS with 18 and 36 ppm of NO. The rise in the right ventricular ejection fraction (RVEF) was similar to that produced by intravenous administration of prostaglandin PGI$_2$. This increase in RVEF was not associated with the increase in cardiac index which was observed with PGI$_2$.

NO can be considered as a pharmacological tool to test the reserve of vasodilatation of the pulmonary circulation in patients with acute respiratory failure or chronic pulmonary hypertension. The correlation shown in Figure 12.4 was obtained in patients during the early phase of ARDS. Most often, patients in whom a decrease in PVRI is observed initially continue to show decreased PVRI after NO inhalation throughout the course of their pulmonary disease. This result supports the hypothesis that a reserve of vasodilatation persists during the course of ARDS although the fixed part of the elevated pulmonary pressure increases with time. In fact, 'NO-responders' become 'NO non-responders' when their basal PVRI returns to normal in the recovery phase of acute lung injury or when pulmonary hypertension becomes 'fixed' due to vascular remodelling.

Tachyphylaxis to inhaled NO is infrequent in patients with ARDS.[16] Experimentally, inhaled NO at a concentration of 100 ppm does not exert a negative feedback inhibition on inducible NO synthase.[67] This result suggests that acute pulmonary hypertension associated with withdrawal of NO in patients chronically inhaling the gas (rebound effect) is not related to a down-regulation of the inducible isoform of NO synthase.

The decrease in PVRI induced by inhaled NO does not seem to be correlated with the initial degree of hypoxaemia and pulmonary shunt.[62] This is due to the fact that, in ARDS, arterial Pao_2 is dependent on many factors other than distribution of PVRI within the lung, e.g. hypoxic pulmonary vasoconstriction in non-ventilated lung areas, extension of the alveolar disease and the haemodynamic and metabolic status. This also applies to static lung compliance, which is a good index of the extension of the alveolar disease[68] and cannot be considered as a predictor of the effect of inhaled NO.[62] Only PVRI, which can be seen as an index of pulmonary vascular disease chracterising acute lung injury, is predictive of a pulmonary vascular effect induced by NO.

In some patients, no decrease, or even a paradoxical increase, in MPAP is observed after inhalation of NO, despite a decrease in PVRI. In severe left ventricular failure associated with pre-capillary pulmonary hypertension, inhaled NO may produce rapid pulmonary vasodilatation with paradoxical increases in MPAP and pulmonary wedge pressure[69] leading to pulmonary oedema.[70] The decrease in right ventricular afterload induced by inhaled NO increases right ventricular output, which in turn increases venous return to the failing left ventricle and produces pulmonary oedema. This feature is not observed with intravenous vasodilators such as sodium nitroprusside which, together with an increase in venous return to the left heart, markedly reduce left ventricular afterload, thus preventing acute increases in left central blood volume and cardiac filling pressure.[71, 72]

Effects on pulmonary arteries and veins

Inhaled NO is potentially both an arterial and a venous vasodilator. Arteries and veins have different pathways inside the secondary pulmonary lobule; arteries follow the bronchovascular axis of the lobule, whereas veins go back to the left atrium with lymphatics within interlobular septa. Since these vessels are surrounded by ventilated alveolar spaces, NO can theoretically reach the vascular structures anywhere along their pathway within pulmonary lobules and interlobular septa. Part of the increase in PVRI during ARDS is due to venous constriction and is reversed after inhalation of NO. Experimental and clinical arguments in favour of venodilatation induced by inhaled NO have been presented recently.[73-75]

Effects on smooth muscle cell proliferation

The diameter of resistive arteries of the human pulmonary circulation varies from 200 to 500 μm. The muscular coat of the arteries is initially circular, and becomes partly muscular before it disappears at the capillary level. 'Intermediate cells' located in partly muscular arteries can change their phenotype during acute lung injury and can be transformed into muscular cells. This mechanism explains in part the observed increase in PVRI during ARDS.[76] Because NO inhibits smooth muscle growth,[77] it can be hypothesised that thickening of pulmonary vascular walls observed in ARDS is related to endothelial dysfunction resulting in insufficient release of endogenous NO. Consequently, inhaled NO could prevent abnormal proliferation of smooth muscle in non-muscular pulmonary vessels during the course of ARDS. Prolonged inhalation of low concentrations of NO reduces vascular smooth muscle proliferation and prevents pulmonary arterial structural changes in newborn rats exposed to chronic hypoxia.[78]

Effects on gas exchange

Effect on arterial oxygenation

In acute respiratory failure, inhaled NO improves arterial oxygenation by reducing lung areas characterised by a low V/Q ratio and by diverting pulmonary blood flow away from unventilated towards ventilated lung areas.[15] Pulmonary vasodilatation induced by inhaled NO selectively involves ventilated lung territories. NO does not inhibit hypoxic pulmonary vasoconstriction present in unventilated lung areas. In contrast to intravenous vasodilators,[58, 59] inhaled NO has no effect on the systemic circulation and does not induce any vasodilatation in pulmonary vessels perfusing unventilated lung areas. As a result, pulmonary shunt does not increase and Pao_2 does not deteriorate following inhalation of NO.[15] The increase in Pao_2 and decrease in pulmonary shunt induced by inhaled NO are dependent on the initial level of PVRI.[62] The greater the baseline PVRI, the greater are the increase in Pao_2 and the decrease in pulmonary shunt. The correlation between baseline PVRI and the increase in Pao_2 induced by inhaled NO, although statistically significant, is weak. The increase in Pao_2 induced by inhaled NO depends on baseline Pao_2 only in severely hypoxaemic patients who also have a very high pulmonary vascular resistance.[16, 62]

Application of positive end-expiratory pressure (PEEP) potentiates the improvement in arterial oxygenation with NO.[62, 79] This beneficial effect of PEEP is observed only when PEEP induces alveolar recruitment (Figure 12.5). When PEEP induces lung distension only, the effect of inhaled NO on arterial oxygenation does not differ in PEEP and zero end-expiratory pressure (ZEEP) conditions. Therefore, the effect of inhaled NO on arterial oxygenation should always be tested after optimisation of alveolar recruitment. Patients considered as 'NO non-responders' in ZEEP conditions might become 'NO-responders' if PEEP is applied.

In contrast, PEEP-induced alveolar recruitment has an unpredictable effect on the decrease in PVR caused by inhaled NO. On average, the decrease in pulmonary vascular resistance induced by NO is similar in ZEEP and PEEP conditions and is not always potentiated by alveolar recruitment. Thus, the increase in Pao_2 induced by inhaled NO depends on alveolar recruitment whereas the vascular effect does not. A possible

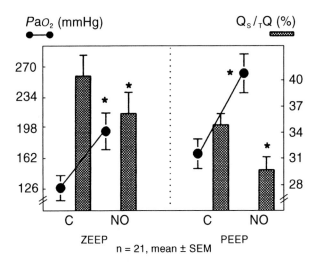

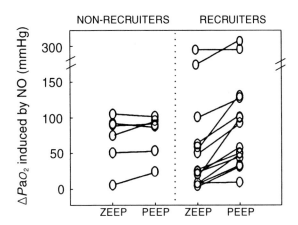

Fig 12.5 Influence of PEEP and alveolar recruitment on inhaled NO-induced improvement in arterial oxygenation. In 20 critically ill patients with severe ARDS, PEEP-induced alveolar recruitment was assessed using a high-resolution thoracic CT scan. Significant alveolar recruitment was found following PEEP 10 cmH$_2$O in 14 patients ('recruiters') whereas no alveolar recruitment was observed in 6 patients ('non-recruiters'). As shown in the upper panel, when considering all patients, inhaled NO-induced changes in Pao$_2$ (Fio$_2$=1) and pulmonary shunt (Q_s/Q_t) are more marked with PEEP 10 cmH$_2$O than without PEEP (ZEEP) ($P<0.01$). Inhaled NO-induced individual changes in Pao$_2$ (ΔPao$_2$) are more marked in PEEP than in ZEEP conditions in recruiters only (lower panel) suggesting that PEEP-induced alveolar recruitment rather than PEEP itself enhances the effect of inhaled NO on arterial oxygenation. (From Puybasset *et al.*, 1995,[62] with permission)

255

explanation for this apparently paradoxical effect could have an anatomical basis. Pulmonary vessels follow a long course within the lung parenchyma; arteries follow the bronchovascular axis of the secondary pulmonary lobules, but veins return to the left atrium within the interlobular septa. Since pulmonary lesions are non-homogeneously distributed in ARDS and pulmonary vessels and alveolar spaces are in contact over a long distance, even under ZEEP, there could be enough ventilated alveolar territories surrounding pulmonary vessels to allow inhaled NO to reach and relax constricted vascular smooth muscle and to increase pulmonary blood flow within the corresponding capillary network. The effect on gas exchange then depends on the V/Q ratio at the alveolar level. For a given secondary pulmonary lobule, V/Q and Pao_2 will increase if this increased pulmonary blood flow is directed towards ventilated acini. By inducing alveolar recruitment, PEEP increases the proportion of ventilated alveolar territories. The increased pulmonary blood flow induced by NO is directed through these newly aerated alveoli. Therefore, for the same vascular effect, an increase in arterial oxygenation is observed.

Inhaled NO may also improve arterial oxygenation in patients with ARDS by closing a patent foramen ovale.[80] The incidence of patent foramen ovale in the general population ranges from 25 to 35%.[81] In this category of patients, pulmonary hypertension associated with ARDS may induce a right-to-left intracardiac shunt. As shown in Figure 12.6, inhaled NO, by reducing pulmonary arterial pressure and unloading the right ventricle, reverses the right-to-left atrial pressure gradient and closes the patent foramen ovale. A dramatic improvement in arterial oxygenation results when the right-to-left intracardiac shunt represents a significant proportion of cardiac output. Patent foramen ovale should be sought systematically in patients with ARDS and severe hypoxaemia. If present, a low concentration of inhaled NO may induce a functional closure of the right-to-left intracardiac shunt and a dramatic improvement in arterial oxygenation.[80] Similar results may be obtained in patients with pulmonary embolism and patent foramen ovale.[82]

Effect on alveolar dead space

Most often, NO inhalation induces an increase in the end-tidal carbon dioxide tension ($Petco_2$) simultaneously with the decrease in pulmonary arterial pressure. These changes are observed independently of any modification in minute ventilation and cardiac output and are generally associated with a small but significant reduction in $Paco_2$ corresponding to a marked decrease in alveolar dead space.[17, 18, 62] The reduction of lung areas with high V/Q ratio, which is related probably to the re-opening of constricted pulmonary arteries in ventilated lung regions, contributes to increased alveolar ventilation. The effect on alveolar dead space does not depend on alveolar recruitment and has a large inter-patient variability. In a minority of patients, the decrease in Paco$_2$ induced by inhaled NO can reach up to 10 mmHg and provides an opportunity to reduce tidal volume and peak airway pressure,[83] thereby decreasing the risk of barotrauma.

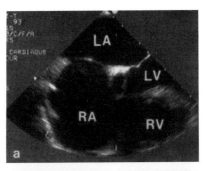

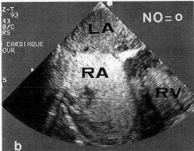

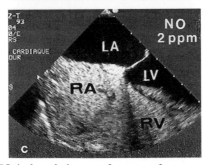

Fig 12.6   Inhaled NO-induced closure of a patent foramen ovale in a patient with severe ARDS following multiple trauma. Echocardiographic views centred on right and left atrium without (a) or with (b and c) contrast echoes in the presence (c) or absence (a and b) of inhaled NO. In the absence of NO, the interatrial septum is curved to the left, suggesting a positive right-to-left pressure gradient (a) and contrast echoes massively move from right to left atrium indicating a right-to-left intracardiac shunt (b). The Pao$_2$ is 7·5 kPa (56 mmHg) with an Fio$_2$ of 1. In the presence of NO 2 ppm, microbubbles are no longer seen in the left atrium (c), indicating closure of the patent foramen ovale. The Pao$_2$ rises from 7·5 kPa (56 mmHg) to 42·4 kPa (318 mmHg). LA, left atrium; LV, left ventricle, RA, right atrium; RV, right ventricle. (From Fellahi et al., 1995,[80] with permission)

257

Bronchial effects

Inhaled NO inhibits methacholine-induced bronchoconstriction in guinea-pigs[84] and rabbits;[85] this bronchodilating effect is dose-dependent in the range of 5–150 ppm. Acute lung injury is associated frequently with increased respiratory resistance which can be caused by two different mechanisms. Part of the increased respiratory resistance is fixed, resulting from the external compression of bronchioles by the surrounding pulmonary oedema and from bronchiolitis; another part is reversible, resulting from the bronchoconstriction induced by circulating inflammatory mediators such as thromboxane-A_2 and leukotrienes.

Inhaled NO does not decrease the respiratory resistance in patients with ARDS between concentrations ranging from 10 to 80 ppm.[86] Reasons for this lack of bronchodilating effect remain speculative. In patients with ARDS, the increased repiratory resistance might be due entirely to the reduction in lung volume, the specific bronchial resistance remaining normal. Therefore, the absence of true bronchoconstriction could explain the lack of a bronchodilator effect resulting from inhalation of NO. Another possibility could be that the bronchodilator effect of NO is offset by a bronchoconstricting effect of NO_2.[33, 56] When using inspiratory NO concentrations greater than 15 ppm and $Fio_2 \geqslant 0.6$, NO_2 concentrations can be above 0·3 ppm[87] and could induce bronchoconstriction.[33]

In spontaneously breathing asthmatic patients, inhaled NO at a concentration of 80 ppm exerts a bronchodilating effect much smaller than that of β_2-agonists.[88] Therefore, in humans with increased bronchial reactivity, inhaled NO appears to be a poor bronchodilating agent.

Effects on platelets

An activation of coagulation, related mainly to platelet aggregation,[89] induces microvascular thrombosis in the pulmonary circulation during ARDS.[64] Endogenous NO causes antiplatelet effects by activating intraplatelet guanylate cyclase and thereby increasing platelet cyclic guanosine monophosphate (cGMP). In turn, cGMP-dependent protein kinase is stimulated, resulting in a decrease in the intracellular Ca^{2+} level by inhibition of agonist-mediated calcium flux.[90] The latter induces: (a) reduction in fibrinogen binding to glycoprotein GP IIb/IIIa; (b) partial inhibition of platelet aggregation; (c) inhibition of phosphorylation of myosin light chains and of protein kinase C; (d) stimulation of phosphorylation of the subunit of glycoprotein I; and (e) modulation of phospholipase-A_2 and C-mediated responses.[91]

Inhibition of platelet aggregation by NO was first demonstrated *in vitro* by Mellion *et al* .[92] and then confirmed by Radomski *et al.*[91] Incubation of human platelet-rich plasma with NO resulted in a concentration-dependent inhibition of platelet aggregation induced by adenosine diphosphate, collagen, and thrombin. NO was two to three times more potent in human washed platelets than in platelet-rich plasma. Inhibition of aggregation of human washed platelets decayed (half-life approximately 2 min) and disappeared completely after 4 minutes.[92] Preincubation of platelets with haemoglobin or Fe^{2+} reduced the anti-aggregating activity of NO. NO was a less potent anti-aggregant agent than prostacyclin. Salvemini *et al.* also demonstrated that *in vitro* NO completely inhibited thrombin-induced platelet aggregation.[93] However, this inhibition was reversed by oxy-haemoglobin administered 30 s to 10 min after thrombin-induced platelet aggregation according to a time-dependent profile.[93] NO is very unstable, especially when stirred in solution[94] as in the aggregometer cuvette.

To date, there has been only one *in vitro* study of the antiplatelet activity of inhaled NO in patients with ARDS.[95] An antithrombotic effect and/or an increase in the bleeding risk might be expected in patients receiving inhaled NO, if the antiplatelet effect is of sufficient magnitude. As shown in Figure 12.7, a dose-independent but statistically significant decrease in *in vitro* platelet aggregation induced by three different aggregating agents was observed following inhaled NO administered at concentrations ranging between 1·5 and 150 ppm. This study excluded patients with septic shock, pre-existing haemostatic disorders (congenital or acquired), platelet count less than $100 \times 10^3/mm^3$, decreased platelet aggregation, and treatment with antiplatelet or anticoagulant agents. In each individual, Ivy bleeding time remained within normal limits and variations following NO did not correlate with changes in platelet aggregation (Figure 12.7). In another study performed in eight patients with ARDS and free of pre-existing coagulation disorders, inhaled NO induced a dose-dependent decrease in platelet aggregation in concentrations ranging from 45 ppb to 1·5 ppm.[96] The antiplatelet effect of NO was associated with a significant increase in intraplatelet cGMP, suggesting activation of the intraplatelet guanylate cyclase metabolic pathway. It can be concluded that in patients with ARDS without pre-existing coagulation disorders, the beneficial effects of inhaled NO on arterial oxygenation and pulmonary circulation are associated with significant inhibition of platelet aggregation at very low NO concentrations (< 1 ppm). This antithrombotic effect is not associated with a significant prolongation of the bleeding time. These results contrast with those of Högman, who found a 33% prolongation of the bleeding time 15 minutes after administration of 30 ppm of NO in the rabbit[97] and in six healthy volunteers.[98] Reasons for these conflicting results are not clear but it can be assumed that factors influencing primary haemostasis might be quite different in rabbits, in healthy volunteers, and in patients with ARDS. Furthermore, there is a general agreement that bleeding time is not sufficiently sensitive or specific for predicting the bleeding risk in many clinical settings.[99]

Because of the lack of a test of haemostasis exploring platelet aggregation

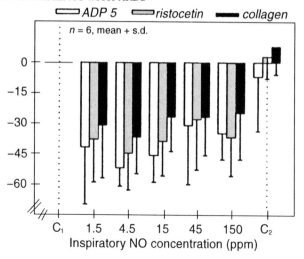

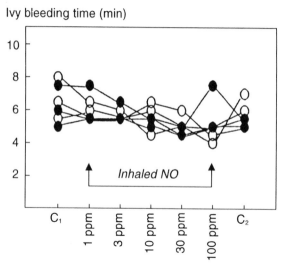

Fig 12.7 Changes in maximal intensity and velocity of platelet aggregation induced by inhaled NO in patients with ARDS. The upper part of the figure shows mean percentage changes of maximal intensity of platelet aggregation induced by 5 μmol adenosine diphosphate (ADP5), ristocetin, and collagen measured in six patients with ARDS. Five increasing concentrations of inhaled NO were administered in a randomised order. Changes are expressed as percentage of variation from the first control value (C_1). Inhaled NO induces a significant dose-independent decrease in maximal intensity of platelet aggregation induced by the three different aggregating agents. Maximal intensity and velocity of platelet aggregation return to control values after the cessation of inhaled NO. The lower part of the figure shows corresponding individual changes in Ivy incision bleeding time. No significant change in Ivy bleeding time was observed whatever the concentration of inhaled NO. (From Samama et al.,[95] with permission)

directly *in vivo*, the true antiplatelet effect of inhaled NO still remains to be documented in humans. However, Golino and Yao and their coworkers[100, 101] have shown that NO, either endogenous or exogenous, can inhibit intravascular platelet aggregation in the Folts model of carotid thrombosis in the rabbit.[102] Soluble NO infused into the carotid atery completely abolished cyclic flow reductions due to recurrent platelet aggregation. These effects were transient and cyclic flow reductions were restored spontaneously within 10 min after cessation of NO infusion. Therefore, in the rabbit, NO was considered as an antithrombotic agent inhibiting platelet aggregation *in vivo* to an extent very similar to aspirin and thromboxane synthase inhibitors. It should be pointed out that this method of NO administration (direct intravascular) is very different from NO inhalation used in humans. Further studies are required to assess whether low concentrations of inhaled NO abolish cyclic flow reductions in experimental animals with and without acute lung injury.

Other effects of potential benefit

Improvement in gas exchange with NO could also be explained by mechanisms other than the diversion of pulmonary blood flow following arterial and venous vasodilatation. Because inhaled NO probably dilates both sides of the pulmonary circulation (arteries and veins), the reduction in pulmonary arterial pressure may be associated with a reduction in pulmonary capillary hydrostatic pressure, which in turn could reduce the amount of pulmonary oedema, resulting in a progressive improvement in arterial oxygenation. Unexpected rapid resolution of pulmonary infiltrates during NO inhalation has been reported.[103] In a clinical study comprising nine patients with acute lung injury,[104] NO at a concentration of 40 ppm decreased pulmonary transvascular flux of ^{99m}Tc-labelled human albumin. In the same study NO decreased pulmonary venous resistance more than pulmonary arterial resistance, a situation which favours resorption of pulmonary oedema. A good correlation was found also between the change in pulmonary vascular resistance and the change in transvascular albumin flux.

Inhaled NO could also limit the remodelling of the pulmonary circulation which occurs following acute lung injury.[76] In response to various types of lung injury, vascular smooth muscle appears rapidly in distal units of the pulmonary vascular bed, increasing the proportion of arteries that are completely muscular. This anatomical remodelling of the pulmonary circulation forms the basis of the increases in pulmonary arterial pressure and pulmonary vascular resistance observed in the late stages of ARDS. Endogenous NO released by pulmonary endothelial cells seems to exert a permanent antitrophic effect on adjacent vascular smooth muscle fibres.[78, 105] Endothelial lesions observed in acute lung injury could prevent the antiproliferative effect of endogenous NO and enhance proliferation of vascular smooth muscle distally in the pulmonary vascular bed. Chronic inhalation of small concentrations of NO could re-establish the antiproliferative effect and prevent structure remodelling of the pulmonary circulation during the course of ARDS, thus reducing pulmonary arterial hypertension.

There is conflicting evidence regarding the effect of NO on oxidant-induced acute lung injury. In isolated rabbit lungs submitted to oxidative stress, inhaled NO partly prevented the development of increased capillary permeability and pulmonary arterial hypertension[14] and dilated the constricted pulmonary vessels despite the presence of pulmonary endothelial injury.[106] However, it has also been shown that endogenous NO probably mediates hyperoxia-induced damage to human lung cells[107] and is an essential intermediary in the production of acute lung injury due to paraquat in guinea-pigs.[108] NO synthase inhibitors totally prevent lung injury due to paraquat and xanthine oxidase. Therefore, administration of inhaled NO to treat patients with paraquat-induced lung injury could be potentially harmful.

Recent evidence also suggests an anti-inflammatory role for NO in ARDS. In one human study, after 4 days of NO inhalation, polymorphonuclear cells from the bronchoalveolar lavage showed a reduction in both spontaneous H_2O_2 production and β_2 integrin CD11b/CD18 expression. In addition, the levels of interleukins IL-8 and IL-6 also decreased after NO inhalation.[28]

Concentration–response curves

In experimental animals, concentration–response curves are reported in the range of 5–150 ppm which appears to be species-dependent and also dependent on the model of pulmonary hypertension.[5, 6, 11, 12, 109, 110] In humans, concentration–response curves to inhaled NO may vary among patients, and may be influenced by the presence of associated septic shock or patent foramen ovale. In patients with ARDS and without septic shock,[18, 32] the maximal effect on Pao_2 and PVRI was observed for inspiratory NO concentrations below 5 ppm (Figure 12.8). In some other patients, there was a dose-dependent response in the range of 20–100 ppb.[18, 111] Maximum haemodynamic and oxygenation responses to NO at very low concentrations have been reported in other studies also. Lowson et al.[112] demonstrated that a dose of 0·1 ppm produced near-maximum decreases in PVRI and MPAP and that there was no dose-response relationship for either PVRI or MPAP over the range 0·1–40 ppm. In contrast, the maximum increase in the Pao_2/Fio_2 ratio was observed at 10 ppm, although this was not significantly different from the response to 1 ppm. The conclusion from this study was that the optimum dose of NO is 1 ppm.

In patients with ARDS treated by extracorporeal oxygenation (ECMO), concentration–response curves for systemic oxygenation and pulmonary hypertension were found in the range of $0\cdot1-100$ ppm.[113] This difference could be related to permanent activation of the pulmonary circulation by ECMO. In patients with ARDS and septic shock receiving a continuous intravenous infusion of noradrenaline and treated by conventional mechanical ventilation, there was a concentration-dependent increase in oxygenation in the range $0\cdot1-150$ ppm, whereas a plateau effect for PVRI was observed at 5 ppm (Figure 12.8).[114] In other words, although the pulmonary vascular effect induced by inhaled NO was similar in patients with and without shock, the improvement in arterial oxygenation was much more pronounced in patients with ARDS and shock. In patients under general anaesthesia, if NO does not change the cardiac output, changes in Sv_{O_2} are closely related to changes in Sa_{O_2}. Consequently, continuous $S_v_{O_2}$ monitoring is an easy means of determining the minimal effective concentration of inhaled NO at the bedside.

In neonates with acute pulmonary hypertension, the decrease in pulmonary arterial pressure induced by NO is much more pronounced than in adults[115, 116] and concentration–response curves for both oxygenation and pulmonary hypertension are likely between 0 and 5 ppm.[117] In a recent study in children with severe lung disease, there was no difference in the effects of 11 and 60 ppm of NO on pulmonary vascular resistance and oxygenation. These results probably imply that concentrations in excess of 10 ppm are not needed for prolonged therapy in children.[118]

Inhaled prostacyclin

Because inhaled NO selectively dilates pulmonary vessels perfusing the ventilated areas, it is considered to be close to the ideal pulmonary vasodilator. However, expensive technology is required to ensure safe administration and to provide continuous monitoring of NO concentrations delivered to the patient. In addition, long-term toxicity is not known. Therefore, inhalation of other vasodilating substances has been proposed recently. Aerosolised prostacyclin in doses as low as 2 ng/kg/min has been shown to induce selective pulmonary vasodilatation in infants[119] and adults with ARDS[120, 121] and in neonates undergoing surgery for congenital heart disease.[122] Prostacyclin is a potent physiological vasodilator released mainly from endothelial cells. It plays an important role in maintaining low pulmonary vascular resistance. It has a short half-life of 2–3 min because it is spontaneously hydrolysed at physiological pH into an inactive metabolite, 6-keto-prostaglandin F1a.[123] Administered by the inhalational route, prostacyclin binds itself to the receptors located on the surface of the vascular smooth muscle cells and increases intracellular levels of cyclic adenosine monophosphate (cAMP) by activating adenylate cyclase. cAMP activates protein kinase A and decreases free intracellular calcium which in

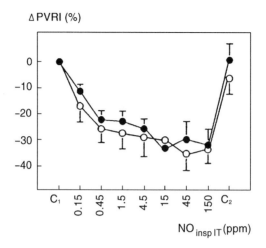

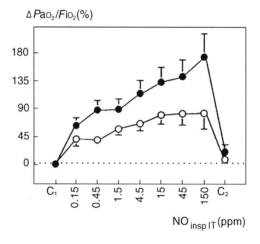

Fig 12.8 Effect of septic shock on dose–response curves of inhaled NO in patients with ARDS. Increasing inspiratory intratracheal concentrations of inhaled NO ($NO_{insp\ IT}$) were administered in a randomised order to eight patients with ARDS with septic shock (closed circles) and eight patients with ARDS without septic shock (open circles). Changes in Pao_2/Fio_2 and PVRI are expressed as percentage of variation. Inhaled NO induces a dose-dependent decrease in PVRI with a plateau effect at 4·5 ppm in both the groups. In contrast, a dose-dependent increase in Pao_2/Fio_2 was observed in patients with septic shock in the range of 0·15–150 ppm whereas in patients without septic shock a plateau effect on arterial oxygenation was observed from NO concentration of 4·5 ppm ($P<0·05$) (From Mourgeon et al., 1997[114] with permission)

turn induces relaxation of the vascular smooth muscle. Prostacyclin appears stable in aerosol form if prepared in a glycine buffer and diluted with saline immediately before use. Aerolised prostacyclin administered by the inhalational route has been reported to have an efficacy profile identical to inhaled NO.[124] PGI_2, administered by the intravenous route, decreases both pulmonary and systemic vascular resistances and increases shunt through non-specific vasodilatation. In contrast, administration by the inhalational route produces an improvement in V/Q matching due to an effect which is restricted only to the ventilated lung regions. The exact dose at which prostacyclin 'spills over' into the pulmonary circulation to increase pulmonary shunt and decrease arterial pressure remains unknown. It appears to be a selective pulmonary vasodilator at concentrations lower than 10 ng/kg/min.[119, 121] In some patients, administration of concentrations as high as 51 ng/kg/min[122] does not induce arterial hypotension or worsening of gas exchange. Because only a small fraction of the administered aerosol reaches the alveolar space, the effective concentration reaching the alveoli can be quite different from the administered concentration. In patients with pulmonary hypertension, community-acquired pneumonia and lung fibrosis, concentrations in the range of 60–80 ng/kg/ min are required to decrease pulmonary artery pressure and are associated with systemic effects and worsening of arterial oxygenation, indicating the lack of pulmonary selectivity.[121] Some patients receiving 10–20 ng/kg/min of aerosolised prostacyclin demonstrate increased pulmonary shunt whereas others do not.[121] Therefore, one of the main problems related to the administration of aerosolised prostacyclin is to determine the exact concentration at which selective pulmonary vasodilation is obtained for a given patient. Because the maximum effect on arterial oxygenation can be obtained at a lower concentration than that required for the maximum effect on pulmonary arterial pressure, it is likely that prostacyclin can reach pulmonary vessels perfusing unventilated lung areas when administered at high concentrations.[119] Apart from the lack of pulmonary selectivity, aerosolised prostacyclin may markedly inhibit platelet aggregation and induce bronchoconstriction.[125] The latter effect could be deleterious in patients with ARDS. Prostacyclin, in contrast to inhaled NO, does not have any toxic metabolites, and has no toxicity *per se*. Further studies are required to determine whether inhaled prostacyclin (or other prostaglandins) represents an attractive alternative to inhaled NO for producing selective pulmonary vasodilatation.

Almitrine

The first description relating to an increase in Pao_2 induced by almitrine in ARDS was reported in the late 1980s.[126] A beneficial effect on arterial oxygenation had been reported 7 years earlier in patients with chronic

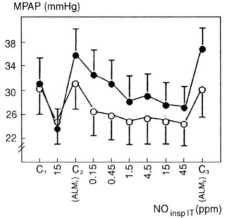

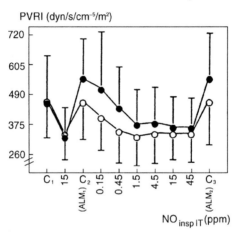

Fig 12.9 Comparative changes in mean pulmonary artery pressure (MPAP) and pulmonary vascular resistance index (PVRI) induced by increasing inspiratory intratracheal concentrations of inhaled NO (NO$_{\text{insp IT}}$) in the presence (closed circles) or absence (open circles) of a continuous intravenous infusion of 16 µg/kg/ min of almitrine in six patients with ARDS. PVRI and MPAP were measured: before NO administration (C$_1$); after the administration of 15 ppm of NO (15); after the cessation of NO, with almitrine (ALM$_1$) or without almitrine (C$_2$); following six randomised concentrations of NO between 0·15 and 45 ppm, with or without almitrine; and after the cessation of NO, with (ALM$_2$) or without almitrine (C$_3$). Almitrine alone induced significant increases in PVRI and MPAP ($P<0·01$). NO alone and almitrine–NO induced significant and dose-dependent decreases in PVRI and MPAP in the range of 0·15–4·5 ppm ($P<0·01$). With regard to PVRI, there was no interaction between almitrine and NO, suggesting that the dose–response relationship of NO is not affected by the presence of almitrine. With regard to MPAP, profiles of the NO dose–response relationship with and without almitrine are significantly different as shown by two-way analysis of variance ($P<0·05$), suggesting that NO does not entirely reverse almitrine-induced pulmonary hypertension. (From Lu et al., 1995,[32] with permission)

obstructive pulmonary disease.[127] The effect of almitrine on Pao_2 in ARDS varies markedly among patients[128] and could not be uniformly reproduced in experimental models of acute lung injury.[129] In contrast, a rise in pulmonary artery pressure has always been described after almitrine administered at 15 µg/kg/min. There is conflicting experimental evidence concerning the effects of almitrine on hypoxic pulmonary vasoconstriction (HPV); both inhibition[130] and potentiation[131] have been reported. Indeed, its effects on the pulmonary circulation depend upon (a) the previous status of HPV and (b) the dose of almitrine. Almitrine seems to re-establish HPV only when it is deficient.[131] At high doses, almitrine constricts the entire pulmonary circulation, including arteries perfusing lung regions normally ventilated and can partly reverse HPV by diverting pulmonary blood flow away from normally oxygenated lung regions towards hypoxic lung areas.[130] At low doses, almitrine has a double selectivity; it constricts only pulmonary arteries to the exclusion of veins and systemic vessels, and acts predominantly in lung areas where HPV is impaired. In lung regions where HPV is already effective, almitrine does not induce any additional constriction.[132] In fact, almitrine mimics HPV and competes with the different stimuli inducing constriction of pulmonary arteries subjected to a hypoxic challenge, i.e. partial pressures of oxygen in the alveoli and in mixed venous blood.[133]

The first report of the combined administration of almitrine and NO in two patients with ARDS was published in 1993.[134] The rationale for this combination was to reinforce HPV in unventilated lung areas by administering almitrine, and at the same time, to reverse the constriction of pulmonary vessels perfusing ventilated lung regions with NO. Potentiation of the redistribution of pulmonary blood flow towards ventilated lung areas, leading to an additional reduction of pulmonary shunt, was expected. In fact, two types of responses may be observed in patients with ARDS who receive a combination of intravenous almitrine and inhaled NO.[27, 135] In 'non-responders' to this combination, Pao_2 following almitrine associated with NO is equal or inferior to Pao_2 following NO alone. In 'responders', Pao_2 following almitrine-NO is higher than Pao_2 following NO alone.

In patients with ARDS, almitrine administered at a dose of 16 µg/kg/min increases pulmonary artery pressure and pulmonary vascular resistance.[32] Because, experimentally, almitrine constricts selectively pulmonary arteries to the exclusion of pulmonary veins,[132] this increase in pulmonary artery pressure should not induce an increase in microvascular pressure and therefore should not exacerbate pulmonary oedema. In patients with pre-existing right heart failure, high doses of almitrine may worsen right venticular failure and decrease cardiac output via an increase in pulmonary artery pressure.

Inhaled NO incompletely reverses almitrine-induced pulmonary hypertension because it acts only on the constricting component of the increased pulmonary pressure and leaves unchanged the almitrine-induced increase in cardiac output observed in some patients. The reasons why almitrine increases cardiac output in some patients with ARDS remain unclear. Concentration–response curves of inhaled NO for reversing almitrine-induced increases in pulmonary artery pressure and pulmonary vascular resistance and for improving arterial oxygenation are represented in Figures 12.9 and 12.10. Concomitant administration of almitrine and NO does not change the concentration–response curves of inhaled NO with respect to pulmonary artery pressure, pulmonary vascular resistance, and arterial oxygenation. A plateau effect is obtained at NO concentrations around 3 ppm whether or not almitrine is administered. The effects of almitrine and NO on arterial oxygenation are additive.[32] In many patients, smaller doses of almitrine (2–4 µg/kg/min) provide the same improvement in arterial oxygenation without increasing markedly pulmonary artery pressure significantly.[136] When used in combination with inhaled NO at a concentration of 5 ppm, almitrine at a dose of 4 µg/kg/min improves arterial oxygenation dramatically via a reduction of intrapulmonary shunt and increases pulmonary artery pressure only slightly.

Septic shock seems to modify the response of patients to almitrine. Maximal effects on Pao_2 and shunt are seen at a dose of 4 µg/kg/min in patients without shock and at 2 µg/kg/min in patients with shock. The basis for this difference seems to lie in the hypoxic pulmonary vasoconstriction which is deficient in patients with septic shock and is, at least, partly operative in ARDS patients without shock. Total absence of HPV in unventilated zones of patients with septic shock probably offers greater scope for almitrine to exert its constricting effect on the pulmonary vessels. In contrast, in patients without septic shock, competition with normal HPV renders almitrine less effective at low doses. Almitrine in a dose of 2–16 µg/kg/min also increases PVRI and decreases alveolar dead space in a dose-dependent manner in patients without shock and in a dose-independent manner in patients with shock.

Prolonged administration of almitrine in patients with ARDS should be regarded with caution. Almitrine is a lipophilic substance which is metabolised by the liver. Its plasma clearance is very low, around 4 ml/kg/min.[137, 138] Due to its very large volume of distribution and low plasma clearance, almitrine has a very long elimination half-life that reaches up to one month if almitrine is administered for 6 months.[139] In patients with ARDS, the administration of almitrine can usually be limited to less than one week and doses of 4 µg/kg/min are sufficient to improve arterial oxygenation markedly. Nausea, vomiting, and diarrhoea are some of the minor complications that can be encountered.[140] Peripheral neuropathies have also been described in patients with chronic obstructive lung disease receiving high-dose almitrine for periods longer than one month.[141-143] These neurological complications were always reversible, although they

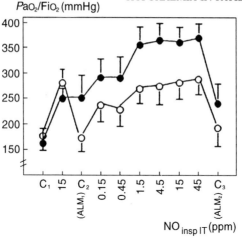

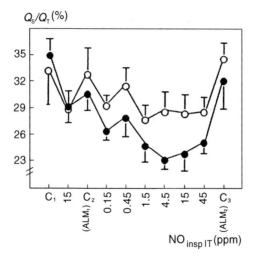

Fig 12.10 Changes in PaO_2/FiO_2 ratio and pulmonary shunt (Q_s/Q_t) induced by increasing inspiratory intratracheal concentrations of inhaled NO ($NO_{insp\ IT}$) in the presence (closed circles) or absence (open circles) of a continuous intravenous infusion of 16 μg/kg/min of almitrine in six patients with ARDS. PaO_2/FiO_2 and Q_s/Q_t were measured: before NO administration (C_1); after the administration of 15 ppm of NO (15); after the cessation of NO, with almitrine (ALM_1) or without almitrine (C_2); following six randomised concentrations of NO between 0·15 and 45 ppm, with or without almitrine; and after the cessation of NO, with (ALM_2) or without almitrine (C_3). NO alone and almitrine–NO induced a significant and dose-dependent increase in PaO_2/FiO_2 and decrease in Q_s/Q_t in the range of 0·15 to 4·5 ppm ($P<0·01$). There is no interaction between almitrine and NO suggesting that the profile of the NO dose–response curve is not affected by the presence of almitrine. PaO_2/FiO_2 ratio was significantly greater and Q_s/Q_t significantly lower during almitrine–NO than during NO alone ($P<0·001$). (From Lu et al., 1995,[32] with permission)

269

significantly lengthened the hospital stay of the patients. It can reasonably be expected that such complications will not be observed in patients with ARDS treated with almitrine if the duration of administration is less than one week and if low doses of almitrine (2–4 μg/kg/min) are used.

NO-synthase and cyclooxygenase inhibitors

Constitutive endothelial NO synthase (cNOS) and cyclooxygenase (COX1) synthesise NO and prostacyclin which vasodilate the underlying smooth muscle cells through the activation of guanylate cyclase and adenylate cyclase, respectively. Both enzymes[144, 145] also have an inducible isoform (iNOS and COX2) that can be expressed in inflammatory cells (macrophages[146] and polymorphonuclear leucocytes) and in vascular cells (endothelial[147] and smooth muscle cells[148]). Non-specific inhibitors of both isoforms may have different effects depending on the presence or absence of the inducible isoform. NO synthase inhibitors reinforce HPV resulting from the inhalation of a hypoxic mixture,[149–151] but not from experimentally induced acute respiratory failure[150, 152] or human ARDS associated with septic shock.[153] NO may oppose HPV in the normal pulmonary circulation because it is synthesised in response to active vasoconstriction induced by HPV through an increase in shear stress. Conversely, during acute respiratory failure, inducible NO synthase could be activated in the entire pulmonary circulation. As a consequence, NO synthase inhibitors will induce a non-specific increase in vascular tone of the entire pulmonary circulation. Thus, they do not help in diverting pulmonary blood flow away from the unventilated areas of the lung. Therefore, NO synthase inhibitors probably should not be used to correct hypoxaemia in ARDS. Furthermore, the inhibition of flow-dependency that they induce is responsible for a marked decrease in organ perfusion which precludes their use in the treatment of septic shock.

Contrasting with NO synthase inhibitors, cyclooxygenase inhibitors reinforce HPV induced by inhalation of a hypoxic mixture or by experimental acute respiratory failure. In dogs, aspirin restores normal HPV when it is deficient and amplifies the normal response when it is not deficient.[154] Indomethacin improves arterial oxygenation through a reduction in true shunt when administered either before and after the onset of oleic acid-induced acute respiratory failure in anaesthetised dogs.[155, 156] In the same experimental model, meclofenamate reduced true shunt measured by the multiple inert gas technique from 48±5% to 30±11%.[157] The reinforcement effect of cyclooxygenase inhibitors on HPV has been confirmed in multiple experimental studies.[158–161] Indomethacin also improves arterial oxygenation in human ARDS.[162, 163] Further studies are required to determine the potential beneficial and detrimental effects of cyclooxygenase inhibitors, in combination with inhaled NO, on gas exchange, coagulation and immunological functions in patients with ARDS.

Permissive hypercapnia

Permissive hypercapnia is a new modality of mechanical ventilation in patients with severe acute respiratory failure. Severe acute respiratory failure is characterised by a major reduction of aerated lung parenchyma as assessed by a decrease in static respiratory compliance.[68, 164] Frequently, more than 50% of the lung is consolidated and remains inaccessible to the respiratory gases. The intrapulmonary shunt induced by these extensive lesions results in severe hypoxaemia which cannot be reversed even by administration of pure oxygen. Concomitantly, perfusion is markedly reduced in normally ventilated areas due to the combination of vascular thrombosis,[165] remodelling of the pulmonary vessels by muscular hypertrophy, pulmonary vasoconstriction, and barotraumatic pulmonary emphysema.[166] This increased proportion of the high V/Q ratio zone enhances the alveolar–arterial CO_2 gradient. In this context, high minute ventilation and high airway pressures are required to maintain normocapnia. Barotraumatic lesions generated as a consequence worsen the acute respiratory failure through increased oedema[167] and alveolar rupture.[166]

A volume- and pressure-limited ventilatory strategy that allows progressive hypercapnia and acidosis while keeping the lung 'open', as the compliance decreases, has been proposed to reduce the contribution of mechanical ventilation to lung damage.[168] The principle of permissive hypercapnia comprises administration of small tidal volumes, so as to keep the peak airway pressure below the distension pressure on the pressure–volume curve during mechanical insufflation. Acceptance of a state of respiratory acidosis is a corollary of such a ventilatory strategy.

Understanding the pathophysiological effects of permissive hypercapnia on the pulmonary circulation must take into account its indirect and direct effects. Both hypercapnia and respiratory acidosis induce central sympathetic stimulation; of the two, hypercapnia is a more potent stimulant of the sympathetic system than acidosis.[169] However, acidosis and hypercapnia have opposite direct effects on the isolated pulmonary circulation: vasoconstriction and vasodilatation, respectively.[170, 171] Due to its direct vasodilating effect, hypercapnia alone, without acidosis, inhibits HPV during experimental acute respiratory failure.[172] Despite the pulmonary vasodilating effect induced by hypercapnia, a marked increase in pulmonary artery pressure is observed in humans during acute permissive hypercapnia.[17] It is related not only to increases in pulmonary vascular resistance and cardiac output resulting from sympathetic stimulation but also to the direct pulmonary vasoconstricting effect of acidosis (Figures 12.11, 12.12). The resulting increase in right ventricular afterload can

271

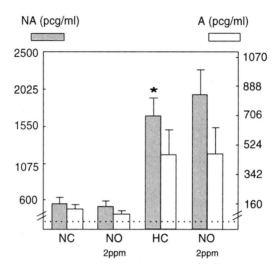

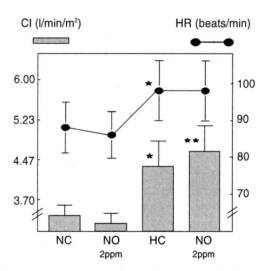

Fig 12.11 Heart rate (HR), cardiac index (CI), noradrenaline (NA) and adrenaline (A) concentrations without and with NO 2 ppm in normocapnic and hypercapnic conditions. HR, CI, plasma noradrenaline and adrenaline concentrations were measured under the following conditions: normocapnia without NC; normocapnia and NO 2 ppm; hypercapnia ($Pao_2 = 65 \pm 15$ mmHg) without HC; hypercapnia and NO 2 ppm. Hypercapnia alone induced increases in HR, CI and in nordrenaline and adrenaline concentrations. NO significantly increased CI in hypercapnic conditions only. (From Puybasset et al., 1994,[17] with permission)

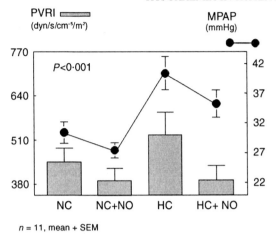

PVRI ▭
(dyn/s/cm⁻⁵/m²)

MPAP
(mmHg)

NC   NC+NO   HC   HC+ NO

n = 11, mean + SEM

Fig 12.12 Pulmonary vascular resistance index (PVRI) and mean pulmonary artery pressure (MPAP) without and with NO 2 ppm in normocapnic and hypercapnic conditions. PVRI and MPAP were measured under the following conditions: normocapnia without NO (NC); normocapnia and NO 2 ppm (NC+NO); hypercapnia ($Pao_2 = 65 \pm 15$ mmHg) without NO (HC); hypercapnia and NO 2 ppm (HC+NO). Hypercapnia alone induced increases in PVRI and MPAP. NO significantly decreased PVRI and MPAP in both conditions. After NO inhalation, PVRI was not significantly different in normocapnic and hypercapnic conditions whereas MPAP remained elevated in hypercapnic but not normocapnic conditions. (From Puybasset et al., 1994,[17] with permission)

induce right ventricular failure. These haemodynamic side effects of acute permissive hypercapnia may potentially reverse its benefits through increases in pulmonary microvascular pressure and pulmonary oedema.

Inhaled NO can partly reverse the deleterious effects on the pulmonary circulation induced by acute permissive hypercapnia during human acute respiratory failure.[17] The increase in pulmonary vascular resistance can be reversed completely by the administration of inhaled NO, thus reducing pulmonary artery pressure and right ventricular afterload.

The reduction in mean airway pressure following the institution of permissive hypercapnia induces an alveolar derecruitment that increases pulmonary shunt. This deleterious effect of permissive hypercapnia on Pao_2 may be masked by the concomitant increase in $S_{\bar{v}}O_2$ (Figure 12.13) and a more efficient PEEP-induced alveolar recruitment.[173] Inhaled NO increases Pao_2 in hypercapnic conditions, although the determinants of the increase in arterial oxygenation are different in normocapnic and hypercapnic conditions. In normocapnic conditions, the increase in Pao_2 induced by inhaled NO is related to a reduction in pulmonary shunt. In hypercapnic conditions, shunt does not decrease following NO whereas $S_{\bar{v}}O_2$ and cardiac index increase. The absence of a significant reduction in shunt is related

273

probably to the alveolar derecruitment induced by acute permissive hypercapnia; the effects of inhaled NO on arterial oxygenation and pulmonary shunt are greatly influenced by the state of lung recruitment.[62]

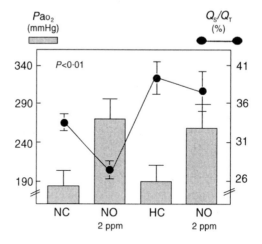

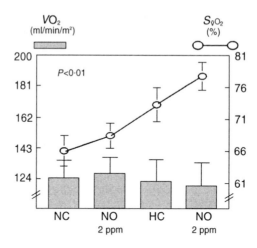

Fig 12.13 Pao_2, pulmonary shunt (Q_s/Q_t), $S_{\bar{v}}O_2$ and VO_2 without and with NO 2 ppm in normocapnic and hypercapnic conditions. Pao_2, Q_s/Q_t, $S_{\bar{v}}O_2$ and VO_2 were measured under the following conditions: normocapnia without NC; in normocapnia and NO 2 ppm; in hypercapnia ($Pao_2 = 65 \pm 15$ mmHg) without NO; in hypercapnia and NO 2 ppm. Hypercapnia alone induced an increase in Q_s/Q_t that did not result in hypoxaemia because of a concomitant increase in $S_{\bar{v}}O_2$. In normocapnic conditions, NO increased Pao_2 through a reduction in Q_s/Q_t. In hypercapnic conditions, the increase in Pao_2 induced by NO results from the combination of a non-significant decrease in Q_s/Q_t and a significant increase in $S_{\bar{v}}O_2$. (Puybasset et al., 1994,[17] with permission)

The improvement in arterial oxygenation induced by inhaled NO appears therefore to be related to the beneficial haemodynamic effect resulting from right ventricular unloading.

Conclusions

The refractory hypoxaemia characterising ARDS has a complex pathophysiology. Far from being an inert anatomical barrier, pulmonary vascular endothelium is an active structure in which various vasoactive substances are synthesised and released into the bloodstream. These locally produced mediators modulate vascular tone and the distribution of pulmonary blood flow between ventilated and unventilated alveolar territories. When hypoxic pulmonary vasoconstriction is inhibited by vasodilating substances released from the endothelium, hypoxaemia worsens as a result of an increase in pulmonary shunt. Inhaled NO is a selective pulmonary vasodilator which relaxes constricted pulmonary vessels perfusing ventilated parts of the lung. It diverts pulmonary blood flow away from unventilated lung areas towards ventilated lung regions. As a consequence, the decrease in pulmonary artery pressure induced by inhaled NO is associated usually with an improvement in arterial oxygenation. Other substances, such as prostacyclin administered by the inhalational route, may also provide selective pulmonary vasodilatation associated with an increased Pao_2.

Almitrine and cyclooxygenase inhibitors improve arterial oxygenation by reinforcing hypoxic pulmonary vasoconstriction, but they tend to increase pulmonary arterial pressure. When combined with inhaled NO, the beneficial effect of almitrine on arterial oxygenation is potentiated while its detrimental effects on the pulmonary circulation are blunted.

All these new treatments have profoundly modified the therapeutic strategies aimed at correction of life-threatening hypoxaemia in patients with severe ARDS. Today, the correction of hypoxaemia cannot be based only on increases in the intrathoracic pressure and Fio_2. Selective pulmonary vasodilators administered by inhalation, alone or in combination with intravenous selective pulmonary vasoconstrictors, may improve ventilation/perfusion ratios and gas exchange. The routine use of these new modalities of therapy should contribute to a decrease in the risk of barotrauma induced by high intrathoracic pressures and should limit the indications for costly and invasive procedures such as extracorporeal membrane oxygenation and extracorporeal CO_2 removal.

1 Furchgott RF, Zawadski JV. The obligatory role of endothelial cells in the relaxation of arterial smooth muscle by acetylcholine. *Nature (Lond)* 1980;**288**:373–6.
2 Palmer RMJ, Ferrige AG, Moncada SA. Nitric oxide release accounts for the biological activity of endothelium-derived relaxing factor. *Nature (Lond)* 1987;**327**:524–6.
3 Higenbottam T, Pepke-Zaba J, Scott J, Woolam P, Coutts C, Wallwork J. Inhaled 'endothelial derived-relaxing factor' (EDRF) in primary hypertension (PPH). *Am Rev*

Respir Dis 1988;**137**(Suppl):A107 (Abstract).

4 Pepke-Zaba J, Higenbottam TW, Dinh-Xuan AT, Stone D, Wallwork J. Inhaled nitric oxide as a cause of selective pulmonary vasodilation in pulmonary hypertension. *Lancet* 1991;**338**:1173–4.

5 Fratacci MD, Frostell CG, Chen TY, Wain JC, Robinson DR, Zapol WM. Inhaled nitric oxide: a selective pulmonary vasodilator of heparin-protamine vasoconstriction in sheep. *Anesthesiology* 1991;**75**:990–9.

6 Frostell C, Fratacci MD, Wain JC, Jones R, Zapol WM. Inhaled nitric oxide: a selective pulmonary vasodilator reversing hypoxic pulmonary vasoconstriction. *Circulation* 1991;**83**:2038–47.

7 Pison U, Lopez FA, Heidelmeyer CF, Rossaint R, Falke K. Inhaled nitric oxide reverses hypoxic pulmonary vasoconstriction without impairing gas exchange. *J Appl Physiol* 1993;**74**:1287–92.

8 Roberts JD, Polaner DM, Lang P, Zapol WM. Inhaled nitric oxide in persistent pulmonary hypertension of the newborn. *Lancet* 1992;**340**:818–19.

9 Freden F, Wei SZ, Berglund JHE, Frostell C, Hedenstrierna G. Nitric oxide modulation of pulmonary blood flow distribution in lobar hypoxia. *Anesthesiology* 1995;**82**:1216–25.

10 Weitzberg E, Rudehill A, Alving K, Lundberg JM. Nitric oxide inhalation selectively attenuates pulmonary hypertension and arterial hypoxia in porcine endotoxin shock. *Acta Physiol Scand* 1991;**143**:451–2.

11 Berger JI, Gibson RL, Redding GJ, Standaert TA, Clarke WR, Truog WE. Effect of inhaled nitric oxide during group B streptococcal sepsis in piglets. *Am Rev Respir Dis* 1993;**147**:1080–6.

12 Dyar O, Young JD, Xiong L, John S. Dose–response relationship for inhaled nitric oxide in experimental pulmonary hypertension in sheep. *Br J Anaesth* 1993;**71**:702–8.

13 Dahm P, Blomquist S, Martensson L, Thoine J, Zoucas E. Circulatory and ventilatory effects of intermittent nitric oxide inhalation during porcine endotoxemia. *J Trauma* 1994;**37**:769–77.

14 Kavanach BP, Mouchawar A, Goldsmith J, Pearl RG. Effects of inhaled NO and inhibition of endogenous NO synthesis in oxidant-induced acute lung injury. *J Appl Physiol* 1994;**76**:1324–9.

15 Rossaint R, Falke KJ, Lopez F, Slama K, Pison U, Zapol WM. Inhaled nitric oxide for the adult respiratory distress syndrome. *N Engl J Med* 1993;**328**:399–405.

16 Bigatello LM, Hurford WE, Kacmarek RM, Roberts JD, Zapol WM. Prolonged inhalation of low concentrations of nitric oxide in patients with severe adult respiratory distress syndrome. *Anesthesiology* 1994;**80**:761–70.

17 Puybasset L, Stewart TE, Rouby JJ, *et al.* Inhaled nitrix oxide reverses the increase in pulmonary vascular resistance induced by permissive hypercapnia in patients with ARDS. *Anesthesiology* 1994;**80**:1254–67.

18 Puybasset L, Rouby JJ, Mourgeon E *et al.* Inhaled nitric oxide in acute respiratory failure: dose-response curves. *Intens Care Med* 1994;**20**:319–27.

19 Young JD, Brampton WJ, Knighton JD, Finfer SR. Inhaled nitric oxide in acute respiratory failure in adults. *Br J Anaesth* 1994;**73**:499–502.

20 Rich FR, Murphy GD, Roos CM, Johns RA. Inhaled nitric oxide: selective pulmonary vasodilation in cardiac surgical patients. *Anesthesiology* 1993;**78**:1028–35.

21 Girard C, Lehot J, Pannetier J, Filley S, French P, Estanove S. Inhaled nitric oxide after mitral valve replacement in patients with chronic pulmonary hypertension. *Anesthesiology* 1992;**77**:880–3.

22 Adnot S, Kouyoumdjian C, Defouilloy C *et al.* Hemodynamic and gas exchange responses to infusion of acetylcholine and inhalation of nitric oxide in patients with chronic obstructive lung disease and pulmonary hypertension. *Am Rev Respir Dis* 1993;**148**:310–16.

23 Moinard J, Manier G, Pillet O, Castaing Y. Effect of inhaled nitric oxide on hemodynamics and VA/Q inequalities in patients with chronic obstructive pulmonary disease. *Am J Respir Crit Care Med* 1994;**149**:1482–7.

24 Stenqvist O, Kjelltoft B, Lundin S. Evaluation of a new system for ventilatory administration of nitric oxide. *Acta Anaesthesiol Scand* 1993;**37**:687–91.

25 Wessel DL, Adatia I, Thompson JE, Hickey PR. Delivery and monitoring of inhaled nitric

oxide in patients with pulmonary hypertension. *Crit Care Med* 1994;**22**:930–8.

26 Nishimura M, Hess D, Kacmarek RM, Ritz R, Hurford WE. Nitrogen dioxide production during mechanical ventilation with nitric oxide in adults. *Anesthesiology* 1995;**82**:1246–54.

27 Wysocki M, Delclaux C, Roupie E *et al*. Additive effect on gas exchange of inhaled nitric oxide and intravenous almitrine bismesylate in the adult respiratory distress syndrome. *Intens Care Med* 1994;**20**:254–9.

28 Cholet-Martin S, Gatecel C, Kerrmarrec N, Gougerot-Pocidalo MA, Payen DM. Alveolar neutrophil functions and cytokine levels in patients with adult respiratory distress syndrome during nitric oxide inhalation. *Am J Respir Crit Care Med* 1996;**153**:985–90.

29 Mourgeon E, Gallart L, Umamheswara Rao GS *et al*. Distribution of inhaled nitric oxide during sequential and continuous administration into the inspiratory limb of the ventilator. *Intensive Care Med* 1997;**23**:in press.

30 Zapol WM, Rimar S, Gillis N, Bosken CH. Nitric oxide and the lung. *Am J Respir Crit Care Med* 1994;**149**:1375–80.

31 Moutafis M, Hatahet Z, Castelain MH, Renaudin MH, Monnot A, Fischler M. Validation of a simple method assessing nitric oxide and nitrogen dioxide concentrations. *Intens Care Med* 1995;**21**:537–41.

32 Lu Q, Mourgeon E, Law-Koune JD *et al*. Dose–response of inhaled NO with and without intravenous almitrine in adult respiratory distress syndrome. *Anesthesiology* 1995;**83**:929–43.

33 Bauer MA, Utell MJ, Morrow PE, Speers DM, Gibb FR. Inhalation of 0·30 ppm nitrogen dioxide potentiates exercise-induced bronchospasm in asthmatics. *Am Rev Respir Dis* 1986;**134**:1203–8.

34 Hazucha MJ, Founsbee LJ, Sead E, Bromberg PA. Lung function response of healthy women after sequential exposures to NO_2 and O_3. *Am J Respir Crit Care Med* 1994;**150**:642–7.

35 Sandström T, Stjernberg N, Eklund A *et al*. Inflammatory cell response in bronchoalveolar lavage fluid after nitrogen dioxide exposure of healthy subjects: a dose–response study. *Eur Respir J* 1991;**3**:332–9.

36 Wennmaln A, Benthin G, Edlund A *et al*. Metabolism and excretion of nitric oxide in humans. An experimental and clinical study. *Circ Res* 1993;**73**:1121–7.

37 Young JD, Dyar O, Xiong L, Howell S. Methaemoglobin production in normal adults inhaling low concentrations of nitric oxide. *Intens Care Med* 1994;**20**:581–4.

38 Isomura K, Chikahira M, Terashini K, Hamada K. Induction of mutations and chromosome aberrations in lung cells following in vivo exposures to nitrogen oxides. *Mut Res* 1984;**136**:119–25.

39 Arroyo PL, Hatch-Pigott V, Mower HF, Cooney RV. Mutagenicity of nitric oxide and its inhibition by antioxidants. *Mut Res* 1992;**281**:193–202.

40 Nguyen T, Brunson D, Crospi CL, Penman BW, Wishnok JS, Tannenbaum SR. DNA damage and mutation in human cells exposed to nitric oxide *in vitro*. *Proc Natl Acad Sci* 1992;**89**:3030–4.

41 Wink DA, Kasprzak KS, Maragos CM *et al*. DNA deaminating ability and genotoxicity of nitric oxide and its progenitors. *Science* 1991;**254**:1001–3.

42 Beckman JS, Beckman TW, Marshall PA, Freeman BA. Apparent hydroxyl radical production by peroxynitrite: implications for endothelial injury from nitric oxide and superoxide. *Proc Natl Acad Sci* 1990;**87**:1620–4.

43 Haddad LY, Crow JP, Yaozu Y, Beckman J, Matalon S. Concurrent generation of nitric oxide and superoxide damages surfactant protein A (SP-A). *Am J Respir Crit Care Med Suppl* 1994;**149**:A549 (Abstract).

44 Greenbaum R, Bay J, Hargreaves MD *et al*. Effects of higher oxides of nitrogen in the anaesthetized dog. *Br J Anaesth* 1967;**39**:393–404.

45 Oda H, Nogami H, Kusumotos S, Nakajima T, Kurata A, Imai K. Long-term exposure to nitric oxide in mice. *J Jpn Soc Air Pollut* 1976;**11**:150–60.

46 Oda H, Nogami H, Kusumoto S, Nakajima T, Kurata A. Lifetime exposure to 2·4 ppm nitric oxide in mice. *Env Res* 1980;**22**:254–63.

47 Mercer R, Costa D, Crapo J. Effects of prolonged exposure to low doses of nitric oxide or nitrogen dioxide on the alveolar septa of the adult rat. *Lab Invest* 1995;**73**:20–8.

48 Gessler P, Nebe T, Birle A, Mueller W, Kachel W. A new side effect of inhaled nitric oxide in neonates and infants with pulmonary hypertension: functional impairment of the neutrophil respiratory burst. *Intens Care Med* 1996;**22**:252–8.

49 Foubert L, Fleming B, Latimer R *et al.* Safety guidelines for use of nitric oxide. *Lancet* 1992;**339**:1615–16.

50 Westfelt U, Lundin S, Stenqvist O. Safety aspects of delivery and monitoring of nitric oxide during mechanical ventilation. *Acta Anaesthesiol Scand*, 1996;**40**:302–10.

51 Mann SFP, Williams DJ, Amy GC, Man CGW, Lien DC. Sequential changes in canine pulmonary epithelial and endothelial cell functions after nitrogen dioxide. *Am Rev Respir Dis* 1990;**142**:199–205.

52 Ranga V, Kleinerman J, Ip MPC, Collins AM. The effect of nitrogen dioxide on tracheal uptake and transport of horseradish peroxidase in the guinea pig. *Am Rev Respir Dis* 1980;**122**:483–90.

53 Guth DJ, Mavis RD. Biochemical assessment of acute nitrogen dioxide toxicity in rat lung. *Toxicol Appl Pharmacol* 1985;**81**:128–38.

54 Stavert DM, Lehnert BE. Nitrogen oxide and nitrogen dioxide as inducers of acute pulmonary injury when inhaled at relatively high concentrations for brief periods. *Inhal Toxicol* 1990;**2**:53–7.

55 Ben-Jebria A, Marthan R, Savineau JP. Effect of *in vitro* nitrogen dioxide exposure on human bronchial smooth muscle response. *Am Rev Respir Dis* 1992;**146**:378–82.

56 Frampton MW, Morrow PE, Cox C, Gibb FR, Speers DM, Utell MJ. Effects of nitrogen dioxide exposure on pulmonary function and airway reactivity in normal humans. *Am Rev Respir Dis* 1991;**143**:522–7.

57 Rose RM, Fugelstad JM, Skornik WA *et al.* The pathophysiology of enhanced susceptibility to murine cytomegalovirus respiratory infection during short-term exposure to 5 ppm nitrogen dioxide. *Am Rev Respir Dis* 1988;**137**:912–17.

58 Radermacher P, Santak B, Becker H, Falke KJ. Prostaglandin E1 and nitroglycerin reduce pulmonary capillary pressure but worsen ventilation-perfusion distributions in patients with adult respiratory distress syndrome. *Anesthesiology* 1989;**70**:601–6.

59 Radermacher P, Santak B, Wüst HJ, Tarnow J, Falke KJ. Prostacyclin for the treatment of pulmonary hypertension in patients with acute respiratory distress syndrome: effects on pulmonary capillary pressure and ventilation–perfusion distributions. *Anesthesiology* 1990;**72**:238–44.

60 Stamler JS, Loh E, Roddy MA, Currie KE, Creager MA. Nitric oxide regulates basal systemic and pulmonary vascular resistance in healthy humans. *Circulation* 1994;**89**:2035–40.

61 Frostell CG, Blomqvist H, Hedenstierna G, Lundberg J, Zapol WM. Inhaled nitric oxide selectively reverses human hypoxic pulmonary vasoconstriction without causing systemic vasodilation. *Anesthesiology* 1993;**78**:427–35.

62 Puybasset L, Rouby JJ, Mourgeon E *et al.* Factors influencing cardiopulmonary effects of inhaled nitric oxide in acute respiratory failure. *Am J Respir Crit Care Med* 1995;**152**:318–28.

63 Langleben D, Demarchie M, Laporta D, Spanier AH, Schlesinger RD, Stewart DJ. Endothelin-1 in acute lung injury and the adult respiratory distress syndrome. *Am Rev Respir Dis* 1993;**148**:1646–50.

64 Zapol WM, Snider MT, Rie MA, Quinn DA, Frikker M. Pulmonary circulation during adult respiratory distress syndrome. In: Zapol WM and Falke KJ (eds). *Acute respiratory failure.* New York: Dekker, 1985:209–26 (*Lung biology in health and disease,* vol. 24).

65 Fierobe L, Brunet F, Dhainaut JF *et al.* Effect of inhaled nitric oxide on right ventricular function in adult respiratory distress syndrome. *Am J Respir Crit Care Med* 1995;**151**:1414–19.

66 Rossaint R, Slama K, Steudel W *et al.* Effects of inhaled nitric oxide on right ventricular function in severe acute respiratory distress syndrome. *Intens Care Med* 1995;**21**:197–203.

67 Kurrek MM, Castillo L, Bloch KD, Tannenbaum SR, Zapol WM. Inhaled nitric oxide does not alter endotoxin-induced nitric oxide synthase activity during rat lung perfusion. *J Appl Physiol* 1995;**79**:1088–92.

68 Gattinoni L, Pesenti A, Avalli L, Rossi F, Bombino M. Pressure–volume curve of total

respiratory system in acute respiratory failure. Computed tomographic scan study. *Am Rev Respir Dis* 1987;**136**:730–6.

69 Loh E, Stamler JS, Hare JM, Loscalzo J, Colucci WS. Cardiovascular effects of inhaled nitric oxide in patients with left ventricular dysfunction. *Circulation* 1994;**90**:2780–5.

70 Bocchi EA, Bacal F, Costa Auter JO, De Carvalho C, Bellotti G, Pileggi F. Inhaled nitric oxide leading to pulmonary edema in stable severe heart failure. *Am J Cardiol* 1994;**74**:70–72.

71 Kieler-Jensen N, Ricksten SE, Stenqvist O *et al.* Inhaled nitric oxide in the evaluation of heart transplant candidates with elevated pulmonary vascular resistance. *J Heart Lung Transplant* 1994;**13**:366–75.

72 Semigran RCS, Cockrill BA, Kacmarek R *et al.* Hemodynamic effects of inhaled nitric oxide in patients with left ventricular dysfunction. *J Am Coll Cardiol* 1994;**24**:982–8.

73 Koizumi T, Gupta R, Banerjee M, Newman JH. Changes in pulmonary vascular tone during exercise. Effects of nitric oxide synthase inhibition, L-arginine infusion and NO inhalation. *J Clin Invest* 1994;**94**:2275–82.

74 Lindeborg DM, Kavanagh BP, Van Meurs K, Pearl RG. Inhaled nitric oxide does not alter the longitudinal distribution of pulmonary vascular resistance. *J Appl Physiol* 1995;**78**:341–8.

75 Benzing A, Geiger K. Inhaled nitric oxide lowers pulmonary capillary pressure and changes longitudinal distribution of pulmonary vascular resistance in patients with acute lung injury. *Acta Anaesthesiol Scand* 1994;**38**:640–5.

76 Jones R, Langleben D, Reid LM. Patterns and mechanisms of remodeling of the pulmonary circulation in acute and subacute lung injury. In: Said SI (ed). *The pulmonary circulation and acute lung injury*. Mount Kisko, NY: Futura, 1991:179–242.

77 Scott-Burden T, Vanhoutte PM. The endothelium as a regulator of vascular smooth proliferation. *Circulation* 1993;**87**:(Suppl V):V51–V55.

78 Roberts JD, Roberts CT, Jones RC, Zapol WM, Bloch KD. Continuous nitric oxide inhalation reduces pulmonary structural changes, right ventricular hypertrophy and growth retardation in the hypoxic newborn rat. *Circ Res* 1995;**76**:215–22.

79 Putensen C, Räsänen J, Lopez FA, Downs JB. Continuous positive airway pressure modulates effect of inhaled nitric oxide on the ventilation–perfusion distribution in canine lung injury. *Chest* 1994;**106**:1563–9.

80 Fellahi JL, Mourgeon E, Goarin JP *et al.* Inhaled nitric oxide-induced closure of a patent foramen avale in a patient with adult respiratory distress syndrome and life-threatening hypoxemia. *Anesthesiology* 1995;**83**:635–8.

81 Hagen PT, Scholz DG, Edwards WD. Incidence and size of patent foramen ovale during first decades of life: an autopsy study of 965 normal hearts. *Mayo Clin Proc* 1984;**59**:17–20.

82 Estagnasié P, Le Bourdeles G, Mier L, Coste F, Dreyfuss D. Use of inhaled nitric oxide to reverse flow through a patent foramen ovale during pulmonary embolism. *Ann Intern Med* 1994;**120**:757–9.

83 Stewart TE, Rouby JJ, Puybasset L, Mourgeon E, Descouls AM, Viars P. Inhaled NO reduces alveolar dead space in patients with ARDS and pulmonary hypertension. *Am J Respir Crit Care Med* 1994;**149**(Suppl):A424 (Abstract).

84 Dupuy PM, Shore SA, Drazen JM, Frostell C, Hill WA, Zapol WM. Bronchodilator action of inhaled nitric oxide in guinea pigs. *J Clin Invest* 1992;**90**:421–8.

85 Högman M, Frostell CG, Arnberg H, Hedenstierna G. Inhalation of nitric oxide modulates metacholine induced bronchoconstriction in the rabbit. *Eur Respir J* 1993;**6**:177–80.

86 Puybasset L, Mourgeon E, Segal E, Bodin L, Rouby JJ, Viars P. Effects of inhaled nitric oxide on respiratory resistance in patients with ARDS. *Anesthesiology* 1993;**79**(Suppl 3A):A299 (Abstract).

87 Law-Koune JD, Roche S, Mourgeon E *et al.* Acute toxicity of inhaled NO in ARDS. *Anesthesiology* 1994;**81**(Suppl 3A):A263 (Abstract).

88 Högman M, Frostell CG, Hedenström H, Hedenstierna G. Inhalation of nitric oxide modulates adult bronchial tone. *Am Rev Respir Dis* 1993;**148**:1474–8.

89 Heffner JE, Sahn SA, Repine JE. The role of platelets in the adult respiratory distress syndrome. Culprits or bystander? *Am J Respir Crit Care Med* 1987;**135**:482–92.

90 Loscalzo J. Antiplatelet and antithrombotic effect of organic nitrates. *Am J Cardiol* 1992;**70**:18B–22B.

91 Radomski MW, Moncada S. Regulation of vascular homeostasis by nitric oxide. *Thromb Haemost* 1993;**70**:36–41.

92 Mellion BT, Ignarro LJ, Ohlstein EH, Pontecorvo EG, Hyman AL, Kadowitz PJ. Evidence for the inhibitory role of guanosine 3í5í monophosphate in ADP induced human platelet aggregation in the presence of nitric oxide and related vasodilators. *Blood* 1981;**57**:946–55.

93 Salvemini D, Radziszewski W, Korbut R, Vane J. The use of oxyhaemoglobin to explore the events underlying inhibition of platelet aggregation induced by NO or NO-donors. *Br J Pharmacol* 1990;**101**:991–5.

94 Furchgott RF. Studies on relaxation of rabbit aorta by sodium nitrite: the basis for the proposal that acid-activatable inhibitory factor from bovine retractor penis is inorganic nitrite and the endothelium-derived relaxing factor is nitric oxide. In: Vanhoutte PM, ed. *Vasodilatation: vascular smooth muscle, peptides, autonomic nerves and endothelium.* New York: Raven Press, 1988:401–14.

95 Samama CM, Diaby M, Fellahi JL *et al.* Inhibition of platelet aggregation by inhaled nitric oxide in patients with adult respiratory distress syndrome. *Anesthesiology* 1995;**83**:56–65.

96 Umamaheswara Rao GS, Lu Q, Diaby M *et al.* Inhibition of platelet aggregation by inhaled nitric oxide in ARDS patients – a dose–effect study. *Br J Anaesth* 1996;**76**(Suppl 2):112,A360 (Abstract).

97 Högman M, Frostell CG, Arnberg H, Sandhagen B, Hedenstierna G. Prolonged bleeding time during NO inhalation in the rabbit. *Acta Physiol Scand* 1994;**151**:125–9.

98 Högman M, Frostell CG, Arnberg H, Hedenstierna G. Bleeding time prolongation and NO inhalation. *Lancet* 1993;**341**:1664–5.

99 Rodgers C, Levin J. A critical reappraisal of the bleeding time. *Serim Thromb Hemost* 1990;**16**:1–20.

100 Golino P, Capelli-Bigazzi E, Ambrosio G *et al.* Endothelium-derived relaxing factor modulates platelet aggregation in an *in vivo* model of recurrent platelet activation. *Circ Res* 1992;**71**:1447–56.

101 Yao SK, Ober JC, Krishnaswami A *et al.* Endogenous nitric oxide protects against platelet aggregation and cyclic flow variations in stenosed and endothelium-injured arteries. *Circulation* 1992;**86**:1302–9.

102 Folts JD. An *in vivo* model of experimental arterial stenosis, intimal damage, and periodic thrombosis. *Circulation* 1991;**83**(S IV):4–14.

103 Blomquist H, Wickert CJ, Andreen M, Ullergberg U, Ortquist A, Frostell C. Enhanced pneumonia resolution by inhalation of nitric oxide. *Acta Anaesthesiol Scand* 1993;**37**:110–14.

104 Benzing A, Brautigam P, Geiger K, Loop T, Beyer U, Moser E. Inhaled nitric oxide reduces pulmonary transvascular albumin flux in patients with acute lung injury. *Anesthesiology* 1995;**83**:1153–61.

105 Garg UC, Hassid A. Nitric oxide-generating vasodilators and 8-bromo cyclic guanosine monophosphate inhibit mitogenesis and proliferation of cultured rat vascular smooth muscle cells. *J Clin Invest* 1989;**83**:1774–7.

106 Rimar S, Gillis CN. Pulmonary vasodilation by inhaled nitric oxide after endothelial injury. *J Appl Physiol* 1992;**73**:2179–83.

107 White CW, Nguyen DH, Tuder R. Nitric oxide modulation of hyperoxic injury. *Am J Respir Crit Care Med* 1994;**149**(Suppl):A548 (Abstract).

108 Berisha H, Pakbaz H, Absood A, Said SI. Excess nitric oxide (NO) production in acute lung injury: role of constitutive vs inducible NO synthase. *Am J Respir Crit Care Med* 1994;**149**:A552.

109 Rovira I, Chen TY, Winkler M, Kawai N, Bloch KD, Zapol WM. Effects of inhaled nitric oxide on pulmonary hemodynamics and gas exchange in an ovine model of ARDS. *J Appl Physiol* 1994;**76**:345–55.

110 Rich FR, Roos CM, Anderson SM, Urich DC, Daugherty MO, Johns RA. Inhaled nitric oxide: dose response and the effects of blood in the isolated rat lung. *J Appl Physiol* 1993;**75**:1278–84.

111 Gerlach H, Pappert D, Lewandowski K, Rossaint R, Falke KJ. Long-term inhalation with evaluated low doses of nitric oxide for selective improvement in oxygenation in patients with adult respiratory distress syndrome. *Intens Care Med* 1993;**19**:443–9.

112 Lowson S, Rich G, McArdle P, Jaidev J, Morris G. The response to varying concentrations of inhaled nitric oxide in patients with acute respiratory distress syndrome. *Anesth Analg* 1996;**82**:574–81.

113 Gerlach H, Rossaint R, Pappert D, Falke KJ. Time-course and dose–response of nitric oxide inhalation for systemic oxygenation and pulmonary hypertension in patients with adult respiratory distress syndrome. *Eur J Clin Invest* 1993;**23**:499–502.

114 Mourgeon E, Puybusset, L, Law-Koune JD *et al.* Inhaled NO in ARDS with and without septic shock: dose–response curves. *Critical Care* 1997 (in press).

115 Journois D, Poulard P, Mauriat P, Malhère T, Vouhé P, Safran D. Inhaled nitric oxide as a therapy for pulmonary hypertension after operations for congenital defects. *J Thorac Cardiovasc Surg* 1994;**107**:1129–35.

116 Sellden H, Winberg P, Gustafsson LE, Lundell BO, Book K, Frostell CG. Inhalation of nitric oxide reduced pulmonary hypertension after cardiac surgery in a 3·2 kg infant. *Anesthesiology* 1993;**78**:577–80.

117 Tiner NN, Etches RC, Kamstra B, Tierney AJ, Peliowski A, Ryan A. Inhaled nitric oxide in infants referred to extracorporeal membrane oxygenation: dose–response. *J Pediatr* 1994;**124**:302–8.

118 Day RW, Guarin M, Lynch JM, Vernon DD, Dean JM. Inhaled nitric oxide in children with severe lung disease: results of acute and prolonged therapy with two concentrations. *Crit Care Med* 1996;**24**:215–21.

119 Pappert D, Busch T, Gerlach H, Lewandowski K, Radermacher P, Rossaint R. Aerosolized prostacyclin versus inhaled nitric oxide in children with severe acute respiratory distress syndrome. *Anesthesiology* 1995;**82**:1507–11.

120 Walmrath D, Schneider T, Pilch J, Grimminger F, Seeger W. Aerosolized prostacyclin reduces pulmonary artery pressure and improves gas exchange in adult respiratory distress syndrome. *Lancet* 1993;**342**:961–2.

121 Walmrath D, Schneider T, Pilch J, Schermuly R, Grimminger F, Seeger W. Effects of aerosolized prostacyclin in severe pneumonia – impact of fibrosis. *Am J Respir Crit Care Med* 1995;**151**:724–30.

122 Zwissler B, Rank N, Jaenicke U *et al.* Selective pulmonary vasodilation by inhaled prostacyclin in a newborn with congenital heart disease and cardiopulmonary bypass. *Anesthesiology* 1995;**82**:1512–16.

123 Kerins DM, Murray R, Fitzgerald GA. Prostacyclin and prostagandin E1: molecular mechanisms and therapeutic utility. *Progr Hemost Thromb* 1991;**10**:307–37.

124 Walmrath D, Schneider T, Schermuly R, Olschewski H, Grimminger F, Seeger W. Direct comparison of inhaled nitric oxide and aerosolised prostacyclin in acute respiratory distress syndrome. *Am J Respir Crit Care Med* 1996;**153**:991–6.

125 Parsargiklian M, Bianco S. Ventilatory and cardiovascular effects of prostacyclin and 6-oxo-PGF2 a by inhalation. *Adv Prostaglandin Thromboxane Res* 1980;**7**:943–51.

126 Reyes A, Roca J, Rodriguez-Roisin R, Torres A, Ussetti P, Wagner PD. Effect of almitrine on ventilation-perfusion distribution in adult respiratory distress syndrome. *Am Rev Respir Dis* 1988;**137**:1062–7.

127 Naeije R, Melot C, Mois P. Effects of almitrine in decompensated chronic respiratory insufficiency. *Bull Eur Physiopath Respir* 1981;**17**:153–61.

128 Dreyfuss D, Djedaini K, Lanore JJ, Mier L, Froidevaux R, Coste F. A comparative study of the effects of almitrine bismesylate and lateral position during unilateral bacterial pneumonia with severe hypoxemia. *Am Rev Respir Dis* 1992;**146**:295–9.

129 Leeman M, Delcroix M, Vachiery JL, Mélot C, Naeije R, Almitrine and doxapram in experimental lung injury. *Am Rev Respir Dis* 1992;**145**:1042–6.

130 Chen L, Miller FL, Malmkvist G, Clergue F, Marschall C, Marschall BE. High-dose almitrine bismesylate inhibits hypoxic pulmonary vasoconstriction in closed chest dogs. *Anesthesiology* 1987;**67**:534–42.

131 Naeije R, Lejeune P, Vachiery JL *et al.* Restored hypoxic pulmonary vasoconstriction by peripheral chemoreceptor agonists in dogs. *Am Rev Respir Dis* 1990;**142**:789–95.

132 Gottshall EB, Fernyak S, Wuertemberger G, Voelkel AF. Almitrine mimics hypoxic

vasoconstriction in isolated rat lungs. *Am J Physiol* 1992;**263**:383–91.

133 Leeman M. The pulmonary circulation in acute lung injury: a review of some recent advances. *Intens Care Med* 1991;**17**:254–60.

134 Payen D, Gatecel C, Plaisance P. Almitrine effect on nitric oxide inhalation in adult respiratory distress syndrome. *Lancet* 1993;**341**:1664.

135 Roche S, Lu Q, Law-Koune JD *et al.* Effects of combining inhaled NO and intravenous almitrine in patients with ARDS. *Anesthesiology* 1994;**81**:A264 (Abstract).

136 Gallart L, Umamaheswara Rao G, Law-Koune J *et al.* Almitrine alone or in combination with inhaled nitric oxide: dose-response curves in patients with ARDS (abstract). *Br J Anaesth* 1996;**76**(Suppl 2):114.

137 Bromet N, Singlas E. Pharmacocinétique clinique du bismésylate d'almitrine. *Presse Méd* 1984;**13**:2071–7.

138 Aubert Y, Baune A, Courbe S, Guillaudeux J, Bromet N. Pharmacocinétique du bismésilate d'almitrine chez l'homme. *Bull Physio Respir* 1982;**18**(Suppl 4):307–14.

139 Tweeny J, Evans TW, Waterhouse JC, Nicoll J, Suggett AJ, Howard P. Long term oxygen therapy and almitrine bismesylate. In: Allegra L and Rizzato G (eds). *Bronch Emphys,* 1985:A171.

140 Stradling JR, Barnes P, Pride NB. The effects of almitrine on the ventilatory response to hypoxia and hypercapnia in normal subjects. *Clin Sci* 1982;**63**:401–4.

141 Wounters EFM, Greve LH, Steenhuis ES, Gimeno F. Almitrine and peripheral neuropathy. *Lancet* 1988;**ii**:336.

142 McLeed CM, Thomas RW, Bartley EA, Parkhurst GW, Bachaud RT. Effect of handling of almitrine bismesylate in healthy subjects. *Eur J Respir Dis* 1983;**64**:275–89.

143 Bouche P, Lacomblez L, Leger JM *et al.* Peripheral neuropathies during treatment with almitrine: report of 46 cases. *J Neurol* 1989;**236**:29–33.

144 Julou-Schaeffer G, Gray GA, Fleming I, Schott C, Parratt JR, Stoclet JC. Loss of vascular responsiveness induced by endotoxin involves L-arginine pathway. *Am J Physiol* 1990;**259** (Heart Circ. Physiol. 28):H1038–1043.

145 Ristimaki A, Garfinkel S, Wessendorf J, Maciag T, Hla T. Induction of cyclo-oxygenase-2 by interleukin-1 alpha. *J Biol Chem* 1994;**269**:11769–75.

146 Fu J, Masferrer JL, Seibert K, Raz A, Needleman P. The induction and suppression of prostaglandin H2 synthase (cyclo-oxygenase) in human monocytes. *J Biol Chem* 1990;**265**:16737–40.

147 Maier JAM, Hia T, Maciag T. Cyclo-oxygenase is an immediate-early gene induced by interleukin-1 in human endothelial cells. *J Biol Chem* 1990;**265**:10805–8.

148 Pritchard KA, O'Banion MK, Miano JM *et al.* Induction of cyclo-oxygenase-2 in rat vascular smooth muscle cells *in vitro* and *in vivo. J Biol Chem* 1994;**269**:8504–9.

149 Liu S, Crawley DE, Barnes PJ, Evans TW. Endothelium-derived relaxing factor inhibits hypoxic pulmonary vasoconstriction in rats. *Am Rev Respir Dis* 1991;**143**:32–7.

150 Leeman M, de Beyl VZ, Delcroix M, Naeije R. Effects of endogenous nitric oxide on pulmonary vascular tone in intact dogs. *Am J Physiol* 1994;**266** (Heart Circ Physiol. 35): H2343–H2347.

151 Sprague RS, Thiemermann C, Vane JR. Endogenous endothelium-derived relaxing factor opposes hypoxic pulmonary vasoconstriction and supports blood flow to hypoxic alveoli in anesthetized rabbits. *Proc Natl Acad Sci* 1992;**89**:8711–15.

152 Putensen C, Räsänen J, Downs JB. Effect of endogenous and inhaled nitric oxide on the ventilation–perfusion relationships in oleic-acid lung injury. *Am J Respir Crit Care Med* 1994;**150**:330–6.

153 Lorente JA, Landin L, de Pablo R, Renes E, Liste D. L-arginine pathway in the sepsis syndrome. *Crit Care Med* 1993;**21**:1287–95.

154 Brimioulle S, Lejeune P, Vachiéry JL *et al.* Stimulus–response curve of hypoxic pulmonary vasoconstriction in intact dogs: effects of ASA. *Am J Physiol* 1994;**77**:476–80.

155 Leeman M, Lejeune P, Hallemans R, Mélot C, Naeije R. Effects of increased pulmonary vascular tone on gas exchange in canine oleic pulmonary edema. *J Appl Physiol* 1988;**65**:662–8.

156 Leeman M, Delcroix M, Vachiéry JL, Mélot C, Naeije R. Blunted hypoxic vasoconstriction in oleic acid lung injury: effect of cyclo-oxygenase inhibitors. *J Appl Physiol*

1992;72:251–8.

157 Schulman LL, Lennon PF, Ratner SJ, Enson Y. Meclofenamate enhances blood oxygenation in acute oleic acid lung injury. *J Appl Physiol* 1988;**64**:710–18.

158 Hales CA, Peterson M, Kong D, Miller M, Watkins WD. Role of thromboxane and prostacyclin in pulmonary vasomotor changes after endotoxin in dogs. *J Clin Invest* 1981;**68**:497–505.

159 Graham LM, Vasil A, Vasil ML, Voelkel NF, Stenmark KR. Decreased pulmonary vasoreactivity in an animal model of chronic pseudomonas pneumonia. *Am Rev Respir Dis* 1990;**142**:221–9.

160 Schuster DP, Sandiford P, Stephenson AH. Thromboxane receptor stimulation: inhibition and perfusion redistribution after acute lung injury. *J Appl Physiol* 1993;**75**:2069–78.

161 Janssens SP, Musto SW, Hutchinson WG, *et al.* Cyclo-oxygenase and lipooxygenase inhibition by BW-755C reduces acrolein smoke-induced acute lung injury. *J Appl Physiol* 1994;**77**:888–95.

162 Hanly PJ, Roberts D, Dobson K. Light RB. Effect of indomethacin on arterial oxygenation in critically ill patients with severe bacterial pneumonia. *Lancet* 1987;**i**: 351–4.

163 Steinberg SM, Rodriguez JL, Bitzer LG, Kelley KA, Flint LM. Indomethacin treatment of human adult respiratory distress syndrome. *Circ Shock* 1990;**30**:375–84.

164 Gattinoni L, Pesenti A, Bombino M, *et al.* Relationships between lung computer tomographic density, gas exchange, and PEEP in acute respiratory failure. *Anesthesiology* 1988;**69**:824–32.

165 Greene R, Zapol WM, Snider MT *et al.* Early bedside detection of pulmonary vascular occlusion during acute respiratory failure. *Am Rev Respir Dis* 1981;**124**:593–601.

166 Rouby JJ, Lherm T, Martin de Lassale E *et al.* Histologic aspects of pulmonary barotrauma in critically ill patients with acute respiratory failure. *Intens Care Med* 1993;**20**:187–92.

167 Dreyfuss D, Soler P, Basset G, Saumon G. High inflation pressure pulmonary edema. Respective effects of high airway pressure, high tidal volume, and positive end-expiratory pressure. *Am Rev Respir Dis* 1988;**137**:1159–64.

168 Hickling KG, Henderson SJ, Jackson R. Low mortality associated with low volume pressure limited ventilation with permissive hypercapnia in severe adult respiratory distress syndrome. *Intens Care Med* 1990;**16**:372–7.

169 Offner B, Czachurski J, König SA, Seller H. Different effects of respiratory and metabolic acidosis on preganglionic sympathetic nerve activity. *J Appl Physiol* 1994;**77**:173–8.

170 Viles PH, Shepherd JT. Relationship between pH, PO_2, and PCO_2 on the pulmonary vascular bed of the cat. *Am J Physiol* 1968;**215**:1170–6.

171 Viles PH, Shepherd JT. Evidence for a dilator action of carbon dioxide on the pulmonary vessels of the cat. *Circ Res* 1968;**22**:325–32.

172 Brimioulle S, Vachiéry JL, Lejeune P, Leeman M, Melot C, Naeije R. Acid-base status affects gas exchange in canine oleic acid pulmonary edema. *Am J Physiol* 1991;**260** (Heart Circ Physiol 29):H1080–1086.

173 Ranieri VM, Mascia LM, Fiore T, Bruno F, Brienza A, Giuliani R. Cardiorespiratory effects of positive end-expiratory pressure during progressive tidal volume reduction (permissive hypercapnia) in patients with acute respiratory distress syndrome. *Anesthesiology* 1995;**83**:710–20.

13: Cardioactive drugs: future directions

PHILIPPE LECHAT

The pharmaceutical industry is still very actively developing new cardio-active drugs. The research of the past 20 years has promoted a high level of knowledge of physiopathological processes and therapeutic targets in the different fields of cardiovascular disease, and therapeutic advances have been achieved. Anaesthesiologists, then, will have to manage patients being treated with such new drugs, giving rise to new questions and possibly producing hitherto unseen interactions with anaesthetic procedures.

Antihypertensive drugs

In the field of hypertension, it is basically the impact of antihypertensive treatment on complicating events such as stroke and myocardial infarction that is currently under evaluation with compounds such as calcium antagonists and ACE inhibitors. Indeed, the main objective of anti-hypertensive treatment is to prevent long-term complications. This was demonstrated in the early 1980s with diuretics or β-blockers. The well-known meta-analysis of MacMahon[1] showed that antihypertensive treatment with diuretics or β-blockers reduced the risk of stroke by 42% as expected, but the risk of coronary events only by 14%. This lower than expected effect on coronary events was interpreted as an insufficient correction of other coronary risk factors such as hypercholesterolaemia, diabetes or tobacco use.

This prompted the development of calcium antagonists and ACE inhibitors as antihypertensive agents acting directly on the function and structure of large systemic vessels and without potential deleterious effects on lipid profile or glucose metabolism. Results of large scale trials with such drugs will be available by the end of the 1990s. They will be particularly important since a controversy has arisen about the potential deleterious effects of some calcium antagonists, especially the short-acting dihydropyr-idines, during long-term treatment in patients with coronary disease.[2, 3]

A new class of antihypertensive drugs has recently emerged: the angiotensin II receptor antagonists such as losartan, valsartan, candesartan etc. The potential therapeutic interest of this group of drugs is twofold: first, they should not induce the bradykinin-related side effects of ACE inhibitors such as cough, which occurs in 10–20% of patients receiving ACE inhibitors. Secondly, since they competitively block angiotensin II receptors (AT_1), they should suppress angiotensin II effects better than ACE. Indeed, blockade of converting enzyme favours other metabolic pathways leading to angiotensin II synthesis, the chymase pathway particularly. However, the real importance of such converting-enzyme-independent angiotensin II synthesis in man is not well known. In addition, since bradykinin breakdown reduction by ACE inhibitors could also participate in their therapeutic effect, angiotensin II receptor antagonists may not provide a similar therapeutic profile.

Combination of both types of drugs may provide a particularly synergic action (if tolerated) in hypertension, but also in heart failure.

Another still unclear point with angiotensin II receptor antagonists is the respective role of the two angiotensin receptor subtypes AT_1 and AT_2.[4] The majority of physiological effects of angiotensin are related to AT_1 receptors but the role of AT_2 receptors is still unclear. Since angiotensin II receptor antagonists selectively compete with AT_1 receptors, and since plasma angiotensin II levels increase during such a treatment, AT_2 receptors will be over-stimulated. Consequences of such a stimulation are so far unknown.

Therefore, many investigations are ongoing to further delineate the most appropriate clinical use of angiotensin II receptor antagonists, while allowing a better understanding of the role and function of the renin–angiotensin system.

Inhibition of neutral endopeptidase preventing the degradation of atrial natriuretic peptide has been a focus of antihypertensive drug development. The observed clinical efficacy has not, however, achieved a sufficient level to prompt the development of such agents. Indeed, renal and vascular atrial natriuretic peptide receptors are rapidly downregulated when plasma ANP concentrations increase, which greatly limits chronic efficacy. Some compounds, such as candoxatril, are still of value, however, especially in heart failure. Since ANP inhibits renin release and reduces angiotensin II effects, compounds inhibiting both angiotensin-converting enzyme and the neutral endopeptidase have been studied but have not yet reached a high level of clinical development. Such compounds may, however, be available for treatment of hypertension and heart failure.

Coronary artery disease

Coronary artery disease has benefitted in the past ten years from the introduction and extensive use of angioplasty of coronary stenosis and, more recently, from the complementary actions of stent application.[5] These developments have led to new therapeutic problems and their active investigation. Breakthroughs are sought in two important areas: the prevention of restenosis and the anti-thrombotic regimen associated with these interventional procedures.

Post-angioplasty restenosis occurs several months after coronary angioplasty and appears to be secondary to a myocyte cell proliferation. The pathophysiology of such a process remains unclear but has triggered very extensive experimental and clinical research to find an effective preventive treatment.[6] Such a therapy has not yet been found, and no medical treatment appears able to prevent the restenosis phenomenon. The only procedure which has provided consistent results is post-angioplasty stent application.[5] The cost of stents has so far prevented extensive application of the technique, but this situation should change in the future. Another very promising strategy is delivery via the angioplasty catheter of substances to the very site of coronary lesions during the dilatation procedure. Anti-thrombotic agents can be delivered by this means to avoid immediate thrombosis complications (heparin-coated balloons for example), but more specifically, the technique has been used for gene therapy, aiming at inhibition of cell proliferation by local delivery of anti-sense coding genetic material using adenovirus as the vector. This exciting research is still in the initial phase, but will very likely lead to future developments.

Anti-thrombotic treatments

The 'interventional' era in the treatment of coronary disease, which followed the tremendous development of angioplasty and stents for the treatment of coronary stenoses, has induced clinical situations associated with a high risk of arterial thrombosis. Aggressive anti-thrombotic treatments have thus been developed, with a search for new anti-thrombotic agents. Thus, after the fibrinolytic era of the 1980s, the 1990s are presently the decade of study of two new therapeutic categories: the anti-thrombin agents and the fibrinogen GP. IIb–IIIa platelet-receptor antagonists.

The potential interest of anti-thrombin agents such as hirudine and hirulog is based on their action on thrombin that is bound to the fibrin clot and still activates fibrinogen clivage into fibrin. In contrast, "standard" anti-thrombin therapy with heparin only neutralises the circulatory thrombin in the plasma.

Efficacy of such compounds in acute coronary syndromes and high-risk angioplasty has been rather disappointing, since it was close to that of heparin with a higher incidence of haemorrhagic complications.[7, 8] Initially, dosages used were too high; lower dose regimens, however, did not change efficacy but only reduced haemorrhagic complications. Therefore, quite apart from their high cost, these compounds are not likely to be extensively used in the future. Experience with the antagonists of the GP IIb–IIIa fibrinogen platelet receptors has been quite the opposite.[9, 10] Several compounds have been developed with the monoclonal antibody 7EC3 (Reo Pro®) which provides a significant reduction of complicating events after high-risk angioplasty and a reduction in the incidence of myocardial infarction following unstable angina. Several other compounds are also under study: integrelin, lamifiban, tirofiban.

These are the drugs of the future, but several questions remain to be answered: what is the role of associated treatments such as aspirin and heparin, that have always been associated with such compounds in the clinical trials, what is the optimal duration of such a treatment (intravenous administration) and what is the optimal level of inhibition of fibrinogen receptors that must be achieved?

Heart failure

Whatever its aetiology, alteration of left ventricular function is the result of an initial myocardial injury which induces an increased stress on remaining viable myocytes. Such a situation progressively alters their function and viability, leading to further loss of contractile tissue and progressive alteration of the disease. This process is accelerated by the deleterious consequences at the cellular level of the action of compensatory mechanisms, mainly represented by stimulation of both the sympathetic and the renin–angiotensin system.

Therapeutic strategy in heart failure is thus directly oriented towards both the reduction of loading cardiac conditions and also the inhibition of all neuro-hormone receptors involved in the actions of compensatory mechanisms. This explains the impressive development of drugs such as ACE inhibitors in heart failure. They reduce cardiac loading conditions and suppress the direct consequences of angiotensin II and aldosterone, namely potential deleterious cardiac effects, especially the stimulation of collagen synthesis.[11, 12]

ACE inhibitors have proved beneficial in all stages of heart failure, and in symptomatic patients such a treatment is combined with diuretics to counteract the sodium retention syndrome.

The question of the next therapeutic step is a matter of intense investigation and results of large-scale trials will tell us the value of additional blockade of adrenergic receptors (α- and especially β-adrenergic receptors), of angiotensin II receptors, of aldosterone receptors, and receptors of other substances whose production is stimulated in heart failure, such as endothelin.

Very promising results on morbidity end points and left ventricular ejection fraction have been obtained with administration of progressively increased doses of β-blockers,[13, 14] but demonstration of prognosis improvement requires the results of ongoing large-scale trials with mortality as a primary end point, such as CIBIS II with bisoprolol and BEST with bucindolol. Then, by the end of the 1990s we will obtain results of large-scale trials on the efficacy of β-blockers, angiotensin II antagonists, and aldosterone blockade in heart failure. Therapeutic strategy will obviously depend on such results.

Antiarrhythmic drugs

Antiarrhythmic drug development has been greatly influenced by the results of the CAST study,[15] which was prematurely stopped because of an increased death rate in the patients treated with class 1 antiarrhythmic therapy. Such patients were initially included if they displayed ventricular arrhythmias after myocardial infarction. The objective of antiarrhythmic therapy was first to suppress all arrhythmias and then to reduce mortality, especially 'arrhythmic' deaths. The overall adverse effect of such anti-arrhythmic treatment on mortality appears to be a consequence of the potential arrhythmogenic effects of these drugs, which becomes pre-dominant in low-risk patients.

In the most recent trials, other antiarrhythmic drugs, such as class 3 antiarrhythmic agents (amiodarane, sotalol), have not proved to be effective on mortality in patients with severe arrhythmias with or without altered ventricular function. This was the case with amiodarone, tested during the EMIAT and CAMIAT trials. No reduction in mortality was obtained. A reduction of presumed arrhythmic deaths was found but such a sub-group analysis does not change the conclusion of these trials and it is now well established that a very large proportion of the so-called sudden deaths in such patients are deaths not secondary to severe arrhythmias, but to electromechanical dissociation and asystole.

Another class 3 antiarrhythmic drug such as D sotalol which is also a weak β-blocker did not provide any benefit in post-myocardial infarction patients with altered left ventricular function and severe arrhythmias. Other antiarrhythmic agents are also under study but their therapeutic benefit is more focused on clinical symptoms and quality of life (especially in supraventricular arrhythmias) than on improved survival.

Most recently, new compounds acting on potassium currents in the autonomic cells of the sinus node have been discovered. They induce a reduction of heart rate and could be beneficial in angina pectoris and heart failure. Clinical development of such drugs is currently under way and they may provide a new therapeutic approach to some cardiac disorders.

Antiatherogenic drugs

Prevention of progression of the atherosclerosis process which induces the majority of cardiovascular ischaemic events through artery stenosis, occlusion or systemic emboli, provides a major therapeutic challenge.

The atherosclerotic process starts with an excess of lipid infiltration of the intimal region of the arterial wall. LDL lipoprotein is subsequently modified, oxidised and taken up by macrophages which degenerate into foam cells. Oxidation of LDL seems to trigger further inflammatory cell accumulation, myocyte migration from the intima toward the sub-endothelial space, and proliferation of such cells. Such a cellular infiltrative process leads to the formation of the atherosclerosis lesion, made of a central lipidic zone surrounded by cell proliferation (smooth muscle cells and monocyte macrophages).

Complications occur when the volume of the lesion reduces arterial flow but also when fissuration of the plaque induces platelet activation and thrombosis. Preventive treatment of such a process is primarily based on reduction of lipid infiltration of the arterial wall through reduction of plasma levels of lipoprotein, especially of low density lipoproteins and very atherogenic small lipid particles, such as lipoprotein Lpa.

The most effective lipid-lowering drugs are the inhibitors of the HMG Co-A reductase enzyme (statins). Large-scale trials have now clearly demonstrated that a reduction of total cholesterol and LDL cholesterol with this group of drugs is effective as primary or secondary prevention of mortality and myocardial infarction in patients with hyperlipidaemia, whatever the intial plasma cholesterol level, age, and sex of the patient.[16, 17] The cost-effectiveness of this long-term therapy, however, is likely to restrict treatment to secondary prevention or to primary prevention in high-risk patients. In the near future, different statins will be developed with still a greater efficacy on blood lipid levels.

Other antiatherogenic treatments have attempted to reduce either the proliferation of smooth muscle cells or the oxidation of lipoproteins in the arterial wall. Inhibition of smooth muscle proliferation is currently evaluated with different ACE inhibitors since angiotensin II induces stimulatory effects on such proliferation and migration. Preliminary results with quinapril, however, are negative. Larger scale trials are ongoing and will not be concluded before the end of the decade. Prevention of the oxidative process with anti-oxidants such as vitamin E is under evaluation and the results of such investigation should be available in the near future.

Conclusions

There is thus a high level of clinical investigation in the cardiovascular field which will give rise to therapeutic advances that the anaesthesiologist will have to face in the near future. For each new treatment, however, clinical research will have to delineate the benefit–risk ratio and define the characteristics of patients who will benefit most from these new treatments.

1 MacMahon S, Peto R, Cutler J, Collins R, Sorlic P, Neaton J *et al.* Blood pressure, stroke and coronary heart disease. *Lancet* 1990;**335**:765–74 (Part I); *Lancet* 1990;**335**:827–38 (Part II).

2 Furberg CD, Psaty BM, Meyer JV. Nifedipine – dose related increase in mortality in patients with coronary artery disease. *Circulation* 1995;**92**:1326–31.

3 Opic LH, Messerli FH. Nifedipine and mortality. Grave defects in the dossier. *Circulation* 1995;**92**:1068–73.

4 Timmermans P, Benfield P, Chiu AT, Herblin WF, Wong PC, Smith RD. Angiotensin II receptors and functional correlates. *Am J Hypertens* 1992;**5**:221S–235S.

5 Serruys PW, de Saegere P, Kiemeneij F *et al*, for the Benestent Study Group. A comparison of balloon expandable stent implantation with balloon angioplasty in patients with coronary artery disease. *N Engl J Med* 1994;**331**:489–95.

6 Serruys PW, Herrman JPR, Simon R *et al*, for the Helvetica investigators. A comparison of hirudin with heparin in the prevention of restenosis after coronary angioplasty. *N Engl J Med* 1995;**333**:757–63.

7 Topol EJ, Fuster V, Harrington R, Califf RM, Kleiman NS, Kereiakes DJ *et al.* Recombinant hirudin for unstable angina pectoris. A multicenter, randomized angiographic trial. *Circulation* 1994;**89**:1557–66.

8 Sharma GVRK, Lapsley D, Vita JA, Sharma S, Coccio E, Adelman B *et al.* Usefulness and tolerability of hirulog, a direct thrombin inhibitor, in unstable angina pectoris. *Am J Cardiol* 1993;**72**:1357–60.

9 Simoons ML, de Boer MJ, van den Brand M *et al*, and The European Cooperative Study Group. Randomized trial of a GP IIb/IIIa platelet receptor blocker in refractory unstable angina. *Circulation* 1994;**89**:596–603.

10 The EPIC investigators. Use of a monoclonal antibody directed against the platelet glycoprotein IIb/IIIa receptor in high risk coronary angioplasty. *N Engl J Med* 1994;**330**(14):956–61.

11 The SOLVD investigators. Effect of enalapril on survival in patients with reduced left ventricular ejection fraction and congestive heart failure. *N Engl J Med* 1991;**325**:293–301.

12 The consensus trial study group. Effects of enalapril on mortality in severe congestive heart failure: results of the cooperative North Scandinavian enalapril survival study. *N Engl J Med* 1987;**316**:1429–35.

13 CIBIS investigators and committees. A randomized trial of beta-blockade in heart failure. The cardiac insufficiency bisoprolol study. *Circulation* 1994;**90**:1765–73.

14 Packer M, Bristow MR, Cohn J, Colucci W, Fowler MB, Gilbert EM *et al*, for the US carvedilol heart failure study group. The effect of carvedilol on morbidity and mortality in patients with chronic heart failure. *N Engl J Med* 1996;**334**:1349–55.

15 The Cardiac Arrhythmia Suppression Trial (CAST) investigators. Increased mortality due to encainide or flecainide in a randomized trial of arrhythmia suppression after myocardial infarction. *N Engl J Med* 1989;**321**:406–12.

16 The Scandinavian Simvastatin Survival Study Group. Randomised trial of cholesterol lowering in 4444 patients with coronary heart disease: the Scandinavian Simvastatin Survival Study (4S). *Lancet* 1994;**344**:1383–9.

17 Sheperd J, Cobbe S, Ford I, Isles CG, Lorimer A, Macfarlane PW *et al*, for the West of Scotland Prevention Study Group. Prevention of coronary heart disease with pravastatin in men with hypercholesterolemia. *N Engl J Med* 1995;**333**:1301–7.

Index

acadesine 169
acebutolol 5–6, 7(table)
acetylcholine 214–15
acute left ventricular dysfunction 182
acute respiratory distress syndrome 241
  pharmacological treatment of
    hypoxaemia 241–75
    almitrine 265–70
    cyclooxygenase inhibitors 270
    nitric oxide, inhaled 242–63
    nitric oxide synthase 270
    pathophysiological basis 241–2
    permissive hypercapnia 271–4
    prostacyclin, inhaled 263–5
    see also adult respiratory distress
      syndrome
Addison's disease 123
adenosine 74, 180, 205–6, 209(fig)
adrenaline 62, 128, 180, 182, 184
  pulmonary endothelial mediator 215
adrenergic neurones 110
adrenergic receptors 182(table)
adult respiratory distress syndrome
    206, 219–20
afterload 180, 188
"aged heart" 202
airway obstruction 8
ajmalin 206, 209(fig)
alecepril 57
aldosterone 54–5
almitrine, hypoxaemia in patients with
    ARDS 265–70
alpha–2-adrenoceptor agonists 108–16,
    205
  analgesic effects 112
  cardiovascular control 110–11
  clinical applications 112–16
  haemodynamic effects 111–12
  mechanism of action 109–10
  pharmacokinetics 108–9
  recovery time 115
  sedative effects 112

  structural characteristics 108–9
alpha-methyldopa 13
alveolar hypoxia 218–20
alveolar ventilation 256
amezinium 128
aminophylline 215
amiodarone 82–4, 89–90, 127, 204–5,
    288
  induced pulmonary toxicity 206
amlodipine 32 (table)
  combined with dantrolene 42
amrinone 181, 188, 189 (table), 191
angina pectoris
  effort 14
    effect of celiprolol 22
    effect of xamoterol 21
  pathogenesis of coronary artery
    spasm 161(fig)
  rebound 4
  recurrence after discontinuation of
    calcium channel blockers 39
  rest 14
  unstable 4, 14
angiotensin I 53(fig)
angiotensin II 52, 53(fig), 127, 219
  as arrhythmogen in ischaemic heart
    disease 61
  compared to noradrenalin 127
  mechanism of action 54–5
  role 55–7
  dual action 56(fig)
angiotensin-converting enzyme 52
angiotensin-converting enzyme (ACE)
    inhibitors 52–67, 180
  acute postoperative hypertension
    153–4
  anaesthesia 61–7
    blood pressure regulation 61–2
    hypotension, risk 62–4
    premedication 64–5
    regional circulation 66
    systemic haemodynamics 65–6

pharmacology 57–61
  effects on systemic
    haemodynamics 58–9
  mechanism of action 57
  pharmacokinetics 57
  regional circulation 59
  therapy 59–61
  renin-angiotensin system, physiology
    53–7
antagonism, competitive 5
antiarrhythmic agents 74–92
  anaesthetic agents, their possible
    interactions 84–8
  complications induced
    implications for anaesthesia 89–92
  pharmacology 74–84
    Vaughan Williams classification
      74–5, 204
  proarrhythmic effects 90
antiatherogenic drugs, future directions
  288–9
anticholinergic drugs 209
antihypertensive drugs
  future directions 284–5
  ideal 142
anxiety 14, 201
aortic cross-clamping
  infrarenal 66
  thoracic 66
aortic stenosis 220
arachidonic acid 214, 220
arginine vasopressin 219
arrhythmia(s)
  cardiac sympathetic activity,
    increased 204
  congenital 202
  perioperative, treatment 201–9
    bradycardic arrhythmias,
      treatment 208–9
    cardiology, lessons 203–4
    drugs, classification 204–8
    intraoperative 202–3
    preoperative 201–2
    tachyarrhythmias, emergency
      treatment 208
ASL–8123 16
aspirin 164, 270, 287
asthma 11
  inhaled nitric oxide 258
atenolol 5–6, 7(table), 22
  chronic hypertension 34
atrial fibrillation 209, 210(fig)

esmolol 17
verapamil 17, 35
atrial flutter 209
atrial myxoma 220
atrial natriuretic factor 217
atropine 12, 86, 111, 131, 209
  resistant bradycardia 87
azepexole 108

barbiturates 38
  arrythmogenic effects 88
baroreceptor reflex 128
baroreflex arc, abnormalities 39
baroreflex responses, halogenated
  anaesthetics 37
benazepril 57
benzodiazepines 14, 32(table), 88
benzothiazepines 29
bepridil 29–30, 37, 90
  paroxysmal supraventricular
    tachycardia 35
  pharmacological properties 31(table)
beta-adrenoceptor antagonists 3–23,
  180, 209(fig)
  absorption 6, 7(table)
  acute postoperative hypertension
    148–52
    anaesthetic practice 12–15
    haemodilution 15
    preoperative anxiety 14
    silent ischaemia 14–15
  antiarrythmic action 6, 11
  cardiac protection 8
  characteristics 4–7
    competitive antagonism 5
    membrane stabilisation 6
    partial agonist activity 5–6
    receptor subtype selectivity 5
    up-regulation 6
  classification 6–7
  complex, effects on alpha-
    adrenoceptors 6
  congestive heart failure 10–11
  contraindications 11–12
  control of sympathetic overactivity
    13–14
  effect of opiates 87
  effect on respiratory function 8
  elimination 6, 7(table)
  haemodynamic effects 7–8
  intravenous / oral use 13
  medical indications 9
  myocardial infarction 9–10, 204

"quinidine-like activity" 5
regional ischaemic dysfunction 10
reversal of blockade 8
up-regulation 13
Vaughan Williams classification
    75(table), 82
withdrawal syndrome 8
beta-blockers *see also* beta-adrenoceptor
    antagonists
beta-thrombin 219
BEST 287-8
Bezold–Jarish reflex 128, 131
bisoprolol 287
bradycardic arrhythmias, drug
    treatment 208-9
bradykinin 57-9, 215
brain, acute hypertensive episodes 140
bretylium 204, 206
bronchoconstriction, methacholine-
    induced 258
bupivacaine 88
bycindolol 288

calcium channel blockers 9, 20, 29-42,
    180, 227
    acute hypertension 34, 145-8
    angina pectoris 34
    antiatherogenic properties 34
    combined with volatile anaesthetics,
        studies 38
    comparative pharmacology 29-34
        cardiac/vascular selectivity 32(fig)
        chemical characteristics 29
        classifications 29
        effects on major determinants of
            left ventricular function 33(fig)
        interactions 30-2
        mechanism of action 29-30
        pharmacodynamic effects 32-4
        pharmacokinetic parameters 30
        pharmacological properties
            31(table)
    coronary artery disease 34
    effect of opiates 87
    effect on coronary arteries
        indications for intravenous use 42
        indications not related to
            anaesthesia 34-5
    pharmacological interactions during
        anaesthesia 36-9
        neuromuscular relaxants 39
        other anaesthetics 38
        volatile anaesthetics 36-8

rebound vasoconstriction 161
renal / carotid blood flows induced
    by volatile anaesthetics 37
Vaughan Williams classification
    75(table), 84
calmodulin 30
CAMIAT trial 288
captopril 57
    myocardial infarction 60
cardiac failure 123
    perioperative, therapeutic triangle
        180(fig)
cardiac index 124(fig)
cardiomyopathy 202
    obstructive 9
cardiovascular system, classification of
    drugs acting on 180
cardioversion 209-10(figs)
cardioverter-defibrillators 91
carotid endarterectomy 140-1
carotid stenosis surgery 140
carvedilol 7(table), 22-3
CAST study 81
catecholamine(s) 201
    actions 183(table)
    down-regulation 187
    ideal, does it exist 186
    pulmonary hypertension 228
    therapy, alternatives 186-8
celiprolol 7(table), 22
cerebral artery spasm 29
cesium 85
chemiluminescence apparatus 247
cibenzoline 75(table), 81-2
CIBIS II 287
cilazapril 57
clonidine 108, 110-11, 114, 169
    abrupt discontinuation 112-13
    acute postoperative hypertension 145
    analgesic effect 112
    effect on MAC 13
    premedication 113
    sedative effect 112
cocaine toxicity 115
congestive heart failure 202
contractility 180
coronary artery bypass grafting
    (CABG) 18, 159, 161
    calcium channel blockers 39
    diltiazem-treated patients 30
    flow, clinical evaluation 166
    spasm, treatment 167-71

coronary artery disease 202
  drugs, future directions 285–7
coronary artery spasm 159, 161–6
  coronary artery graft flow, clinical
    evaluation 166
  gastroepiploic artery, relativity 163–4
  internal mammary artery spasm
    161–3
  radial artery reactivity 164–5
  saphenous vein reactivity 165–6
coronary blood flow
  calcium channel blockers 33
  redistribution 9
cor triatrium 220
cromakalin 216
cyanide ions 142–3
  toxicity 145
cyclooxygenase inhibitors 270

dantrolene 42
delivalol 7(table), 22
depression 12
desflurane 113
  induced hypotension 131
dexmetedomidine 108, 110–11, 115,
    169
  effect on MAC 13
diazepam 14
diastole, duration 8
digitalis 74, 181, 205, 209(fig)
  combined with amiodarone 84
  combined with propafenone 81
digoxin 17, 77, 209(fig)
  combined with flecainide 81
  combined with xamoterol 21
dihydralazine 142
dihydroergotamine 128
dihydropyridines 29, 32(table)
  effects on cerebral circulation 33
diltiazem 29–30, 32(table), 34, 85, 88,
    164, 170
  acute hypertension 34
    postoperative 146, 148, 154(table)
  angina pectoris 34
  atrioventricular block with enflurane
    37
  combined with halothane 36
  complete heart block with halothane
    or isoflurane 37
  effect on glomerular blood flow 33
  intravenous use 42
  onset of cardiopulmonary bypass 30
  paroxysmal supraventricular

  tachycardias 35
  pharmacological properties 31(table)
  potentiation of suxamethonium 39
diphenylhydantoin 75(table)
disopyramide 75(table), 76–8, 189, 204
dobutamine 5, 8, 128, 163, 171, 182,
    184–6
  down-regulation 187
dopamine 128, 180, 182, 185,
    186(table)
  pulmonary endothelial predictor 215
dopexamine 180, 185–6
  splanchnic perfusion 192
doxorubicin 64
droperidol 88
dynorphine 87

edrophonium 87
EMIAT trial 288
enalapril 57–8,
  myocardial infarction 60
enalaprilat 64, 193
  acute postoperative hypertension
    153–4
encainide 90–1, 204
endothelin 54, 215, 219
endothilium-derived relaxing factor
    214–17
end-tidal carbon dioxide tension 256
enflurane 86
  combined with calcium channel
    blockers 36
  coronary artery bypass grafting 18
  effect on
    sinus node and atrioventricular
      node 84
    slow calcium channels 37
enkephalins 57
enoximone 181, 188–9, 190
  effect on cardiac output 192
ephedrine 125–6, 128–9, 130(fig), 180
epidural anaesthesia 62, 127–31
  phenylephrine 125
epinephrine 219
ergonovine 162
esmolol 7(table), 16–19, 160, 204, 206
  acute hypertensive episodes 151
  atrial fibrillation 17
  effect on MAC for halothane 13
  hypertension 17
    deliberate 18
  myocardial revascularisation 18
  pheochromocytoma 19

tachycardia 17
tetralogy of Fallot 18–19
thyrotoxicosis 19
etidocaine 88
etilefrine 126, 128
etomidate 113
European Society of Cardiology 75

felodipine 32(table)
fentanyl 64
    antiarrhythmic action 86–7
    calcium channel blockers 38
    combined with clonidine 113
    high doses 18
fibrinogen GP 286
First International Study of Infarct
    Survival (ISIS – I) 9
fisinopril 57
flecainide 75(table), 76, 80–1, 90–1,
    204
flunarizine 29
flunitrazepam 63
forskolin 181
free fatty acids 9

ganglionic-blocking agents 215
gastroepiploic artery relativity 163–4
glibenclamide 216
glyceryl trinitrate 41, 142–5, 149(fig),
    167–71, 180, 193
    acute postoperative hypertension
        154(table)
    intracoronary infusion 162
G-protein 3–4, 109, 112
    inhibitory 187
    regulatory 187
    stimulatory 187
growth factor 219

haemoglobin, fetal 248
halogenated volatile anaesthetics,
        interactions with antiarrhythmic
        drugs 84–6
haloperidol 88
halothane 12, 86
    cardiac output reduction 131
    combined with
        amiodarone 85
        calcium channel blockers 36
    effect on
        sinus node and atrioventricular
            node 84
        slow calcium channels 37
heart failure

acute, therapy 181
angiotensin-converting enzyme
        inhibitor therapy 60–1
classification 178
congestive 177
drugs, future directions 287–8
perioperative, pathogenesis 177–9
    monitoring 179
heparin 287
    combined with amiodarone 84
hirudine 286
hirulog 286
histamine 215
hydralazine 180, 228
hydroquinidine 76–8
hypercapnia 215
    permissive 271–4
hypertension 202
    acute / chronic, calcium channel
        blockers 34
    angiotensin-converting enzyme
        inhibitor therapy 59–60
    calcium channel blockers 40–2
    essential, haemodynamic
        characteristics 137–9
    rebound 8, 13
    postoperative, pathophysiological
        mechanisms 137–55
        essential hypertension,
            haemodynamic characteristics
            137–9
        ideal antihypertensive drug 142
        impact on organ systems 140–1
        promoting factors 139–40
        treatment of acute hypertensive
            episodes 141–54
hyperthyroidism 4, 201
hypokalaemia 91, 201
hypomagnesaemia 91, 201
hypotension
    deliberate
        calcium channel blockers 20, 41–2
        esmolol 18
        labetalol 20
        sodium nitroprusside 20
        trimetaphan 20
    during central neural blockade
        127–31
    epidural anaesthesia 125
    induced by inhalational anaesthetics
        131
    intraoperative

postural 125, 131
treatment, see intraoperative
hypotension, treatment
mesenteric traction syndrome 125,
133
spinal anaesthesia 125
hypoxia 201, 214–5, 218–20
hypoxic pulmonary vasoconstriction
223
effect of calcium channel blockers
33–4
rats, verapamil and halotane 37
hypoxic vasoconstriction reflex 214

imidazoles 108
indomethacin 270
inodilator 188
inotropic drugs 123–4
cardiovascular effects 184(table)
classification 181
intravenous, proarrhythmic potential
192(table)
positive 182–6
mechanism 188(fig)
negative effects 191–3
pulmonary hypertension 228
inotropic depressors 180
insulin-dependent diabetes mellitus 12
integrelin 287
interleukin-1 219
internal mammary artery spasm 161–3
intraaortic baloon pump 194
counterpulsation 164
intraoperative hypotension, treatment
123–33
clinical applications 127–33
factors related to
anaesthesia 124
patient's condition 124
surgical procedure 124
frequently used substances 125–7
intravascular volume depletion 124
intrinsic sympathomimetic activity 5–6
ipratropium bromide 209
ischaemia, silent 14–15
isoflurane 86
combined with calcium channel
blockers 36
effect on sinus node and
atrioventricular node 84
induced hypotension 131
cerebral aneurysm surgery 154
isoprenaline 5, 128, 180, 209

pulmonary endothelial mediator 215
isradipine 32(table)
antiatherogenic properties 34
intravenous use 42
myocardial revascularisation 41

ketamine 113
ketanserin 153
kidney, acute hypertensive episode 141

labetalol 7(table), 19–20
acute hypertensive episodes 151–2
postoperative 149(fig), 154(table)
hypotension, stable 20
lacidipine 32(table)
lamifiban 287
left-to-right intra/extra cardiac shunts,
congenital 219
left ventricular ejection fraction 60, 187
left ventricular dysfunction 202
invasive monitoring data 123–4
mechanical assist devices 194–5
perioperative, treatment 177–97
left ventricular end – systolic wall stress
126, 128, 129(fig)
left ventricular filling pressure 194
left ventricular stroke work index 190
leukotrienes 214
lidoflazine, after cardiac arrest 35
lignocaine 38, 75(table), 76, 79, 88–9,
204, 206–7
Lilly Cyanide Antidote Kit 145
local anaesthetic drugs 75(table), 88
combined with calcium channel
blockers 38
systemic actions 128
locus coeruleus 112
low output syndrome 177, 179–86
treatment, phosphodiesterase III
inhibitors 189(table)

magnesium 74, 207, 209–10(figs)
malignant hyperthermia, calcium
channel blockers 42
mass flow regulators 243
mechanical assist devices 194–5
meclofenamate 270
mepivacaine 88
mesenteric traction syndrome 124, 133
methaemoglobin 142, 247
methanol 16
methoxamine 128, 180
methyldopa 108
metoprolol 5–6, 7(table), 204

combined with diazepam 14
compared with esmolol 16
doses reduction, combined with
    propafenone 81
ischaemia, silent 14
mexiletine 75(table), 80, 89, 204, 207
milrinone 181, 189(table), 191
minimum alveolar concentration
    (MAC) 13
mitral stenosis 220
mivazerol 108–9, 169
monoclonal antibody 7EC3 (ReoPro)
    287
morphine 86–7
multiple organ dysfunctioning
    syndrome (MODS) 181
muscarinic–M2 receptors 88, 215
muscle relaxants
    action on cardiac electrophysiology
        87–8
    non-depolarising, effect of quinidine
        77
myocardial depressant factor 59
myocardial hypertrophy, hypertension-
    induced 138
myocardial ischaemia
    angiotensin-converting enzyme
        inhibitors 61
    calcium channel blockers 39–42
    intraoperative (suspected), treatment
        160–1, 167(table)
    prevention 167–71
    treatment 167–71
myocardial oxygen consumption 6,
    8–9, 168, 189
    alpha-2-agonists 111–12
    amiodarone 83
    calcium channel blockers 32
    shivering 115
myocardial revascularisation, use of
    inotropic drugs 171–2
myocarditis 202
myocardium, acute hypertensive
    episodes 140

nadolol 6, 7(table)
naloxone 86
NAPA 78
neostigmine 39
neuromuscular relaxants, potentiation
    by calcium channel blockers 39
nicardipine 33, 170–1
    acute postoperative hypertension
        145–7, 149(fig), 154(table)
    chronic hypertension 34
    combined with isoflurane 36
    effect on glomerular blood flow 33
    intravenous use 42
    pharmacological properties
        31–2(tables)
    pheochromocytoma 41
    potentiation of pancuronium 39
nifedipine 9, 29, 34, 170
    acute hypertension 34
    postoperative 145–7, 154(table)
    acute renal failure 33
    analgesic effect of narcotics
        potentiated 34
    angina pectoris 34
    pharmacological properties
        31–2(tables)
    sublingual 162
nimodipine
    acute pulmonary hypertension
        35
    after cardiac arrest 35
    cerebral blood flow 35
    pharmacological properties
        31(table)
    subarachnoid haemorrhage 35
nitrates 228
nitrendipine 32(table)
    chronic hypertension 34
    intrevenous use 42
nitric oxide 54, 59, 214–17, 223–5
    inhaled 242–63
        administration 243–7
        bronchial effects 258
        concentration-response curves
            262–3
        effects on alveolar dead space
            256–8
        effects on gas exchange 254–6
        effects on platelets 258–61
        effects on pulmonary
            circulation 250–4
        metabolism 247–50
        monitoring 243–7
        other effects 261–2
        tachyphylaxis 252
        toxicity 247–50
    pulmonary hypertension,
        therapy 230–4
nitric oxide synthase inhibitors 270
nitroglycerine 221, 228

nitroprusside (sodium) 20, 142–5,
    164, 180, 193, 222, 228
  compared with esmolol 17
  hypotension, deliberate 18
nitrous oxide 88
noradrenaline 128, 131, 138,
    162–3, 165, 180, 182–4
norfenefrine 127–8

ondansetron 34
opiates
  antiarrhythmic action 86–7
  combined with vecuronium
    bromide 87
  effects on
    beta-adrenergic antagonists 87
    calcium channel blockers 87
oral anticoagulants
  combined with
    amiodarone 84
    quinidine 77
orthostatic syncope 123
orciprenaline 209
ouabain 86
oxalozepines 108
oxprenolol 6, 7(table)
oxygen 222–6
  consumption 123
  delivery 123
  supplementation 227
oxyhaemoglobin 247

pacing 209–10(fig)
pain 201
pancuronium bromide 39, 87
papaverine, intracoronary infusion
    162
perhexiline 29
pericarditis, constrictive 220
perioperative arrhythmias see
    arrhythmia(s)
peripheral neuropathies 123
phenylalkylamines 29, 32(table)
phenylephrine 125–6, 128, 162,
    165–6, 180
  isoflurane-induced hypotension
    131
  postural hypotension, effect of
    intravenous bolus 132(fig)
phenylethylamines 108
pheochromocytoma 4, 9
  alpha-blockade
    combined with beta-blockade
    19
  preoperatively 19
phosphodiesterase III inhibitors
    188–91
  actions 188
  indications 191
  "lusitropic" action 189
  pulmonary hypertension 230
  treatment of low output
    syndrome 189(table)
physostigmine 87
pindolol 6, 7(table), 11
plasma converting enzyme activity
    64
platelet activating factor 215
plexogenic arteriopathy 219
positive end–expiratory pressure
    254–5
post-angioplasty restenosis 286
potassium chloride 162, 164–5
practolol 12
prazosin 109, 166
preload 180, 188
procainamide 75(table), 78–9,
    204, 207, 209(fig)
promethazine 88
propafenone 75(table), 76, 81,
    204, 208
propofol 88, 113
propranolol 5–6, 7(table)
  chronic hypertension 34
  combined with flecainide 81
  compared with esmolol 16
  effect on MAC for halothane 13
  sedation 13
  syndrome X 10
prorenin 54
prostaglandin(s) 215
  E1-pulmonary hypertension 229
prostacyclin 133, 215
  inhaled 263–5
    hypoxaemia in patients with
      ARDS 263–5
  pulmonary hypertension 229–30
pulmonary artery pressure 226
pulmonary capillary wedge
    pressure 63–4, 124(fig)
  effect of xamoterol 21
pulmonary embolism 219
pulmonary endothelial mediators
    215
pulmonary fibrosis, amiodarone

induced 84
pulmonary hypertension 33–4
    neurogenic pathways 224
    of the newborn 222–3, 233
    pathophysiology 218–22
    pharmacological agents 228–34
    postcapillary 220
    treatment, methods 222–8
pulmonary vascular resistance 221,
    226
    index 251

quanabenz 108
quinapril 289
quinidine 6–7, 75(table), 76–8, 81,
    89, 204

radial artery, reactivity 164–5
radiofrequency ablation 91
ramipril, myocardial infarction 61
rauwolscine 109
Raynaud's syndrome 12
receptor operated channels 30
renal blood flow, calcium channel
    blockers 33
renin 53(fig)
    activity / effective volaemia
        relationship 55(fig)
    epidural anaesthesia 62
    release, effect of beta–2 receptor
        blockade 8
renin-angiotensin system (RAS) 61
    activation, thoracic aortic cross-
        clamping 66
    physiology 53–7
        angiotensin II action,
            mechanism 54–5
        angeotensin II, role 55–7
        biochemistry 53–4
        mechanisms of activation 54
reserpine 13, 86
resetting of the baroreflex 139
right ventricle 220–22
    dysfunction 202
        volume expansion 228
Riley-Day syndrome 123
rilmenidine 108

saphenous vein reactivity 165–6
septic shock 123
serotonin 162–3, 215, 220
shivering 115
Shy-Drager syndrome 123
Sicilian Gambit 205

sodium nitroprusside *see*
    nitroprusside (sodium)
sotalol 7(table), 11, 90, 204, 208,
    288
spinal anaesthesia 124, 127–31
    asystole, resuscitation 131
    hypotension 123
subarachnoid haemorrhage,
    nimodipine 35
sufentanyl 87, 160, 169
supraventricular dysrrhythmia 77
supraventricular tachycardia 205,
    208
supraventricular
        tachyarrhythmia(s)
    calcium channel blockers 42
    paroxysmal 209
suxamethonium 39
sympathetic outflow blockade 127
sympathomimetics 123
syndrome X 10

tachyarrhythmia(s)
    emergency treatment 208
    with
        broad QRS complex,
            algorithm for treatment
            210(fig)
        narrow QRS complex,
            algorithm for treatment
            209(fig)
Task Force of the Working Group
    on Arrhythmias of the
    European Society of
    Cardiology 205
tetanus, sympathetic overactivity 9
tetralogy of Fallot 18–19
theodrenaline 128
theophylline 81
thiopentone 38
thiosulphate 145
thrombin III 286
thromboxane-A2 165, 215
thyroid crisis 9
timolol 6, 7(table)
tirofiban 287
tocainide 204
torsades de pointes 11, 78, 83, 88,
    90, 210(fig)
treprotide 58
tri-iodothyronine 181
trimetaphan, hypotension,
    deliberate 20

urapidil 152–3
utero-placental perfusion, during
    hypotension 129

vascular pulmonary bed 218
vascular pulmonary tone, factors
    influencing 213–17
    atrial natriuretic factor 217
    autonomic control 213–14
    carbon dioxide 214–15
    endothelium-derived relaxing
        factor 214–17
    oxygen 214–15
    physical factors 217
    pulmonary endothelial
        mediators 215
vasodilators 123, 141, 180, 193–4
    pulmonary hypertension 228
vasopressin 58, 61, 63
    receptor (V1) antagonists 62
vasopressors 123–4, 180
Vaughan Williams classification of
    antiarrhythmic effects 74–5,
    204–5
vecuronium bromide 39, 87
ventilation-perfusion mismatch
    241, 256
ventricular arrhythmia 78–9
ventricular tachycardia 210(fig)
verapamil 29–30, 32–3, 85, 170,
    204, 208–9
    atrial fibrillation 17, 35
    atrioventricular block with

    enflurane 37
    chronic hypertension 34
    combined with
        enflurane 36
        glyceril trinitrate 165
        halothane 36
    complete heart block, with
        halothane or isoflurane 37
    contraindications 209(fig)
    effect on halothane MAC 37
    intravenous use 42
    obstructive cardiomyopathy 35
    paroxysmal supraventricular
        tachycardia 35
    pharmacological properties
        31(table)
    platelet aggregability 34
    potentiation of suxamethonium
        39
videodensitometry by Rutishauser
    166
vitamin E 289
voltage operated channels 30

warfarin 81
Wolf-Parkinson-White syndrome
    77, 81–2, 88, 206,

xamoterol 6, 7(table), 20–2

yohimbine 109, 166

zero end-expiratory pressure 254,
    255(fig)